Endocrine Dependent Tumors

Comprehensive Endocrinology

Editor-in-Chief: Luciano Martini

Endocrine Control of Sexual Behavior. *Carlos Beyer, Editor. 1979.*

The Adrenal Gland. *Vivian H. T. James, Editor. 1979.*

Gastrointestinal Hormones. *George B. Jerzy Glass, Editor. 1980.*

The Thyroid Gland. *Michel de Visscher, Editor. 1980.*

The Endocrine Functions of the Brain. *Marcella Motta, Editor. 1980.*

The Testis. *Henry Burger and David de Kretser, Editors. 1981.*

Pediatric Endocrinology. *R. Collu, J. Ducharme, and H. Guyda, Editors. 1981.*

Endocrinology of Calcium Metabolism. *John Parsons, Editor. 1982.*

The Ovary. *Giovan Serra, Editor. 1983.*

Endocrine Mechanisms in Fertility Regulation. *G. Benagiano and E. Diczfalusy, Editors. 1983.*

The Pineal Gland. *Russel J. Reiter, Editor. 1984.*

The Pituitary Gland. *Hiroo Imura, Editor. 1985.*

Endocrinology of Aging. *James R. Sowers and James V. Felicetta, Editors. 1988.*

Pediatric Endocrinology, *Second Edition. R. Collu, J. R. Ducharme, and H. J. Guyda, Editors. 1989.*

The Testis, *Second Edition. Henry Burger and David de Kretser, Editors. 1989.*

Endocrine Hypertension. *Edward G. Biglieri and James C. Melby, Editors. 1990.*

The Thyroid Gland Second Edition. *Monte A. Greer, Editor. 1990.*

Endocrine Dependent Tumors. *Klaus-Dieter Voigt and Cornelius Knabbe, Editors. 1991.*

The Endocrine Pancreas. *Ellis Samols, Editor. 1991.*

Comprehensive Endocrinology

Endocrine Dependent Tumors

Editors

Klaus-Dieter Voigt, M.D.
Department of Clinical Chemistry
Medical Clinic
University of Hamburg
Hamburg, Federal Republic of Germany

Cornelius Knabbe, M.D.
Department of Clinical Chemistry
Medical Clinic
University of Hamburg
Hamburg, Federal Republic of Germany

Raven Press 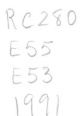 New York

Raven Press, Ltd. 1185 Avenue of the Americas, New York, New York 10036

Made in the United States of America.

Library of Congress Cataloging-in-Publication Data

Endocrine dependent tumors / editors, Klaus-Dieter Voigt, Cornelius
  Knabbe.
        p.   cm. — (Comprehensive endocrinology)
    Includes bibliographical references.
    Includes index.
    ISBN 0-88167-721-3
    1. Endocrine glands—Tumors.   2. Cancer—Endocrine aspects.
  I. Voigt, Klaus-Dieter.   II. Knabbe, Cornelius.   III. Series.
    [DNLM: 1. Breast Neoplasms.   2. Neoplasms, Hormone-Dependent.
  3. Urogenital Neoplasms.   WJ 160 E56]
  RC280.E55E53   1991
  616.99′4—dc20
  DNLM/DLC
  for Library of Congress   90-9055
                                                                  CIP

The material contained in this volume was submitted as previously unpublished material, except in the instances in which credit has been given to the source from which some of the illustrative material was derived.

Great care has been taken to maintain the accuracy of the information contained in the volume. However, neither Raven Press nor the editors can be held responsible for errors or for any consequences arising from the use of the information contained herein.

Materials appearing in this book prepared by individuals as part of their official duties as U.S. Government employees are not covered by the above-mentioned copyright.

9   8   7   6   5   4   3   2   1

Preface

The clinical importance of endocrine-dependent tumors like breast and prostate cancer is very well known because of the high frequency with which they occur and the poor prognosis. It was only in the middle of our century, however, that Charles Huggins published his famous articles on the effect of androgen withdrawal on the growth of human prostatic carcinoma, thus providing the first insights into hormone action. The therapeutic principles derived from these early observations still represent the basis for treatment of hormone-dependent cancer. With the advances of cellular and molecular biology during the last decade, newer and deeper insights have been obtained into how steroids regulate the growth of malignant cells. It can be expected, therefore, that better strategies for prevention, diagnosis, and cure of these diseases will be available before the turn of the millennium.

Given this situation, it seemed necessary to compile the present knowledge in this field. Consequently, various experts from different countries have reviewed the current state-of-the-art, with particular emphasis on important and promising new developments in epidemiology, basic research, and clinical application in breast, prostate, endometrium, and renal and bladder carcinoma. Shorter contributions concern questions of special scientific and clinical impact. In all chapters, significant attention has been paid to the *biology*, i.e., the relevance of the data obtained both for tumor growth and patient care.

We hope that this volume will be a valuable contribution to the series "Comprehensive Endocrinology." The book will be of interest to clinicians and basic researchers. As the mechanism of growth control identified in hormone-dependent tumors should hold true for other types of malignancy, this volume will be valuable for all scientists working in cancer research.

K-D. Voigt
C. Knabbe

Contents

Contributors

Max Bressel
Department of Urology
Harburg General Hospital
D-2100 Hamburg 90
Federal Republic of Germany

P. Davies
Tenovus Institute for Cancer Research
University of Wales College of Medicine
Heath Park, Cardiff CF4 4XX
United Kingdom

Jean B. deKernion
Division of Urology
UCLA School of Medicine
Los Angeles, California 90024

G. Dhom
Cancer Center
University of the Saarland
6650 Homburg/Saar
Federal Republic of Germany

C. L. Eaton
Tenovus Institute for Cancer Research
University of Wales College of Medicine
Heath Park, Cardiff CF4 4XX
United Kingdom

K. Griffiths
Tenovus Institute for Cancer Research
University of Wales College of Medicine
Heath Park, Cardiff CF4 4XX
United Kingdom

M. E. Harper
Tenovus Institute for Cancer Research
University of Wales College of Medicine
Heath Park, Cardiff CF4 4XX
United Kingdom

Richard A. Hiipakka
The Ben May Institute
Departments of Biochemistry
*   and Molecular Biology*
*   and Medicine/Dermatology*
The University of Chicago
Chicago, Illinois 60637

John T. Isaacs
James Buchanan Brady Urological
*   Institute and*
The Johns Hopkins Oncology Center
The Johns Hopkins Medical Institutions
Baltimore, Maryland 21205

V. Isomaa
Biocenter and Department of Clinical
*   Chemistry*
University of Oulu
SF-90220 Oulu Finland

Hartwig Kastendieck
Department of Pathology
Harburg General Hospital
D-2100 Hamburg 90
Federal Republic of Germany

Hartmut Klein
Department of Clinical Chemistry
Medical Clinic, University of Hamburg
D-2000 Hamburg 20
Federal Republic of Germany

Cornelius Knabbe
Department of Clinical Chemistry
Medical Clinic, University of Hamburg
D-2000 Hamburg 20
Federal Republic of Germany

Natasha Kyprianou
James Buchanan Brady Urological
*   Institute and*
The Johns Hopkins Oncology Center
The Johns Hopkins Medical Institutions
Baltimore, Maryland 21205

Tehming Liang
The Ben May Institute
Departments of Biochemistry
 and Molecular Biology
 and Medicine/Dermatology
The University of Chicago
Chicago, Illinois 60637

Shutsung Liao
The Ben May Institute
Departments of Biochemistry
 and Molecular Biology
 and Medicine/Dermatology
The University of Chicago
Chicago, Illinois 60637

Paula Martikainen
James Buchanan Brady Urological
 Institute and
The Johns Hopkins Oncology Center
The Johns Hopkins Medical Institutions
Baltimore, Maryland 21205

William L. McGuire
Department of Medicine/Oncology
The University of Texas Health Science Center
San Antonio, Texas 78284

W. B. Peeling
Department of Urology
St. Woolos' Hospital
Newport, Gwent, United Kingdom

Jeffrey A. Scott
Department of Medicine/Oncology
The University of Texas Health Science Center
San Antonio, Texas 78284

Susumu Seino
The Ben May Institute
Departments of Biochemistry
 and Molecular Biology
 and Medicine/Dermatology
The University of Chicago
Chicago, Illinois 60637

Arnulf Stenzl
Division of Urology
UCLA School of Medicine
Los Angeles, California 90024
Current Address:
University of Bern
CH-3010 Bern
Switzerland

A. Turkes
Tenovus Institute for Cancer Research
University of Wales College of Medicine
Heath Park, Cardiff CF4 4XX
United Kingdom

R. Vihko
Biocenter and Department of Clinical
 Chemistry
University of Oulu
SF-90220 Oulu, Finland

Klaus-Dieter Voigt
Department of Clinical Chemistry
Medical Clinic, University of Hamburg
D-2000 Hamburg 20
Federal Republic of Germany

Comprehensive Endocrinology

Endocrine Dependent Tumors

Endocrine Dependent Tumors, edited by
Klaus-Dieter Voigt and Cornelius Knabbe.
Raven Press, Ltd., New York © 1991.

1

Epidemiology of Hormone-Depending Tumors

G. Dhom

*Cancer Center, University of the Saarland, 6650 Homburg/Saar,
Federal Republic of Germany*

PROSTATE CANCER

Descriptive Epidemiology

Although androgen dependency of prostate carcinomas is probably the same throughout the world, incidences differ greatly. The highest incidence is 120 times the rate of the lowest one (1). The black population of the United States has the highest rates by a wide margin (2). In the United States prostate cancer constitutes 21% of all cancer cases in men and occurs more frequently than bronchial carcinomas (3). The West European countries are within the upper and the mean group; Norway, Sweden, and Switzerland occupy a top position. Incidence of prostate cancer is significantly lower in East European countries. Rates from the USSR, the Islamic countries, and the entire African continent (2) are not available. At the bottom of the list of frequency are the Asian populations of China and of India (2) (Table 1).

The worldwide extreme differences cannot be explained by different qualities of data recording or by different life expectancy (age-standardized incidences). The worldwide incidence rates show an increasing tendency (Table 2) (1). The Asian populations showing low primary incidence display a very high annual rate of increase of 6% to 9%. This reaches 4% in countries of high incidence, such as Sweden, the increase can be observed in all Scandinavian countries (Fig. 1) (4). The incidence of prostate carcinomas once again increased by 20.1% in white men and by 21.4% in the black population of the United States from 1974 to 1983 (Table 3). The age-specific incidences of prostate carcinomas show a pronounced increase in patients over 60 years old (5). The rates from San Francisco and from Detroit reveal how the incidences between whites and blacks differ greatly in all age groups (6) (Table 4).

1

TABLE 1. *Prostate cancer incidence in five continents (136 populations)*

ICD 185 - Prostate - ASR World	
USA—Georgia, Atlanta: Black	91.2
USA—Michigan, Detroit: Black	91.1
USA—Alameda County: Black	87.8
USA—California, Los Angeles: Black	82.6
USA—California, San Francisco Bay: Black	82.5
USA—Connecticut: Black	72.3
USA—Louisiana, New Orleans: Black	71.8
USA—Utah	70.2
USA—Washington, Seattle	63.7
USA—Hawaii: White	58.3
Canada—Saskatchewan	57.6
USA—New Mexico: other White	56.7
USA—Georgia, Atlanta: White	53.4
USA—New Mexico: Hispanic	53.4
USA—Iowa	51.3
USA—Michigan, Detroit: White	51.2
Switzerland—Basel	50.1
France—Martinique	50.1
USA—California, San Francisco Bay: White	49.6
USA—Alameda County: White	49.6
Canada—British Columbia	49.5
USA—Connecticut: White	46.8
Sweden	45.9
Switzerland—Zürich	45.8
Canada—Alberta	45.3
Canada—Manitoba	44.4
New Zealand—Polynesian Islanders	44.3
Brazil—Pernambuco Recife	44.2
Canada—National Cancer Inc. Rep. System	43.7
USA—California, Los Angeles: Latino	43.0
USA—New York State	42.6
USA—Louisiana, New Orleans: White	42.0
Norway	42.0
Australia, South Australia	41.9
USA—New York City	41.7
Canada—Ontario	41.6
Canada—Quebec	41.5
Australia, Victoria	41.1
USA—Hawaii: Hawaiian	40.9
Switzerland—Geneva	39.6
Australia—Queensland	38.8
Australia—Capital Territory	38.7
Canada—New Brunswick	38.5
Iceland	36.2
New Zealand—Maori	35.4
Switzerland—Vaud	35.2
Brazil—Porto Allegre	34.8
Finland	34.2
Australia—New South Wales	33.8
Canada—Maritime Provinces	33.6
New Zealand—Non-Maori	33.2
Brazil—Sao Paulo	33.0
Switzerland—Neuchâtel	32.7
Canada—Prince Edward Island	32.2

TABLE 1. *Continued.*

ICD 185 - Prostate - ASR World	
Australia—Western Australia	32.1
Australia—Tasmania	31.5
USA—Hawaii: Japanese	31.2
USA—California, Los Angeles: Filipino	31.2
Brazil—Fortaleza	30.8
USA—Puerto Rico	30.7
USA—Hawaii: Filipino	30.6
Colombia—Cali	30.6
USA—California, San Francisco Bay: Filipino	29.6
USA—New Mexico: American Indian	29.2
Canada—Nova Scotia	29.2
FR Germany—Saarland	28.7
Netherlands—Eindhoven	28.3
Denmark	27.7
Canada—Northwest Territories	27.7
France—Bas Rhin	27.4
Canada—Newfoundland	27.4
France—Calvados	26.8
Netherlands—Antilles	26.6
Scotland—South East	26.5
FR German—Hamburg	26.5
Costa Rica	26.1
Scotland—North East	26.0
Scotland—East	25.2
USA—Hawaii: Chinese	25.2
France—Doubs	24.9
UK—South Western Region	24.8
Israel—Jews born Israel	24.3
UK—Oxford Region	23.7
France—Isère	23.6
Scotland	23.3
UK—Trent Region	22.9
USA—California, Los Angeles: Japanese	22.8
Israel—Jews born Europ./America	22.5
Scotland—West	21.5
UK—South Thames Region	21.4
Spain—Catalona Tarragona	21.2
UK—England, Wales	20.9
UK—Northwestern Region	20.8
Spain—Navarra	20.5
Ireland—Southern	20.3
Italy—Lombardy Region	20.3
German Democratic Republic	19.9
Scotland—North	19.3
England—Wales, Mersey Region	19.2
UK—Birmingham and West Midland	18.9
Israel—all Jews	18.8
Italy—Ragusa	18.8
Yugoslavia—Slowenia	18.7
Italy—Parma	17.6
Spain—Zaragoza	17.0
Hungary—County Vas	16.9
USA—California, Los Angeles: Chinese	16.9
Israel—Jews born Africa/Asia	16.8
USA—California, San Franciso Bay: Japanese	16.5

(Table continues.)

TABLE 1. *Continued.*

ICD 185 - Prostate - ASR World	
Czechoslovakia—Slovakia	15.8
USA—California, San Francisco Bay: Chinese	14.9
Kuwait—Non-Kuwaitis	13.8
Poland—Cracow City	13.8
Hungary—County Szabolcs	12.6
USA—California, Los Angeles: Korean	11.7
Poland—Warsaw City	11.5
Philippines—Rizal Province	11.1
Poland—Nowy Sacz Rural	10.3
Romania—County Cluy	9.8
Singapore: Indian	8.9
Japan—Nagasaki City	8.8
India—Bombay	8.2
Singapore: Malay	7.6
Japan—Hiroshima City	6.7
Singapore: Chinese	6.6
Israel—Non-Jews	6.5
Japan—Miyagi Prefecture	6.3
Hong Kong	6.2
Kuwait: Kuwaitis	6.0
Japan—Osaka Prefecture	5.1
India—Bangalore	4.9
India—Nagpur	4.8
India—Poona	4.8
India—Madras	3.1
China—Shanghai	1.8
China—Tianjin	1.3

(From Muir C, Waterhouse J, Mack T, Powell J, Whelan S. Cancer incidence in five continents. *IARC Scientific Pub*. 1987;5:88, Lyon.)

ICD, International Classification of Diseases; ASR, Age-specific morbidity rates; World-World standard population.

The mortality rates for prostate cancer are remarkably lower than those of the incidence (Tables 3 and 5) proving that prostate carcinomas are the cause of death only in a small part of the incidences recorded. Although in most countries the mortality rates also have increased, the rate of increase is distinctly lower than that of incidence (Table 6) (1); the trend graphs diverge.

The incidence and mortality rates for prostate cancer can vary regionally and among different ethnic groups from the same region. Taking into account the native countries of the Israeli population, the incidence of prostate cancer differs. This rate is the highest in migrants from Greece and from Bulgaria and the lowest in Jews hailing from Jemen (7). There is a pronounced distinction among the different ethnic groups in San Francisco and in Los Angeles (Table 7) (2). In this study, the Asian population shows the lowest rates, although this rate is higher than for those of the respective native countries. The mortality rates for prostate carcinomas in the United States show a certain geographic variation with preference of the northern and central regions compared with the southern areas (8). Some northwestern departments and the central massif of France display mortality rates above the average

TABLE 2. *Annual increase rate of incidence of prostate carcinoma, 1960–1975*

Registry	Percentage of annual increase rate
Canada, Alberta	+ 4.2
Manitoba	+ 2.3
Newfoundland	+ 5.2
Quebec	+ 3.9
Saskatchewan	+ 2.1
Colombia, Cali	− 0.2
Jamaica, Kingston	+ 4.7
Puerto Rico	+ 3.2
USA, Alameda White	+ 0.9
Alameda Black	+ 2.7
Bay area White	+ 1.2
Bay area Black	+ 3.7
Bay area Chinese	+ 0.5
Connecticut	+ 1.5
New York State	+ 3.4
Hawaii, Hawaiian	+ 5.5
Caucasian	+ 2.5
Chinese	+ 6.6
Japanese	+ 6.9
Filipino	+ 4.4
Asia	
India, Bombay	+ 0.5
Israel, all Jews	+ 1.6
Born Israel	+ 1.8
Born Amer./Europe	− 0.6
Born Africa/Asia	+ 1.8
Non-Jews	+ 4.6
Japan, Miyagi	+ 1.8
Singapore, Chinese	+ 8.5
Europe	
Denmark	+ 1.5
Finland	+ 3.4
FRG, Hamburg	+ 3.9
German Dem. Rep.	+ 3.7
Hungary, Szabolcs	+ 6.5
Vas	− 3.4
Norway	+ 3.0
Poland, Katowice	+ 4.7
Cracow	+ 8.3
Sweden	+ 4.0
UK, Birmingham	+ 0.5
Mersey	+ 0.4
Oxford	+ 0.7
S. Thames	+ 2.2
Yugoslavia	+ 2.4

(From Zaridze D, Boyle P, Smans M. International trends in prostatic cancer. *Int J Cancer* 1984;33:223–230.)

TABLE 3. *Incidence of prostate carcinoma in whites and blacks in the United States from 1974 to 1983*

	Whites	Blacks
1974	64.2	98.2
1975	68.0	110.4
1976	71.7	108.4
1977	73.3	120.1
1978	72.0	114.0
1979	75.5	121.3
1980	76.6	123.3
1981	78.9	124.2
1982	78.6	126.2
1983	80.3	126.9
Increase in percentage	20.1	21.4

(From Byar, ref. 8.)

(9). The cancer map of the Federal Republic of Germany presents rather slight variations for mortality of prostate carcinomas; no striking cluster can be seen (10).

Considering geographic and ethnic differences, the comparative geographic pathology of latent prostate carcinomas only detected at autopsy plays an important role (11–16). It appears that the prevalence of latent carcinomas is associated with

TABLE 4. *Age-specific incidence rates, by race, of 100,000 men, from 1969 to 1971*

Age group	All races	White	Black
San Francisco/Oakland SMSA			
35–39	—	—	—
40–44	1.4	1.7	—
45–49	5.0	4.3	14.3
50–54	15.1	13.7	37.3
55–59	65.7	59.6	145.2
60–64	141.8	138.4	241.6
65–69	263.6	261.4	328.8
70–74	485.9	470.8	992.6
75–79	710.7	708.9	1,002.5
80–84	893.7	909.9	1,486.2
85 +	888.9	927.6	961.5
Detroit, Michigan SMSA			
35–39	0.6	0.4	1.8
40–44	0.5	0.3	1.6
45–49	4.3	3.9	6.2
50–54	19.3	14.5	45.5
55–59	56.9	49.1	99.9
60–64	131.8	105.8	276.3
65–69	294.4	255.7	509.5
70–74	456.3	406.6	767.4
75–79	584.9	552.2	843.7
80–84	818.6	787.2	1,142.2
85 +	741.1	726.3	877.2

(Compiled from Third National Cancer Survey: Incidence Data, NCI).

PROSTATE

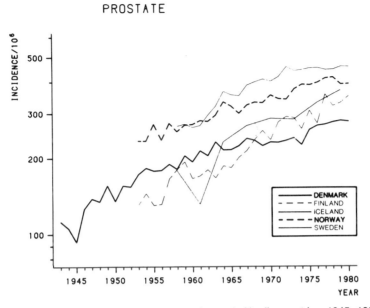

FIG. 1. Increasing incidence of prostate carcinoma in Nordic countries, 1945–1980.

the mortality rates: Populations with high mortality rates also show a higher number of latent prostate carcinomas found at autopsy (in cases where the organ has been submitted to a careful histologic examination by step-section). However, the differences disappear if only small foci are counted. They are again significant if larger foci are exclusively considered (13). It has been concluded from these examinations that the initiation of malignant transformation does not differ in populations with high versus low mortality, but that promoting factors must be responsible for the

TABLE 5. *Mortality rates for prostate carcinoma in whites and blacks in the United States from 1974 to 1983*

	Whites	Blacks
1974	20.2	39.5
1975	20.1	40.4
1976	20.6	40.6
1977	20.6	41.0
1978	21.0	42.3
1979	21.0	42.9
1980	21.1	44.5
1981	21.0	45.4
1982	21.3	44.3
1983	21.7	46.1
Increase in percentage	6.7	13.1

(From Byar, ref. 8.)

TABLE 6. *Annual increase of age-standardized mortality rates for prostate carcinoma, 1950–1975*

Country	Annual percentage increase
North, South and Central America	
Canada	+ 0.6
Chile	+ 2.5
Colombia	+ 1.4
Mexico	+ 3.0
Panama	+ 1.7
Trinidad and Tobago	+ 6.4
United States	+ 0.2
Uruguay	+ 2.2
Venezuela	+ 1.8
Asia	
Hong Kong	+ 6.6
Israel—Jews	+ 0.4
Japan	+ 7.8
Sri Lanka	+ 1.3
Europe	
Austria	+ 1.3
Belgium	+ 1.3
Bulgaria	0.0
Czechoslovakia	+ 2.2
Denmark	+ 1.5
Fed. Rep. Germany	+ 1.8
Finland	+ 2.1
France	+ 2.0
Greece	+ 2.8
Hungary	+ 3.5
Iceland	+ 2.3
Ireland	+ 2.2
Italy	+ 3.0
Netherlands	+ 1.1
Norway	+ 2.2
Poland	+ 5.9
Portugal	+ 1.9
Spain	+ 2.1
Switzerland	+ 1.0
Sweden	+ 2.4
UK, England and Wales	+ 0.4
Northern Ireland	+ 2.2
Scotland	+ 0.3
Yugoslavia	+ 3.5
Oceania	
Australia	+ 0.3
New Zealand	+ 0.8

(From Zaridze D, Boyle P, Smans M. International trends in prostatic cancer. *Int J Cancer* 1984;33:223–230.)

different findings in latent carcinomas and for the mortality rates. A recent study by Yatani and associates (16) shows that in Japan latent carcinomas increase in a parallel fashion to the increase of mortality rates. Applying identical examination methods, the frequency was 22.5% in the collecting period from 1965 to 1979, but 34.6% from 1982 to 1986, with a parallel increase with age (Fig. 2). The larger,

TABLE 7. *Differences in incidence (ASR World Standard) of prostate carcinoma in ethnically different populations living in the same area*

USA, California	Incidence
San Francisco Bay Area	
Black	82.5
White	50.0
Filipino	29.6
Japanese	16.5
Chinese	14.9
Los Angeles	
Black	82.6
other White	49.6
Latino	43.0
Japanese	22.8
Chinese	16.9
Korean	11.7

(From Muir C, Waterhouse J, Mack T, Powell J, Whelan S. Cancer incidence in five continents. *IARC Scientific Pub.* 1987; 5:88, Lyon.)

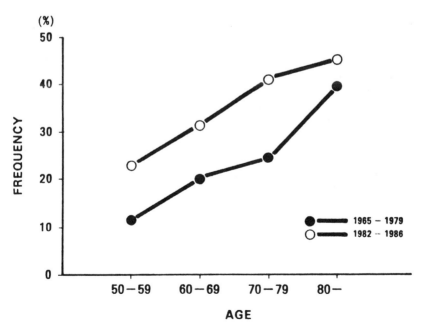

FIG. 2. Rising prevalence of latent carcinoma in Japan, according to age (From Yatani et al., ref. 16).

TABLE 8. *Age-corrected incidences of latent prostate carcinoma in Japan during two observation periods*

Histology	1965–1979 (%) (n = 576)	1982–1986 (%) (n = 660)	Significance
All cases	22.5	34.6	$p = 0.0001$
Infiltrative type	9.8	17.8	$p = 0.0001$
Noninfiltrative type	12.7	16.8	$p = 0.45$

(From Yatani R, et al. Trends in frequency of latent prostate carcinoma in Japan from 1965–79 to 1982–86. *JNCJ* 1988;80:683–687.)

infiltrating carcinomas are greatly relevant to this change of findings in Japan (Table 8). Thus, the rate of latent carcinomas in Japan has reached the values of the white population of the United States (34.6%) (12) or those of a West European population (Saarland 36.4%) (6).

Analytical Epidemiology

The causal pathogenesis of prostate carcinomas is largely unknown. The results of numerous case-control studies are not logical and often contradictory. Studies have shown that the incidence of prostate carcinomas increases when populations from low-risk areas immigrate to high-risk countries (e.g., Japanese in the United States, Japanese in Hawaii) (17). The findings confirm the importance of exogenic influences. The incidence and mortality rates of the Asian populations in the United States, however, remain remarkably under those of the black and the white populations. This difference in incidence and in mortality rates of the black and the white populations of the United States and the further increasing trend in blacks cannot be explained. Whether a difference in the socioeconomic status might be the reason for the high rate for prostate cancer in blacks has been investigated, but a significant gradient could not be found (18). The question of whether the black population of the United States has a genetically higher risk for prostate cancer cannot definitely be answered, because incidence and mortality of prostate cancer is low in most African populations (Table 9). Some regions, for example, Bulawajo, show the same incidence rates as those of the white population of the United States (1), however, Donn and Muir (19) point out that high autopsy rates influence the incidence in Bulawajo.

Case-control studies trying to analyze sexual behavior history show controversial results. It is speculated that sexual continence increases the risk factor of prostate cancer (3,20), and increased sexual activity is said to be responsible for a higher risk factor (21–24). A cohort study undertaken in 500 deceased Catholic priests from the archdiocese of Los Angeles displayed 13 deaths as the result of prostate cancer, compared with eight expected (25). The marital status of the patient (married, unmarried, divorced, widowed) is differently related with the risk of prostate cancer in the case-control studies. In some studies, no relationship can be found (26–28); others show that singles are at a lower risk (29,30) or at a higher risk (18,31).

TABLE 9. *Incidence of prostate carcinoma in blacks in the United States and in Africa*

San Francisco Bay	77.0
Alameda County	75.0
Detroit	67.1
Washington D.C.	59.8
Nigeria	10.2
South Africa	9.4
Uganda	4.4

(From Kovi J et al. Cancer of the prostate and aging: An autopsy study in black men from Washington D.C., and selected African cities. *Prostate* 1982;3:73–80.)

All these studies neither explain the considerable differences of incidence of prostate cancer between the white and the black populations of the United States nor those of the Asian populations who have an extremely low risk of prostate cancer. Viral etiology or sexually transferred viral infection have not yet been proven as a cause of prostate cancer (32). Ross et al. (33) state that circumcision diminishes the risk of prostate cancer. This finding has not been confirmed by other authors (33,34). Virus-like particles were seen in the urine of prostate cancer patients (35), and particles of herpes virus were found in cells of prostate carcinomas (36). In three studies, a higher prevalence of antibodies against herpes virus type 2 was observed in patients compared with controls (37–39). The importance of these findings must remain unclarified.

Studies on the influence of diet on the risk of prostate cancer are more relevant, because nutrition influences the hormone balance, in particular that of androgen steroids. The western diet, with a relatively high meat and fat intake, raises the plasma concentration of androgens (40). Several case-control studies show that increased supply of protein and of fat raises the risk of prostate cancer. Ecologic studies state that populations of high cancer risk show a higher proportion of animal fat in their daily caloric intake than those of low risk (27,41–45). The fact that different ethnic groups from Hawaii have a different risk of prostate cancer shows a positive correlation between relative cancer risk and fat consumption (44,46). Some case-control studies say that being overweight means having an increased risk of prostate cancer (26,47–49), whereas other case control studies do not confirm this finding (23,27,50). Yu and colleagues (28) find a moderate increase of risk in overweight whites, but not in blacks. In this study the cholesterol values do not greatly differ in patients and in controls. The incidence of prostate cancer is low in American Seventh-Day Adventists who are vegetarians (51,52). However, this incidence is negatively influenced by the fact that more than half become Adventists after the age of 40 (53). In Japan, the mortality from prostate cancer is positively correlated with the high consumption of milk, meat, and eggs compared with a low intake of green and yellow vegetables (54). Mettlin (55,56) was not able to prove a risk factor of prostate cancer for higher fat consumption in American blacks compared with the white population of the United States.

Studies on the relationship between the socioeconomic status and the incidence of mortality of prostate cancer have shown contradictory findings, but predominantly no relationship could be proved (18,51). Yu and coworkers (28) observed a slightly augmented but statistically significant risk in whites with high school education and with skilled professions. This study does not reveal any association with marital status, alcohol consumption, or cigarette smoking. Blacks with university education also have an increased risk of prostate cancer compared with blacks with only an elementary school education. It stands to reason that the socioeconomic status is only an indirect indicator that need not be representative for other, real risk factors (28).

A correlation between religion and risk of prostate cancer has been cited. This might be related to the life-style, for example, in Seventh-Day Adventists who practice a lacto-vegetarian diet (52). Some authors speculate whether circumcision is the reason for the lowered incidence of carcinomas in Jews living in the United States (28,33,57). The reason for the low incidence for Jews living in Israel might be related to food habits (27).

Several studies report on an augmented familial risk (22,24,58–60). An unequivocal differentiation between a real genetic risk and influences of the life-style cannot be made (51). Meikle and Stanish (61) state there is a four times higher risk of prostate cancer in brothers compared with brothers-in-law and the male population in general. In this study prostate cancer was diagnosed before the age of 62. Significantly lower values of plasma testosterone were seen in patients and their brothers with carcinomas than in controls.

Radiation exposure from the atom bomb in Hiroshima and Nagasaki has not influenced the frequency of latent carcinomas or the biologic activity of manifest prostate cancer (62).

Among the professional noxae only cadmium is of relevance. This has been confirmed by four studies proving a higher risk of prostate carcinomas following cadmium exposure (63–66). According to these studies, cadmium has to be considered as a carcinogenous substance for human prostate cancer. There might be a relationship between cadmium concentration in the air and zinc, which is a common component of the seminal fluid (18).

It could not be proven that any known chemical carcinogen is the cause of prostate cancer up to now so that the professional risk of prostate cancer should be of secondary importance.

BREAST CANCER

Descriptive Epidemiology

Breast cancer is the most prevalent of all cancer diseases in women throughout the world. In high-incidence areas, 25% to 30% of all malignant female tumors are breast cancers. In populations with low incidence, that is, in the Asian populations of Japan, China and India, as well as in some South American areas, breast cancer

TABLE 10. *Frequency of breast cancer in registry: Populations with low breast cancer incidence*

Registry population	1st position		2nd position	
	ICD	%	ICD	%
New Zealand, Maori	162:	22.9	174:	20.0
Brazil, Fortaleza	180:	31.2	174:	18.1
India, Nagpur	180:	27.3	174:	17.9
India, Poona	180:	24.3	174:	17.7
India, Madras	180:	38.5	174:	17.4
Costa Rica	180:	20.4	174:	16.9
Japan, Hiroshima	151:	21.5	174:	16.8
Singapore, Indian	180:	16.4	174:	16.1
Colombia, Cali	180:	21.8	174:	15.8
Japan, Miyagi	151:	24.8	174:	15.2
India, Bangalore	180:	29.3	174:	14.5
Japan, Osaka	151:	23.8	174:	13.0
China, Tianjin	162:	20.0	174:	12.7
China, Shanghai	151:	15.9	174:	12.4
Japan, Nagasaki	151:	21.8	174:	12.2

(From Muir C, Waterhouse J, Mack T, Powell J, and Whelan S. Cancer incidence in five continents, *IARC Scientific Pub.* 1987; 5:88, Lyon.)

only occupies the second position of cancer frequency with less than 20% (Table 10). In Japan, stomach cancer ranks first; in India and in South America, cervical carcinomas are the most frequent tumors.

The incidence of breast cancer (67) varies between 93.9 and 14/100,000 world standard population (Table 11). Hawaiian women and those from San Francisco rank at the top. The European areas of Geneva and Eindhoven show incidences over 70 and thus are still in the top group. A broad mean group showing incidence rates from 70 to 50/100,000 involves 70 of 137 populations recorded in a recent study (67). Most of the Central and North European populations belong to this group. Furthermore, the Canadian and Australian populations and the black women of the United States are in this mean group.

Some East European, Spanish, and Italian registries, and the Asian populations of the United States are at the bottom of the list. The populations of Japan, China, and India also are in this group.

Among American women there is a difference in rates among different ethnic groups, that is, those from Los Angeles or San Francisco (Table 12). The rates among the Asian populations in the United States, however, are higher than those of comparable populations of Asians in their native countries.

The worldwide incidence of breast cancer is increasing. The largest study of cancer incidence rates in the United States comes from Connecticut, which established cancer registration in 1935. The increase from 53.3 in 1935/1939 to 86.7 in 1975/1978 means an average rate of increase of about 1.2% per annum (68). The rate of 1975/1978 decreased slightly in the subsequent years. The incidence was probably influenced by special early detection activities in 1975/1978. When con-

TABLE 11. *Breast cancer incidence in five continents ICD 174 ASR World (137 populations)*

USA—Hawaii, Hawaiian	93.9
USA—San Francisco Bay, White	87.0
USA—Hawaii, White	84.4
Australia—Pacific Polynesian	80.3
USA—Alameda County, White	78.4
USA—Connecticut, White	77.8
USA—Los Angeles, White	77.3
USA—Washington, Seattle	76.2
USA—Atlanta, White	75.4
USA—Michigan, Detroit, White	74.9
Canada—Manitoba	76.6
Switzerland—Geneva	72.2
USA—New York State	72.2
Netherlands—Eindhoven	71.6
USA—New Mexico, White	71.2
Israel—Jews born Israel	70.2
Israel—Jews born Europe/America	69.8
USA—Iowa	68.7
USA—New York City	68.7
USA—Alameda County, Black	68.4
Canada—Quebec	68.4
USA—New Orleans, White	67.8
Switzerland—Basel	67.8
Switzerland—Neuchâtel	66.9
Canada—British Columbia	66.7
USA—San Francisco, Black	66.4
Canada—National Rep. System	66.4
Canada—Prince Edward Island	66.2
Canada—Saskatchewan	65.6
Brazil—Sao Paulo	65.5
Australia—Capital Territory	65.4
Canada—Ontario	64.7
Scotland—South East	64.3
Switzerland—Vaud	64.0
USA—Utah	63.8
USA—Michigan, Detroit, Black	63.4
Denmark	63.1
Australia—Victoria	62.9
Israel—Jews born Africa/Asia	62.8
France—Bas Rhin	62.4
USA—New Orleans, Black	61.7
Israel—all Jews	61.3
USA—Connecticut, Black	61.3
UK—Oxford	61.3
Scotland—North	60.8
Sweden	60.7
Brazil—Porto Allegre	60.6
Canada—North West Territories	60.5
Canada—Alberta	60.1
Iceland	60.1
Ireland, Southern	59.7
Scotland	59.6
Switzerland—Zurich	59.6
Italy—Lombardy	59.6
New Zealand—Maori	59.1
UK—England, Trent Region	59.1

TABLE 11. *Continued.*

UK—England, Mersey	59.1
USA—Los Angeles, Black	59.1
Canada—New Brunswick	58.9
Scotland—West	58.7
Canada—Maritime Provinces	58.5
Italy—Parma	58.4
Fed. Repub. Germany—Hamburg	58.0
France—Isère	57.7
New Zealand—Non-Maori	57.7
USA—Hawaii, Chinese	57.5
Canada—Nova Scotia	57.1
Scotland—East	56.8
Fed. Repub. Germany—Saarland	56.8
USA—Atlanta, Black	56.6
UK—England, South Western	56.3
Scotland—North East	56.0
Australia—Queensland	55.7
France—Calvados	55.1
UK—England, Birmingham	55.0
UK—England, South Thames	54.6
UK—England, North Western Region	54.6
UK—England and Wales	54.0
Australia—South Australia	53.7
Australia—New South Wales	53.1
France—Doubs	52.9
Australia—Western Australia	52.5
Norway	51.8
Australia—Tasmania	51.3
USA—Hawaii, Japanese	50.1
Brazil—Fortaleza	50.0
USA—San Francisco, Japanese	48.9
Brazil—Pernambuco	48.2
Canada—Newfoundland	46.7
Italy—Ragusa	46.7
USA—New Mexico, Hispanic	45.3
Spain—Catalonia	45.2
Finland	44.7
USA—San Francisco, Chinese	43.7
USA—Los Angeles, Latino	41.8
German Democratic Republic	41.4
USA—Los Angeles, Chinese	39.6
Poland—Cracow City	39.6
Spain—Navarra	38.7
Yugoslavia—Slovenia	37.7
USA—San Francisco, Filipino	37.2
Hungary—County Vas	36.4
USA—Los Angeles, Japanese	36.2
USA—Los Angeles, Filipino	35.7
Netherlands—Antilles	35.2
USA—Puerto Rico	35.1
Colombia—Cali	34.8
Spain—Zaragoza	34.7
Poland—Warsaw City	32.4
USA—Hawaii, Filipino	32.0
Czechoslovakia—Slovakia	31.2
France—Martinique	31.1
Costa Rica	30.7

(Table continues.)

TABLE 11. *Continued.*

Romania—County Cluj	30.4
Philippines—Rizal Prov.	29.8
Hong Kong	28.7
Japan—Hiroshima City	28.0
Singapore—Indian	27.6
Singapore—Chinese	27.1
Kuwait—Non-Kuwaitis	26.3
India—Poona	25.6
India—Bombay	24.1
USA—New Mexico, Amer. Indian	23.8
Hungary—County Szabolcs	22.9
Japan—Miyagi Pref.	22.0
Singapore—Malay	21.1
India—Madras	20.8
Japan—Nagasaki City	20.3
India—Bangalore	19.9
Japan—Osaka Pref.	19.7
India—Nagpur	19.2
China—Shanghai	19.1
Poland—Nowy Sacz, rural	18.4
China—Tianjin	18.2
Kuwait—Kuwaitis	15.9
USA—Los Angeles, Korean	14.1
Israel—Non-Jews	14.0

(From Muir C, Waterhouse J, Mack T, Powell J, Whelan S. Cancer incidence in five continents. *IARC Scientific Pub.* 1987;5:88, Lyon.)

sidering such trends, it should be investigated whether there are age-specific developments. The incidence rate significantly increased by 22% in young women in Washington State (69) from 1974/1977 to 1982/1984 thus showing a yearly rate of increase of 2.5%. During the same period, the incidence of breast cancer in women aged 45 to 54 decreased by 12%; the group over the age of 55, however, showed an increase by 9%. Because this study could not reveal any trend to earlier tumor stages in younger women, the rising incidence apparently is not related to early detection of breast cancer. According to the Danish Cancer Registry (70), breast cancer incidence increased in all age groups between 1948 and 1982, the increase being most pronounced in women less than 55 years old.

The results of the statistical analysis indicated that the increase was mostly because of a cohort effect. Within the same period, breast cancer mortality changed comparatively little and there was no evidence of a cohort effect. In Scandinavian countries the incidence rate increases yearly between 0.50 (Denmark) and 0.94/100,000 (Iceland) (71,72). The longest observation periods in Canada are those from Saskatchewan. There the incidence increased from 45 to 65/100,000 between 1950 and 1970, resulting in a yearly rate of increase of 1.9%. Japan shows a comparable increase in incidence (1.4% annual increase, Miyaga Prefecture; 1.2% Osaka) (68). Before 1960, the Asian populations of Hawaii displayed a 2.4 times higher incidence than the Chinese and Japanese populations in their native

TABLE 12. *Incidence rates of breast cancer in different ethnic populations of the same region*

Los Angeles	
White	77.3
Latino	41.8
Black	59.1
Japanese	36.2
Chinese	39.6
Filipino	35.7
Korean	14.1
San Francisco Bay	
White	87.0
Black	66.4
Japanese	48.9
Chinese	43.7
Filipino	37.2
Japan	
Hiroshima City	28.0
Miyagi	22.0
Nagasaki	20.3
Osaka	19.7
China	
Tianjin	18.2
Shanghai	19.1

(From Muir C, Waterhouse J, Mack T, Powell J, Whelan S. Cancer incidence in five continents. *IARC Scientific Pub.* 1987;5:88, Lyon.)

countries. From 1960/1964 to 1973/1977 the incidence increased from 21.1% to 41.5% in the Japanese population of Hawaii and from 40.2% to 79.7% in the Chinese population in Hawaii. The highest incidence, however, has been observed in Hawaiians, with an increase from 44.2% to 79.7%. This rate has now reached 93.9% (Table 13) (67).

The Jewish population of Israel displays different rates of increase (Table 14). A complete assimilation of incidences has taken place with a remarkably high rate of increase in Israelis having migrated from African and Asian countries.

TABLE 13. *Increasing breast cancer incidence rates in Hawaii*

	1960/64	1973/77	1978/82
Caucasian	48.1	75.8	84.4
Japanese	21.1	41.5	50.1
Chinese	36.4	49.5	57.5
Hawaiian	44.2	79.7	93.9

(From Muir C, Waterhouse J, Mack T, Powell J, Whelan S. Cancer incidence in five continents. *IARC Scientific Pub.* 1987;5:88, Lyon.)

TABLE 14. *Increasing breast cancer incidence rates in Israel*

	1960/66	1967/71	1977/81
Jews born in Europe/America	55.5	60.8	69.8
Jews born in Israel	35.9	53.6	70.2
Jews born in Africa/Asia	22.2	26.7	62.8

(From Muir C, Waterhouse J, Mack T, Powell J, Whelan S. Cancer incidence in five continents. *IARC Scientific Pub.* 1987;5:88, Lyon.)

Analytical Epidemiology

Risk factors for developing breast cancer have been investigated in numerous epidemiologic studies. Genetic risks are compared with risk factors related to reproduction. Special attention has been dedicated to whether nutrition plays a role in the etiology of breast cancer.

Familial Breast Cancer Risk

"Breast cancer has been the subject of an impressive number of extensive genetic studies, perhaps more than any other neoplasm" (73). In the majority of the studies, a two- to three-times risk is calculated in first-degree relatives. The results are different, however, when the development of premenopausal and postmenopausal carcinomas in mothers and sisters is compared with that of bilateral carcinomas (73). In cases of unilateral, premenopausal carcinoma of the mother, the daughter has a three times higher risk of developing carcinoma compared with that of controls with no familial risk. If the mother suffers from postmenopausal cancer, however, the risk for the daughter is statistically insignificantly higher. In premenopausal bilateral carcinoma of the mother the risk is nine times higher, in postmenopausal bilateral cancer it is four times higher. Genetic factors thus play a more important role in bilateral breast cancer, especially in premenopausal carcinoma of the mother. The probability of a second carcinoma developing in the contralateral breast is increased when there is a positive familial history (74,75), reaching 28% compared with 13% in unselected control groups. In premenopausal cancer, the probability rises to 35% to 38% (74).

In Iceland, where there has been a nationwide complete cancer registration since 1955, there is a clear gradient of risk with degree of relativeness risk decreasing from sisters and mothers to aunts, to cousins, to unrelated (145). The observed family risk cannot be explained by familial patterns of reproductive behavior (72). The relative risk is found to be 2.59 for mothers and 2.56 for sisters. Maternal breast cancer is significantly more frequent in medullary breast carcinoma than in other types of breast cancer (76). There is no difference in familial risk between small and large invasive tumors (77).

TABLE 15. *Reproductive risk factors for female breast cancer (case-control studies)*

Case-control studies	Relative risk
Bilateral oophorectomy at age 50+ versus <40 (79)	8.0
Bilateral oophorectomy via surgery or radiation at age 37 + versus <37 (80)	5.6
Natural menopause at age 50 + versus <40 (79)	3.3
Birth of first child at age 30 + versus < 20 (86,87)	2.0
Birth of first child at age 30 + versus < 20	
For premenopausal and perimenopausal women combined	2.7
For postmenopausal women (83)	1.7
No versus any children (82,86,87)	1.4/1.5
Menarche at age < 12 versus 15 + for premenopausal and	
perimenopausal women (83)	1.8

(From Roush GC, Holford TR, Schymura MJ, White C. *Cancer risk and incidence trends.* Washington: Hemisphere Publishing.)

Reproduction and Breast Cancer Risk

Reproductive variables have been consistently associated with female breast cancer. Table 15 (78) shows the relative risk of these variables according to the results of different case-control studies. Accordingly, early menarche and late menopause increase the risk of developing breast cancer by 1.4 to 3.3 times. The onset of menarche plays only a role in premenopausal and perimenopausal carcinomas. Bilateral ovarectomy before the age of 40, that is, an early, surgically induced, menopause, significantly reduces the risk of development of breast cancer (79–85).

Nulliparity raises the risk only 1.4 to 1.5 times (82,86,87); however, birth of the first child after the age of 30 causes a risk of 2.2 to 2.7 times (77). The crucial point is the age of approximately 35 years: Before this age any full-time pregnancy confers some degree of protection (88). If breast cancer is inversely related to high parity independent of age at first birth, the effect is a modest one (79).

Neither postmenopausal estrogens nor oral contraceptives are consistently associated with breast cancer (82,89–93). Long-term athletic training might lower the risk of breast cancer and cancers of the reproductive system (94,95). Athletic activities might delay menarche, which might have relevance for reducing the risk of breast cancer (96).

Diet and Breast Cancer Risk

The rapidly expanding scientific literature on the relationship between diet and cancer etiology is complex and frequently contradictory (97). Human epidemiologic studies of diet as a causal factor in cancer have been generally of four types:

1. Ecologic (correlation) studies
2. Case-control studies
3. Prospective studies
4. Intervention studies.

Ecologic studies are inquiries in which cancer rates for defined populations are correlated with rates of suspected risk factors as measured in the same populations.

Goodwin and Boyd (98) provide a crucial appraisal of the evidence that dietary fat intake is related to breast cancer risk in humans. Twenty-seven correlation studies were identified. Ten of 13 international studies examined the relationship between total dietary fat and breast cancer risk and all demonstrated an association between breast cancer mortality or breast cancer incidence and per capita intake of fat. Six national or regional studies examined the relationship between total fat intake and breast cancer risk. Four demonstrated a positive association, while two did not. Five time-trend studies also examined the relationship between total fat intake and breast cancer risk and the two that tested this association for statistical significance (99–101) found it to be a significant factor. The correlation between breast cancer risk and dietary fat was stronger, if diet 10 or 12 years previously was used in the analysis.

Conclusions from correlation studies always should be drawn with the utmost caution; this already results from the methodical approach. The habits of populations and not those of individuals are estimated. Furthermore, it is difficult to calculate the fat consumption per capita. Of four prospective cohort studies, two American studies do not show any association between fat or meat intake and breast cancer risk (102,103). On the contrary, two studies from Japan, where fat intake is lower and probably more heterogenous, were able to show an association between intake of meat and fatty foods and breast cancer risk (104,105). The large Japanese cohort study showed that women who eat meat daily experience higher breast cancer rates than those who do not. Interestingly, this effect was seen only in those women aged 55 and over (97). Goodwin and Boyd (98) summarize 14 case-control studies that examined the relationship between intake of total fat or fat-containing foods and breast cancer risk. Eight studies examined the relationship between total fat intake and breast cancer risk, but the results of these case-control studies are inconsistent and provide only weak evidence in support of an association between total fat intake and breast cancer risk.

Six study groups demonstrated significant associations between breast cancer risk and one or more specific dietary sources of fat—in particular meat, butter, and margarine. By using hard fat (margarine, butter, or shortening) for frying versus oil, the risk factor was 2.0 in a cohort study in Seventh-Day Adventists (106), whereas a Canadian study (107) shows a risk factor of 2.2 in people who consume pork four to six times weekly versus those who consume pork less than three times weekly (78).

Whether obesity and fat intake are independently associated with breast cancer risk has not been consistently reported (78), although it is important to note that total caloric intake had no effect in the study of Seventh-Day Adventists (106). In two case-control studies by Dubin and associates (108,109) the epidemiologic risk factor differences between minimal breast cancer (*in situ* and small invasive carcinomas) and all other breast carcinomas were examined. Unlike clinical breast cancer, minimal breast cancer was not associated with either family history of breast cancer or obesity. These results could not be explained by any plausible diagnostic bias.

In a study from Sweden, Toernberg and colleagues (110) reported on a statistically significant positive correlation between height, weight, and systolic blood pressure and breast cancer risk. In the group of younger women, a high serum β-lipoprotein level was associated with an increased risk of breast cancer. This relationship became even stronger when studied in a multivariate analysis, which also showed a negative correlation between serum cholesterol and cancer risk. Prospective studies of breast cancer mortality and serum cholesterol and serum lipids show no differences in risk between women with high levels of cholesterol and serum lipids compared with women with low levels (111).

The precise mechanism of the increased risk observed with obesity in postmenopausal years is not clear (97). It is hypothesized that increased risk might be related to the phenomenon of estrone production in adipose tissue from the androstenedione precursor. Adipose tissue in the obese menopausal female is therefore a significant source of estrogen. This raises the possibility that excess caloric intake leading to obesity might be etiologically important in postmenopausal breast cancer indirectly by affecting body fat levels (97).

Other Risk Factors

Racial Differences

Ethnic differences in incidence of breast cancer are particularly evident in American areas where white, black, and Asian populations are living, for example in Los Angeles and in San Francisco (see Table 12). The Asian populations—Chinese and Japanese—display distinctly lower incidence rates than white and black women, but the incidence rates are remarkably higher than those of women in the Asian native countries. Both genetic and life-style factors are probably responsible for such differences. Kolonel and coworkers (112–114) determined that the different ethnic groups of Hawaii showed good correlations with the ethnic-specific incidence rates of breast cancer regarding their food consumption and intake of total fat.

On the other hand, the histopathology of breast cancer is different between white and Japanese women (115).

Breast tumors seen in native Japanese women are more often *in situ* carcinomas, more frequently showing a uniform nuclear pattern and displaying a more extensive infiltration of lymphocytes. Lymph node metastases are rare. A genetic modulation of hormonal balance and/or of immunologic response might be the basis for these differences.

The study of Hoel and associates (116) shows genetic and life-style differences between American and Japanese women. The onset of menarche takes place at the age of 14.4 years in Japanese girls. Differences were observed in age of first birth and nulliparity rates. Age at menopause was similar for the two groups; American women also have a considerably higher rate of surgically induced menopause.

There is a 20% higher mortality rate in blacks than in white American women (117). This higher rate in this study was because breast cancer in blacks was not discovered as early as in white women, tumors were larger in the black women, and there was greater frequency and greater extent of nodule involvement (118,119). Premenopausal and postmenopausal estrogen receptor-positive tumors were found significantly less frequently in blacks compared with whites. No statistically significant difference was observed in the use of hormones between black and white patients; 13.5% of the blacks compared with 18.6% of the whites had one or more affected relatives. No difference exists at the age of menarche, however, 25.3% of the blacks compared with 13.0% of the whites reported cessation of menses before 40 years of age.

Significant differences exist at the age of first pregnancy: 38.5% of the black women, versus 14.5% of the white women, were less than 20 years of age at the first pregnancy; the mean age is 21.8 in blacks, 24.7 in whites ($p = 0.001$) (117).

The immigration study of Haenszel and Kurihara already has shown the low incidence rate of breast cancer among Japanese women in the United States, with no apparent tendency to rise to the host population level, suggesting a role for genetic factors. On the other hand, Staszewski (121) has shown that Polish immigrants both in the United States and in Australia have a higher breast cancer mortality rate than Polish women in their native country despite a decrease in the percentage of nulliparous women. In this case socioeconomic changes resulting in American nutrition style are the more likely candidates for the observed disease trend (122).

Alcohol

Alcohol consumption is a relative risk factor for breast cancer. Case-control and cohort studies (123–127) have shown a relative risk between 1.5 and 2.5. Adjustment for known breast cancer risk factors and a variety of nutritional variables did not materially alter this relation (103).

Smoking

Smoking is not related to breast cancer. As compared with women who had never smoked, the estimated risk of breast cancer was 1.1 for current smokers of any amount and 1.0 for heavy smokers (128). A 1-year reduction at age of menopause was associated with a 0.97 reduction in the risk of breast cancer. However, there was no indication that the overall effect of smoking on breast cancer was protective (129).

Bilateral Breast Cancer Risk

Breast cancer patients have a higher risk for a second carcinoma in the contralateral breast (130). The relative risk of developing a second primary cancer was 2.9. However, the risk is 9.9 before the age of 50; after that age it is only 1.9 (130). The incidence ratio of bilateral to unilateral disease was used in this study as an estimate of the lifetime risk of developing a second primary cancer. The cumulative risk is 13.3% for women younger than 50 and 3.5% for women older than 50 years at first diagnosis.

Chaudary and associates (131) reported in a British study that the incidence of nonsimultaneous bilateral disease was 7.6 second cancers per thousand patients at risk per year. Women whose first breast cancers developed when they were under the age of 40 had three times the risk of a second breast cancer developing. The risk of contralateral cancer developing is significantly higher in lobular carcinomas than in ductal carcinomas (132).

Seasonal Variation in Breast Cancer Detection

In Australia, there was a significant seasonal variation observed in the incidence of breast cancer with a peak in spring (November) and a low in winter (July) (133). Seasonality in the occurrence of breast cancer was also observed in Israel (134) and in England (135). Peaks occurred during spring and troughs appeared during autumn. Unlike primary tumors, there was no significant seasonal variation in the time of recurrence (136). A distinct seasonal deviation was detected in the birth of women who became breast cancer patients in Japan (137). A major peak of birth occurred during spring to autumn and a trough appeared in winter. Differences exist between premenopausal and postmenopausal women and histologic subtype.

Possibly exogenous seasonal factors act as the fetal or neonatal stages in the etiology of breast cancer. In Greek women, seasonal variations in the frequency distribution according to the month of their birth also were observed (138). Two high-frequency peaks in the spring and in the autumn were detected—significantly higher than those of the remaining months.

Radiation Exposure

Fewer than 1% of all cases of breast cancer result from diagnostic radiography. The evaluations of Evans and colleagues (139) reveal that such tumors probably in general occur late in life. The incidence of radiation-induced breast cancer was highest at 76 years. Diagnostic radiography has only a small influence on the occurrence of breast cancer. The higher risk for breast cancer among atomic bomb survivors from Hiroshima and Nagasaki is well known (140). In a recent study of cases between 1950 and 1980 the dose response appeared to be roughly linear and did not differ between the two cities (143). The most remarkable new finding was the emergence of a radiation-related excess among women under 10 years of age at exposure. The risk of radiogenic breast cancer appears to decrease with increasing age at exposure. A 3.6 relative risk for breast cancer after radiation for postpartum-mastitis with 20–34-year follow-up was shown by Shore and associates (144).

TABLE 16. *Endometrial cancer incidence in five continents.*
ICD 182—Corpus uteri—ASR world (137 populations)

USA—New Mexico, other white	29.9
Canada—Maritime Provinces	29.2
USA—Washington, Seattle	28.8
USA—San Francisco, white	25.7
USA—Hawaii, Hawaiian	25.2
USA—Alameda, white	24.8
USA—Los Angeles, other white	24.1
USA—Hawaii, white	23.4
USA—Michigan, Detroit, white	22.0
USA—Utah	21.4
Canada—Manitoba	19.8
Australia—Pacific Polynesian Islanders	19.6
USA—San Francisco, Japanese	19.6
USA—Iowa	19.3
USA—Connecticut, white	19.3
USA—Atlanta, white	18.9
USA—Hawaii, Chinese	18.7
Canada—Ontario	17.4
Canada—Quebec	17.1
Switzerland—Zurich	16.9
Switzerland—Neuchâtel	16.8
USA—New York State	16.7
Canada—Nat. Rep. Syst.	16.7
Canada—Saskatchewan	15.8
Canada—Alberta	15.6
USA—Hawaii, Japanese	15.5
New Zealand—Maori	15.4
Hungary—County Vas	15.3
Denmark	15.3
Switzerland—Geneva	15.2
USA—San Francisco, Chinese	14.8
Canada—British Columbia	14.7
Fed. Repub. Germany—Saarland	14.3
German Democratic Republic	13.9
Switzerland—Basel	13.7
Czechoslovakia—Slovakia	13.7
Brazil—Sao Paulo	13.7
Iceland	13.4
Italy—Parma	13.4
Sweden	13.2
USA—Los Angeles, Latino	12.9
Canada—New Brunswick	12.9
Switzerland—Vaud	12.8
France—Bas Rhin	12.7
Italy—Lombardy	12.5
USA—Los Angeles, Japanese	12.5
USA–Connecticut, Black	12.5
Israel—Jews born Europe/America	12.5
Spain—Navarra	12.5
Italy—Ragusa	12.3
Finland	12.2
USA—New York City	12.2
Canada—Nova Scotia	12.2
Norway	12.1
Canada—Prince Edward Island	11.9
USA—Los Angeles, Chinese	11.8

TABLE 16. *Continued.*

USA—Atlanta, Black	11.6
Yugoslavia—Slovenia	11.6
Scotland—North	11.5
USA—San Francisco Bay, Black	11.5
Fed. Repub. Germany—Hamburg	11.3
Spain—Catalonia	11.3
USA—Los Angeles, Black	11.1
Brazil—Porto Allegre	11.1
Australia—South Australia	11.0
USA—Hawaii, Filippino	11.0
USA—Alameda, Black	10.8
USA—New Orleans, black	10.6
USA—New Orleans, white	10.4
UK—England, Oxford	10.4
Netherlands—Eindhoven	10.3
Australia—Western Australia	10.2
New Zealand—Non-Maori	10.0
USA—Michigan, Detroit, Black	10.0
UK—England, South Western	9.9
Australia—Queensland	9.9
Israel—all Jews	9.8
Canada—Newfoundland	9.7
France—Isère	9.7
USA—New Mexico, Hispanic	9.6
France—Doubs	9.6
Australia—Victoria	9.6
France—Calvados	9.4
Poland—Warsaw City	9.3
UK—England, Trent Region	9.2
UK—England, South Thames	9.2
Poland—Cracow City	9.2
UK—England, Birmingham	9.1
Israel—Jews born Israel	8.9
USA—Los Angeles, Filippino	8.5
Australia—New South Wales	8.3
UK—England and Wales	8.2
USA—Puerto Rico	8.0
Australia—South Australia	7.9
Scotland—South East	7.8
Hungary—County Szabolcs	7.8
France—Martinique	7.7
Scotland—North East	7.6
Spain—Zaragoza	7.5
UK—England, Mersey region	7.4
USA—San Francisco, Filippino	7.3
Australia—Capital Territory	7.3
Brazil	7.1
Scotland—East	6.8
Scotland	6.8
Brazil—Pernambuco	6.6
Hong Kong	6.3
Israel—Jews born Africa/Asia	6.1
Colombia—Cali	6.0
Kuwait—Non-Kuwaitis	5.9
Scotland—West	5.7
Costa Rica	5.6
UK—North Western region	5.5

(Table continues.)

TABLE 16. *Continued.*

Ireland—Southern	5.4
Netherlands—Antilles	5.2
Singapore—Chinese	5.1
Romania—County Cluj	4.4
Poland—Nowy Sacz, rural	4.3
USA—New Mexico, American Indian	3.9
Singapore—Malay	3.9
Japan—Hiroshima City	3.7
Philippines—Rizal Prov.	3.5
Canada—North West Territories	3.5
China—Tianjin	3.4
India—Poona	3.2
USA—Los Angeles, Korean	3.1
Israel—Non-Jews	3.1
China—Shanghai	3.0
Japan—Nagasaki City	3.0
Japan—Miyagi Pref.	2.8
Singapore—Indian	2.7
Japan—Osaka Pref.	2.4
India—Bangalore	2.1
India—Bombay	2.0
India—Madras	1.9
Kuwait—Kuwaitis	1.8
India—Nagpur	1.2

(From Muir C, Waterhouse J, Mack T, Powell J, Whelan S. Cancer incidence in five continents. *IARC Scientific Pub.* 1987;5:88, Lyon.)

ENDOMETRIAL CANCER

Descriptive Epidemiology

The relationship of endometrial cancer incidence to breast cancer incidence varies worldwide between 1:2 and 1:4. In the United States, cancer of the corpus uteri is the third most common cancer in women, with about 40,000 new cases diagnosed annually (14). The incidence rates, however, differ worldwide by about 25 times between 29.9 and 1.2 (Table 16) (2).

The white women of the United States occupy a top position of incidence rates for women over 20. Hawaiian women in Hawaii and women from a Canadian province belong to this top group. Sixty-four populations displaying incidence rates from 10 to 20 constitute a broad mean group. Most Canadian and European populations, as well as the black and Asian populations of the United States, are represented in this group. The Asian populations of Japan, China, and India show low incidence rates, but British, East European, Canadian, and South American populations have incidence rates below 10.

Comparing the rank order of incidence rates of breast and endometrial cancer the following similarities reveal: 19 of 30 populations at the top of breast cancer inci-

TABLE 17. Ethnic differences in incidence in the same area

	ASR World
Los Angeles	
White	24.1
Latino	12.9
Japanese	12.5
Chinese	11.8
Black	11.1
Filippino	8.5
Korean	3.1
San Francisco	
White	25.7
Japanese	19.6
Chinese	14.8
Black	11.5
Hawaii	
Hawaiian	25.2
White	23.4
Chinese	18.7
Japanese	15.5
Filippino	11.0

(From Muir C, Waterhouse I, Mack T, Powell J, Whelan S. Cancer incidence in five continents. *IARC Scientific Pub.* 1987;5:88, Lyon.)

dence also occupy a top position in endometrial cancer. Fifteen of 20 populations with low breast cancer incidence are reversely also represented at the bottom of the list of endometrial cancer. In this context it should be taken into account that the variability of incidence in endometrial carcinomas amounts to 25 times, but in breast cancer only to six times.

Ethnic differences in endometrial cancer in the same area of the United States also can be observed (Table 17): White women show distinctly higher incidence rates than black and Asian women. In Hawaii, white women are still surpassed by the native Hawaiian women. Chinese and Japanese women in the United States display much higher incidence rates than those in their native countries (Table 18). The incidence rates in Los Angeles and San Francisco are from 11 to 19.6, whereas they are lower than 4 in China and in Japan, with the exception of Hong Kong.

The mortality rate from endometrial cancer is much lower than that of incidence. In the Cancer Surveillance, Epidemiology and End Results (SEER) areas for the years 1973–1977, the age-adjusted mortality rate was 4.4/100,000, the annual age-adjusted incidence rate was 29.7. In a West German population (146) the ratio incidence to mortality is 16.7:4.3. The mortality rates throughout the world differ only relatively slightly (147). The European mortality figures lie between 2.9 (Norway) and 7.3 (Romania). The Federal Republic of Germany (FRG) occupies a midposition up to 4.7. According to Segi (147), Japan lies higher (5.6) and both the United States (3.4) and Israel (3.3) are somewhat lower (2).

TABLE 18. *Incidence of endometrial cancer in China and Japan*

	ASR World
China	
Shanghai	3.0
Tianjin	3.4
Hong Kong	6.3
Japan	
Hiroshima City	3.7
Miyagi Prefecture	2.8
Nagasaki City	3.0
Osaka Prefecture	2.4

(From Muir C, Waterhouse J, Mack T, Powell J, Whelan S. Cancer incidence in five continents. *IARC Scientific Pub.* 1987;5:88, Lyon.)

Time Trends

The time trends of incidence and mortality are influenced by different factors:

- Rate of hysterectomy
- Proportion of ICD 179: Uterine cancer not otherwise specified (NOS)
- Criteria of histologic diagnosis by the pathologist
- Rate of latent endometrial carcinoma only detected at autopsy.

Rate of hysterectomy. Between 1970 and 1975 the hysterectomy rate/1,000 women over 40 years rose by 33% and by 1975 almost one-third of American women over 50 years had had a hysterectomy (148). In England and Wales, 10% of the women at the age of 44 and 18% of those at the age of 64 had had a hysterectomy in 1976 (149). The denominators for incidence and mortality rates should thus ideally include only women with intact uteri, but this has not always been done (150). The incidence rate—adjusted for prior hysterectomy—in 1960 is about 5 points higher, but in 1975 already 15 points higher than that of the unadjusted incidence rate in Connecticut (151) (Fig. 3).

Proportion of ICD 179: uterine cancer NOS. In descriptive epidemiology ICD 179 means "uterine cancer not otherwise specified" which can include death from either cancer of the cervix or cancer of the corpus uteri. Weiss (152) points out that uterine cancer NOS death outnumbers corpus cancer death in the ratio 1.6:1.0. In the Connecticut Tumor Registry (153) the proportion of cases classified as primary to the uterus but NOS more precisely was 48% in 1940 and 5% in 1970, respectively (154). Investigators addressing this problem have concluded that trends in corpus cancer mortality are best estimated on the basis of the sum of cancer of the corpus uteri and uterine cancer NOS death with adjustment for the decreasing numbers of death in the uterine cancer NOS category that are attributable to cervical cancer (150).

Criteria of histologic diagnosis by the pathologist. Many carcinomas arise from

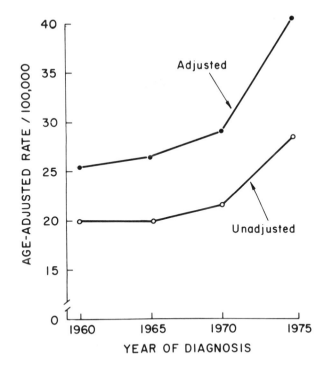

FIG. 3. Rising incidence of endometrial cancer, adjusted versus unadjusted for prior hysterectomy (From Lilienfeld et al., ref. 29).

hyperplastic endometrial tissue (155,156). The development of invasive carcinomas from the following prestages—glandular-cystic hyperplasia, adenomatous hyperplasia, early noninvasive cancer—leads to histologic findings whose diagnosis is difficult and that is subject to individual assessment by the pathologist. Since 1970, pathologists increasingly have diagnosed lesions as early endometrial carcinoma that used to be interpreted as adenomatous hyperplasia up to that time. Slide reviews by expert pathologists have suggested that 20% of the increase in incidence rates can be attributed to changing criteria of pathologists in 1970 (150). It is still unknown whether those figures also can be related to European conditions.

Rate of latent endometrial carcinoma only detected at autopsy. Endometrial carcinomas can remain without symptoms and thus undetected during the patient's lifetime. The proportion of women who have undergone necropsy and with previously undiagnosed endometrial carcinoma at the Yale-New Haven Hospital was about 1/450, and at the Massachusetts General Hospital about 1/325 (157). This proportion is relatively small in comparison to the lifetime risk of diagnosed endometrial cancer among women with intact uteri and it has been estimated on the basis of these and other figures that between 10% and 20% of endometrial cancer are never diagnosed (158).

There is evidence that both incidence and mortality of endometrial carcinoma are influenced—partly contrary—by the four factors mentioned previously. Thus it will be difficult to calculate "true" trends in incidence and mortality rates with international comparison. In many countries, however, rising incidence rates are observed: The Connecticut Tumor Registry shows an increase of incidence rates from 25 to about 40 from 1960 to 1975—adjusted for prior hysterectomy. The increase appeared first in California around 1966 and then in 1970 in the rest of the country with particularly steep increase noted from 1970 to 1974. The increase was greatest for localized disease (159). There is an increasing incidence in different regions of the United States: In postmenopausal women, rates in corpus cancer in the early 1970s show sharp increases that were similar in Hawaii, Los Angeles county, New Mexico, Oregon, the San Francisco Bay area, Seattle, and Utah (160,161). The increase was greatest for localized stage and was limited primarily to postmenopausal ages, particularly women in the 50 to 59 age group. The rates achieved a plateau in 1975, followed by a modest decline (162).

In Denmark, the incidence has been increasing steadily. The trend in the incidence rates varies in different age groups and examination of birth cohorts show higher rates after the age of 50 for more recent generations (163). The rates also have increased in all other Nordic countries (Fig. 4) (164). The increase has been most pronounced in the postmenopausal age groups over 50 years. In Denmark and Sweden, the incidence decreased in the premenopausal women in 1970. The incidence rate among Scottish women is lower than the rates in other parts of Britain and in most European countries. The incidence has been decreasing slowly since the mid1960s (165).

The mortality time trends are decreasing in many countries. The mortality decreased drastically from 12.5 to 4.0 in the Federal Republic of Germany from 1950

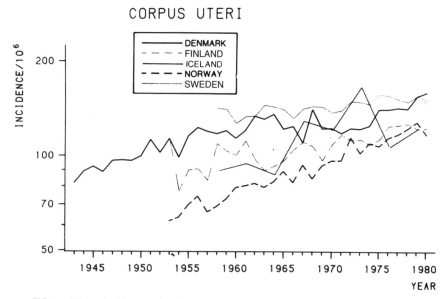

FIG. 4. Rising incidence of endometrial cancer in Nordic countries, 1945–1980 (From Servadio et al., ref. 7).

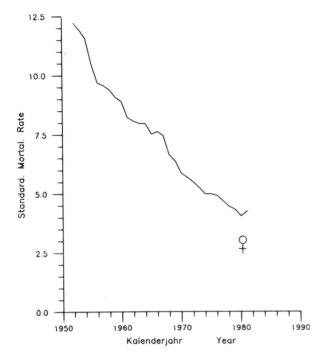

FIG. 5. Decreasing mortality rate of endometrial cancer in the Federal Republic of Germany, 1950–1980 (From Muir et al., ref. 2).

to 1980 (Fig. 5) (166). In the United States, after considering the effect of hysterectomy and unspecified uterine cancers, Weiss (152) concluded that there had been a real decrease in mortality during the years of 1950 and 1960.

Analytical Epidemiology

Most of the major risk factors for endometrial cancer identified to date can be explained by the mechanism of exposure to estrogen without sufficient exposure to progesterone (150).

Weight

Heavy body weight is a strong risk factor for endometrial cancer (167). The American Cancer Society prospective study on 419,060 women who were followed from 1959 to 1972 shows a significant increase of endometrial cancer mortality with increase in body weight (168,169). The relative risk for endometrial cancer in Connecticut women of ages 45 to 74 years is correlated to body weight (Table 19) (170). Heavy body weight is a risk factor regardless of menopausal status.

Endometrial cancer in women aged 45 years or less also show a positive correlation with body weight (Table 20) (171). The study provides clear evidence that the risk of endometrial cancer in young women is markedly increased by obesity.

TABLE 19. Relative risk for endometrial cancer in Connecticut women of ages 45–74 years

Weight (lb.)	Relative risk
≤ 125	1.0
126–145	1.3
146–165	1.3
≥ 166	2.3

(From Kelsey JL, Livolsi VA, Holford TR. A case-control study of cancer of the endometrium. *AMJ Epidemiol* 1982;116:333–343.)

A retrospective study from Denmark showed that 73.4% of patients with endometrial cancer were overweight and 55.8% were obese (172). The patients had a significantly greater absolute and relative weight than normal control subjects. Both premenopausal and postmenopausal obese women convert more plasma androstenedione to estrone than nonobese women (150,173,174). Sex hormone binding globulin (SHBG) concentration in the serum is lower in obese women. Thus, obese women not only have greater concentrations of circulating estrogens, but the estradiol might be more available to estrogen-responsive tissue (171). Several conditions related to body weight, such as hypertension or diabetes mellitus, were more common in cases than in controls (175).

Diet

Endometrial cancer is positively correlated in ecological studies with per capita fat consumption, with coefficients of the same order of magnitude as for breast cancer (168,176). Obesity is obviously linked to diet, but the role of diet independent of its effect on nutritional status has not yet been thoroughly studied. Death rates for

TABLE 20. Postitive correlation with body weight of endometrial cancer patients aged 45 years or younger

Current weight (lb.)	Relative risk
129	1.0
130	1.45
150	1.95
170	9.60
190 +	17.70

(From Henderson BE, Casagrande JT, Pike MC, Mak T, Rosario J, Duke A. The epidemiology of endometrial cancer in young women. *Br J Cancer* 1983;47:749–756.)

endometrial cancer are lower than expected among Californian Seventh-Day Adventists who tend to be lacto-ovo-vegetarians (177). In a case-control study (175) the risk of endometrial cancer was elevated in subjects reporting greater fat (butter, margarine, oil) intake; these people reported less frequent intake of green vegetables, fruit, and whole-grain foods. Endometrial cancer patients drank more wine and other alcoholic beverages with a trend of increasing risk with larger consumption.

In different ethnic groups of Hawaii, Kolonel and associates (178) found significant positive associations between fat intake and risk for endometrial cancer.

Reproduction

Nulliparous women are at higher risk than parous women. Increasing parity is strongly associated with decreased risk (Table 21) (171). The age of the woman at the birth of her first child does not appear to be related to risk for endometrial cancer (150). Infertility, however, might be related to an increased risk for endometrial cancer and is often associated with anovulation. Infertile women with polycystic ovaries or with ovarian stromal hyperplasia tend to have high plasma androstenedione levels (150, 179). Amenorrhea has a relative risk of 5.33 in the case-control study by Henderson and associates (171). Several reports indicate that about 20% of endometrial cancer patients under the age of 40 years have the Stein-Leventhal syndrome. In light of the rarity of both the Stein-Leventhal syndrome and endometrial cancer in young women, it is likely that a high risk exists among women with this syndrome (150,180). Age of menopause and relative risk for endometrial cancer are positively correlated (Table 22) (150). Longer exposure to estrogens in association with anovulatory cycles might be responsible for this correlation.

In some studies, early menarche is weakly correlated with an increased risk for endometrial cancer (170). Women with menarche at age 12 or older were at less risk for endometrial cancer than those with earlier age at menarche, but no further decrease in risk was noted for ages at menarche greater than 12 years (150).

TABLE 21. *Pregnancies and risk for endometrial cancer*

Full-term pregnancies	Relative risk
0	1.0
1	0.54
2	0.22
3	0.12
4 +	0.06

(From Henderson BE, Casagrande JT, Pike MC, Mak T, Rosario J, Duke A. The epidemiology of endometrial cancer in young women. *Br J Cancer* 1983;47:749–756.)

TABLE 22. *Age at menopause and risk for endometrial cancer*

Age at menopause (years)	Relative risk
<40	1.0
41–45	1.2
46–50	1.8
>50	3.1

(From Kelsey JL, Hildreth NG. Breast and gynecological cancer epidemiology. Boca Raton, FL: CRC Press, Inc. 1983.)

Estrogen-Replacement Therapy and Oral Contraceptives

Most investigators have found an increased risk for endometrial cancer among women who have used estrogen-replacement therapy (for the literature, see 150); however, most of this therapy consists of conjugated estrogens in the United States. The relative risk is increasing with time since first used (Table 23) (181). After 15 years, it is not clear whether there is any further increase in risk. Cessation of use appears to be associated with a relatively rapid decrease in risk (150,182–184). The association between estrogen-replacement therapy and endometrial cancer is strongest with cancer of stage I. In this case, however, the differential diagnostic criteria of the pathohistologic diagnosis play a role when demarcating adenomatous hyperplasia from carcinoma (see Time Trends, criteria of histologic diagnosis by the pathologist earlier in this chapter). In Europe, estrogen-replacement therapy with conjugated estrogens has been far less important than in the United States. In Finland, where compounds with estriol or estradiol generally have been used rather than conjugated estrogens, no association between estrogens and endometrial can-

TABLE 23. *Estrogen-replacement therapy and risk of endometrial cancer*

Time since first used (years)	Relative risk
Never used	1.0
1–2	1.2
3–4	5.4
5–7	4.7
8–10	11.7
11–14	24.2
15–19	10.2
≥20	8.3

(From Weiss NS, Szekely DR, English DR, Schweid AJ. Endometrial cancer in relation to patterns of menopausal estrogen use. *JAMA* 1979;242:261.)

TABLE 24. *Combination oral contraceptives and risk of endometrial cancer*

Combination oral contraceptives years	Relative risk
0	1.0
≤ 2	0.75
2 –	0.79
4 –	0.28
6 +	0.14

(From Henderson BE, Casagrande JT, Pike MC, Mak T, Rosario J, Duke A. The epidemiology of endometrial cancer in young women. *Br J Cancer* 1983;47:749–756.)

cer has been found, suggesting that it is only conjugated estrogens that are carcinogenic in the endometrium (185). Oral contraceptives partly increase and partly decrease the risk of endometrial cancer: Use of sequential oral contraceptives is strongly associated with increased risk of endometrial cancer (171,186). Combination oral contraceptive (COC) use, on the other hand, is associated with a decreased risk, correlated with duration of COC-use (Table 24) (171).

Other Risk Factors

Positive family histories of cancer are relatively rare, but have been reported in some studies (14). Women with breast cancer have a slightly increased incidence of corpus cancer (187,188); previous endometrial cancer also is correlated with a higher incidence of breast cancer (189,190). The interval between the diagnosis of endometrial cancer and breast cancer averaged 4.6 years in the study of Doberneck and Garcia (189). Estrogen-producing tumors of the ovary (theca cell and granulosa cell tumors) also are associated with an increased risk for endometrial cancer, especially in postmenopausal women (150,191,192). Women who smoke heavily might have a lower risk of endometrial cancer than nonsmokers. In a hospital-based case-control study the relative risk for current smokers as compared with women who had never smoked was 0.7 (193). Cigarette smoking reduces the estrogen excretion in the urine.

REFERENCES

Prostate Cancer

1. Zaridze DG, Boyle P, Smans M. International trends in prostatic cancer. *Int J Cancer* 1984;33: 223-230.
2. Muir C, Waterhouse J, Mack T, Powell J, Whelan S. Cancer incidence in five continents. *IARC Scientific Pub* 5:88, Lyon. 1987.
3. Rotkin JD. Distribution and risk of prostatic cancer. *Cancer epidemiology in the USA and USSR.* NJH Pub. 80:2044, US Gov. Printing Office, 1980.

4. Hakulinen T, Andersen AA, Malker B, Pukkala E, Schon G, Tulinius H. *Trends in cancer incidence in the Nordic countries.* The Nordic Cancer Registries. Copenhagen: Munksgaard, 1986.

5. Seitz G, Kolles H, Niemeyer AH, Wernert N, Dhom G. Zur Epidemiologie des Prostatakarzinoms in Saarland. *Verh Dtsch Ges Urol* 1988;39:199–200.

6. Dhom G. Epidemiologic aspects of latent and clinically manifest carcinoma of the prostate. *J Cancer Res Clin Oncol* 1983;106:210–218.

7. Servadio C, Mukamel E, Kahan E. Carcinoma of the prostate in Israel: some epidemiological and therapeutical considerations. *Prostate* 1984;5:375–382.

8. Byar DP. Incidence, mortality and survival statistics for prostate cancer. In: *Current Concepts and Approaches to the Study of Prostate Cancer.* New York: Alan R. Liss.

9. Berlie J, Rezvani A, Hacene K, et al. Cancer de la prostate, bilan épidémiologique, fréquence, tendance, en particulier en France. *Bull Cancer (Paris)* 1985;72:391–404.

10. Becker N, Frentzel-Beyme R, Wagner G. *Krebsatlas der bundesrepublik deutschland. 2 Aufl* New York: Springer, 1984.

11. Akazaki K. Comparative studies on the prevalence of latent prostate cancer among Japanese, American and Colombian males. Director's report 1968/69. Aichi Cancer Center Research Institute, Nagoya, 1973.

12. Akazaki K, Stemmermann GN. Comparative study of latent carcinoma of the prostate among Japanese in Japan and Hawaii. *J Natl Cancer Inst* 1973;50:1137–1144.

13. Breslow N, Chan CW, Dhom G, et al. Latent carcinoma of prostate at autopsy in seven areas. *Int J Cancer* 1977;20:680–688.

14. Guileyardo JM, Johnson WD, Welsh RA, Akazaki K, Correa P. Prevalence of latent prostate carcinoma in two US populations. *J Natl Cancer Inst* 1980;65:311–316.

15. Kovi J, Jackson MA, Rao MS, et al. Cancer of the prostate and aging: an autopsy study in black men from Washington, D.C., and selected African cities. *Prostate* 1982;3:73–80.

16. Yatani R, Shiraioshi T, Nakakuki K, et al. Trends in frequency of latent prostate carcinoma in Japan from 1965–79 to 1982–86. *JNCJ* 1988;80:683–687.

17. Haenszel W, Kurihara M. Studies of Japanese migrants. I. Mortality from cancer and other diseases among Japanese in the United States. *J Natl Cancer Inst* 1968;40:43–68.

18. Ernster VL, Seluin S, Sacks ST, Austin DF, Brown SM, Winkelstein W. Prostatic cancer: mortality and incidence rates by race and social class. *Am J Epidemiol* 1978;107:311–320.

19. Donn AS, Muir CS. Prostatic cancer. Some epidemiologic features. *Bull Cancer (Paris)* 1985;72:381–390.

20. Holman CDJ, James JR, Segal MR, Armstrong BK. Recent trends in mortality from prostate cancer in male populations of Australia and England and Wales. *Br J Cancer* 1981;44:340–348.

21. King M, Diamond E, Lilienfeld AM. Some epidemiological aspects of cancer of the prostate. *J Chron Dis* 1963;16:117–153.

22. Krain LS. Some epidemiologic variables in prostatic carcinoma in California. *Prev Med* 1974;3:154–159.

23. Ross RK, McCurtis JW, Henderson BE, Menck HR, Mack TM, Martin SP. Descriptive epidemiology of testicular and prostatic cancer in Los Angeles. *Br J Cancer* 1979: 39:284–292.

24. Steele R, Lees REM, Kraus AS, Rao C. Sexual factors in the epidemiology of cancer of the prostate. *J Chron Dis* 1971;24:29–37.

25. Ross RK, Deapen DM, Casagrande JT, Paganini-Hill A, Henderson BE. A cohort study of mortality from cancer of the prostate in catholic priests. *Br J Cancer* 1981;43:233–235.

26. Talamini R, Vecchia CL, Decarli A, Negri E, Franceschi S. Nutrition, social factors and prostatic cancer in a northern Italian population. *Br J Cancer* 1986;53:817–821.

27. Wynder EL, Mabuchi K, Whitmore WF. Epidemiology of the prostate. *Cancer* 1971;28:344–360.

28. Yu H, Harris E, Wynder EL. Case-control study of prostate cancer and socioeconomic factors. *Prostate* 1988;13:317–325.

29. Lilienfeld AM, Levin ML, Kessler J. Mortality and marital status. *Cancer in the United States.* Cambridge: Harvard Univ. Press, 1972;123–149.

30. Newell GR, Pollack ES, Spitz MR, Sider JG, Fueger JJ. Incidence of prostate cancer and marital status. *J Natl Cancer Inst* 1987;79:259–262.

31. Swanson GM, Belle SH, Satariano WA. Marital status and cancer incidence: Differences in the black and white population. *Cancer Res* 1985;45:5883–5889.

32. Zeigel RF, Arya SK, Horszewicz JJ, Carter WA. A status report. Human prostatic carcinoma, with emphasis on potential for viral etiology. *Oncology* 1977;34:29–44.

33. Ross RK, Shimizu H, Paganini-Hill A, Honda G, Henderson BE. Case-control studies of prostate cancer in blacks and whites in Southern California. *J Natl Cancer Inst* 1987;78:869–874.
34. Kaplan GW, O'Connor VJ. The incidence of carcinoma of the prostate in Jews and gentiles. *JAMA* 1966;196:123–124.
35. Cuatico W, Cheung CH, Sy F. Detection of viral-like cores from the urine of patients with genitourinary malignancies. *Cancer* 1978;41:706–711.
36. Centifano YM, Kaufman HE, Zam ZS. Herpes virus particles in prostatic cancer cells. *J Virol* 1973;12:1608–1611.
37. Baker LH, Mebust WK, Chin TDY, et al. The relationship of herpes virus virus to carcinoma of the prostate. *J Urol* 1981;125:370–374.
38. Herbert JT, Birkhoff JD, Feorino PH. Herpes simplex virus type 2 and cancer of the prostate. *J Urol* 1976;116:611–612.
39. Lüleci G, Sakizli M, Günalp A. Herpes simplex type 2 neutralization antibodies in patients with cancers of urinary bladder, prostate and cervix. *J Surg Oncol* 1981;16:327–331.
40. Hill P, Wynder EL, Garbaczewski L, Walker ARP. Effect of diet on plasma and urinary hormones in South African black men with prostatic cancer. *Cancer Res* 1982;42:3864.
41. Armstrong B, Doll R. Environmental factors and cancer incidence and mortality in different countries, with special reference to dietary practices. *Int J Cancer* 1975;15:617–631.
42. Berg JW. Can nutrition explain the pattern of international epidemiology of hormone-dependent cancers? *Cancer Res* 1975;35:3345–3350.
43. Boing H, Martinez L, Frentzel-Beyme R, Oltersdorf V. Regional nutritional pattern and cancer mortality in the Federal Republic of Germany. *Nutr Cancer* 1985;7:121–130.
44. Heshmat MY, Kaul L, Kovi J, et al. Nutrition and prostate cancer: a case-control study. *Prostate* 1985;6:7–17.
45. Howell MA. Factor analysis of international cancer mortality data and per capita food consumption. *Br J Cancer* 1974;29:328–336.
46. Kolonel LN, Nomura AMY, Hinds MW, Hirobata T, Hankin JH, Lee M. Role of diet in cancer incidence in Hawaii. *Cancer Res* (Suppl) 1983;43:2397–2402.
47. Garfinkel L. Overweight and mortality. *Cancer* 1986;58:1826–1829.
48. Lew EA, Garfinkel L. Variations in mortality by weight among 750,000 men and women. *J Chron Dis* 1979;32:563–579.
49. Snowdon DA, Phillips RL, Choi W. Diet, obesity and risk of fatal prostate cancer. *Am J Epidemiol* 1984;120:244–250.
50. Graham S, Haughey B, Marshall J, et al. Diet in the epidemiology of carcinoma of the prostate gland. *J Natl Cancer Inst* 1983;70:687–692.
51. Flanders WD. Review: Prostate cancer epidemiology. *Prostate* 1984;5:621–629.
52. Phillips RL. Role of life style and dietary habits in risk of cancer among Seventh Day Adventists. *Cancer Res* 1975;35:3513–3522.
53. Rose DP. The biochemical epidemiology of prostatic carcinoma. In: *Dietary, Fat and Cancer*. New York: Alan R. Liss, 1986.
54. Hirayama T. Epidemiology of prostate cancer with special reference to the role of diet. *Natl Cancer Inst Monogr* 1979;53:149–155.
55. Mettlin C. Nutritional habits of blacks and whites. *Prev Med* 1980;9:601–606.
56. Mettlin C. Cancer of the prostate and testis. In: Bonike GJ, ed. *The epidemiology of cancer*, London: Croon Helm, 1983;245–259.
57. Newill VA. Distribution of cancer mortality among ethnic subgroups of the white population of New York City 1953–1958. *J Natl Cancer Inst* 1961;26:405–417.
58. Lynch HT, Larsen AL, Magnuson CW, Krush AJ. Prostate carcinoma and multiple primary malignancies; study of a family and 109 consecutive prostate cancer patients. *Cancer* 1966;19:1891–1897.
59. Schuman LM, Mandel J, Blackard C. Epidemiologic study of prostatic cancer: preliminary report. *Cancer Treat Rep* 1977;61:181–186.
60. Woolf CM. An investigation of the familial aspect of carcinoma of the prostate. *Cancer* 1960;13:739–744.
61. Meikle AW, Stanish WM. Familial prostatic cancer risk and low testosterone. *J Clin Endocrinol Metab* 1982;54:1104–1108.
62. Bean MA, Yatani R, Liu PJ, Fukazawa K, Ashley W, Fujita S. Prostatic carcinoma at autopsy in Hiroshima and Nagasaki Japanese. *Cancer* 1973;32:498–506.
63. Kipling MD, Waterhouse JAH. Cadmium and prostate carcinoma. *Lancet* 1967;1:730–731.

64. Kolonel L, Winkelstein W. Cadmium and prostatic cancer. *Lancet* 1977;2:566–567.
65. Lemen RA, Lee JS, Wagoner JK. Cancer mortality among cadmium production workers. *Ann NY Acad Sci* 1979;271:273–279.
66. Potts CL. Cadmium proteinuria—The healths of battery workers exposed to cadmium oxide dust. *An Occup Hyg* 1965;8:55–61.
67. Muir C, Waterhouse I, Mack T, Powell J, Whelan S. Breast cancer incidence in five continents. *IARC Scientific Pub* 5:88, Lyon, 1987.
68. MacMahon B. Incidence trends in North America, Japan and Hawaii. In: Magnus K, ed. *Trends in cancer incidence*, New York: Hemisphere Publishing, 1982;249–262.
69. White E, Daling JR, Norsted TL, Chu J. Rising incidence of breast cancer among young women in Washington State. *J Natl Cancer Inst* 1987;79:239–243.
70. Ewertz M, Carstensen B. Trends in breast cancer incidence and mortality in Denmark 1943–1982. *Int J Cancer* 1988;41:46–51.
71. Miller AB. Cancer of the breast. In: Magnus K, ed. *Trends in cancer incidence*, New York: Hemisphere Publishing, 1982;231–234.
72. Tulinius H, Sigvaldson H. Trends in incidence of female breast cancer in the Nordic countries. In: Magnus K, ed. *Trends in cancer incidence*, New York: Hemisphere Publishing, 1982a;235–247.
73. Anderson DE. A genetic study of human breast cancer. *J Natl Cancer Inst* 1972;48:1029–1034.
74. Anderson DE, Badzioch D. Bilaterality in familial breast cancer patients. *Cancer* 1985;56:2092–2098.
75. Harris RE, Lynch HT, Guirgis HA. Familial breast cancer: risk to the contralateral breast. *J Natl Cancer Inst* 1978;60:955–960.
76. Rosen PP, Lesser ML, Senie RT, Kinne DW. Epidemiology of breast carcinoma. III. Relationship of family history to tumor type. *Cancer* 1982;50:171–179.
77. Brinton A, Hoover R, Fraumeni JF Jr. Epidemiology of minimal breast cancer. *JAMA* 1983;249:483–487.
78. Roush GC, Holford TR, Schymura MJ, White C. *Cancer risk and incidence trends*. Washington: Hemisphere Publishing, 1987.
79. Helmrich SP, Shapiro S, Rosenberg L. Risk factors for breast cancer. *Am J Epidemiol* 1983;117:35–45.
80. Hirayama T, Wynder EL. A study of the epidemiology of cancer of the breast. II. Influence of hysterectomy. *Cancer* 1962;15:28–38.
81. Irwin KL, Lee NC, Peterson HB, Rubin GL, Wingo PA, Mandel MG. Hysterectomy, tubal sterilization and the risk of breast cancer. *Am J Epidemiol* 1988;127:1192–1201.
82. Kelsey JL, Fischer DB, Holford TR. Exogenous estrogens and other factors in the epidemiology of breast cancer. *J Natl Cancer Inst* 67:327–333.
83. Paffenberger RS, Kampert JB, Chang HG. Characteristics that predict risk of breast cancer before and after the menopause. *Am J Epidemiol* 1980;112:258–268.
84. Talamini R, La Vecchia C, Franceschi S, Colombo F, Decarli A, Grattoni E. Reproductive and hormonal factors and breast cancer in a Northern Italian population. *Int J Epidemiol* 1985;14:70–74.
85. Trichopoulos D, MacMahon B, Cole P. Menopause and breast cancer risk. *J Natl Cancer Inst* 1972;48:605–613.
86. Lilienfeld AM, Coombs J, Bross JDJ. Marital and reproductive experience in a community-wide epidemiological study of breast cancer. *Johns Hopkins Med J* 1975;136:157–162.
87. MacMahon B, Cole P, Lin TM. Age at first birth and breast cancer risk. *Bull WHO* 1970;43:209–221.
88. Trichopoulos D, Hsieh CC, MacMahon B, et al. Age at any birth and breast cancer risk. *Int J Cancer* 1983;31:701–704.
89. Gambrell RD Jr, Maier RC, Sanders BJ. Decreased incidence of breast cancer in postmenopausal estrogen-progesteron-users. *Obstet Gynecol* 1983;62:435–443.
90. Hennekens C, Speizer FE, Lipnick RJ. A case-control study of oral contraceptive use and breast cancer. *J Natl Cancer Inst* 1984;72:39–42.
91. Schlesselman JJ, Stadel BV, Murray P, Wingo PA, Rubin GL. Consistency and plausibility in epidemiologic analysis: application to breast cancer in relation to use of oral contraceptives. *J Chron Dis* 1987;40:1033–1039.
92. Schlesselman JJ, Stadel BV, Murray P, Lai S. Breast cancer in relation to early use of oral contraceptives. No evidence of a latent effect. *JAMA* 1988;259:1828–1833.

93. Vessey MP, McPherson K, Yeates D. Oral contraceptive use and abortion before first term pregnancy in relation to breast cancer risk. *Br J Cancer* 1982;45:327– 331.

94. Frisch RE, Wyshak G, Albright NL, et al. Lower prevalence of breast cancer and cancers of the reproductive system among former college athletes compared to nonathletes. *Br J Cancer* 1985;52: 885–891.

95. Frisch RE, Wyshak G, Albright NL, et al. Lower life-time occurrence of breast cancer and cancers of the reproductive system among former college athletes. *Am J Clin Nutr* 1987;45:328–335.

96. Vihko RK, Apter DL. The epidemiology and endocrinology of the menarche in relation to breast cancer. *Cancer Surv* 1986;5:561–571.

97. Byers T, Graham S. The epidemiology of diet and cancer. *Adv Cancer Res* 1984;41:1–69.

98. Goodwin PJ, Boyd NF. Critical appraisal of the evidence that dietary fat intake is related to breast cancer risk in humans. *J Natl Cancer Inst* 1987;79:473–485.

99. Herns G. The contribution of diet and childbearing to breast cancer rates. *Br J Cancer* 1978;37: 974–982.

100. Herns G. Associations between breast cancer mortality rates, child-bearing and diet in the United Kingdom. *Br J Cancer* 1980;41:429–437.

101. Ingram DM. Trends in diet and breast cancer mortality in England and Wales 1928–1977. *Nutr Cancer* 1981;3:75–80.

102. Phillips RL, Snowdon DA. Association of meat and coffee use with cancers of the large bowel, breast and prostate among Seventh-Day Adventists: Preliminary results. *Cancer Res* 1983;43 (Suppl):2403–2408.

103. Willett WC, Stampfer MJ, Colditz GA. Dietary fat and risk of breast cancer. *New Engl J Med* 1987b;316:22–28.

104. Hirayama T. Epidemiology of breast cancer with special reference to the role of diet. *Prev Med* 1978;7:173–195.

105. Hirayama T. Diet and cancer. *Nutr Cancer* 1979;1:67–81.

106. Phillips RL. Role of life-style and dietary habits in risk of cancer among Seventh-Day Adventists. *Cancer Res* 1975;35:3513–3519.

107. Lubin JH, Burns PE, Blot WJ. Dietary factors and breast cancer risk. *Int J Cancer* 1981;28:685–689.

108. Dubin N, Pasternack BS, Strax P. Epidemiology of breast cancer in a screened population. *Cancer Dectect Prev* 1984a;7:87–102.

109. Dubin N, Hutter RV, Strax P, et al. Epidemiology of minimal breast cancer among women screened in New York City. *J Natl Cancer Inst* 1984b;73:1273–1279.

110. Toernberg SA, Holm LE, Carstensen JM. Breast cancer risk in relation to serum cholesterol, serum beta-lipoprotein, height, weight and blood pressure. *Acta Oncol* 1988;27:31–37.

111. Mettlin C. Diet and the epidemiology of human breast cancer. *Cancer* 1984;53 (Suppl 3):605–611.

112. Kolonel LN, Hankin JH, Lee I. Nutrient intakers in relation to cancer incidence in Hawaii. *Br J Cancer* 1981a;44:332–339.

113. Kolonel LN, Hankin JH, Nomura AM, Chu SY. Dietary fat intake and cancer incidence among five ethnic groups in Hawaii. *Cancer Res* 1981b;41:3727–3728.

114. Kolonel LN, Nomura AM, Hinds MW. Role of diet in cancer incidence in Hawaii. *Cancer Res* 1983;43 (Suppl):2397–2402.

115. Stemmermann GN, Catts A, Fukunaga FH, Horie A, Nomura AM. Breast cancer in women of Japanese and Caucasian ancestry in Hawaii. *Cancer* 1985;56:206–209.

116. Hoel DG, Wakabayashi T, Pike MC. Secular trends in the distributions of the breast cancer risk factors, menarche, first birth, menopause, and weight in Hiroshima and Nagasaki, Japan. *Am J Epidemiol* 1983;118:78–89.

117. Natarajan N, Nemoto T, Mettlin C, Murphy GP. Race related differences in breast cancer patients. Results of the 1982 national survey of breast cancer by the American College of Surgeons. *Cancer* 1985;56:1704–1709.

118. Ownby HE, Frederick J, Russo J, et al. Racial differences in breast cancer patients. *J Natl Cancer Inst* 1985;75:55–60.

119. Polednak AP. Breast cancer in black and white women in New York State. Case distribution and incidence rates by clinical stage at diagnosis. *Cancer* 1986;58:807–815.

120. Haenszel W, Kurihara M. Studies of Japanese migrants. I. Mortality from cancer and other diseases among Japanese in the United States. *J Natl Cancer Inst* 1968;40:43–68.

121. Staszewski J. *Epidemiology of cancer of selected sites in Poland and Polish migrants.* Cambridge, MA: Ballinger, 1976.
122. de Waard F. Breast cancer trends in Europe and Israel. Implications for the nutritional etiology of breast cancer. In: Magnus K, ed. *Trends in cancer incidence,* New York: Hemisphere Publishing, 1982;263–266.
123. Hiatt RA, Bawol RD. Alcoholic beverage consumption and breast cancer incidence. *Am J Epidemiol* 1984;120:676–683.
124. Monique GL, Hill C, Kramar A. Alcoholic beverage consumption and breast cancer in a French case-control study. *Am J Epidemiol* 1984;120:350–357.
125. Schatzkin A, Jones DY, Hoover RN, Taylor PR, Brinton LA, Ziegler RG. Alcohol consumption and breast cancer in the epidemiologic follow-up study of the first National Health and Nutrition Examination Survey. *New Engl J Med* 1987;316:1169–1173.
126. Talamini R, La Vecchia C, Decarli A, et al. Social factors, diet and breast cancer in a Northern Italian population. *Br J Cancer* 1984;49:723–729.
127. Willett WC, Stampfer MJ, Colditz GA, Rosner BA, Hennekens C, Speizer FE. Moderate alcohol consumption and the risk of breast cancer. *New Engl J Med* 1987a;316:1174–1180.
128. Rosenberg L, Schwingl PJ, Kaufman DW, et al. Breast cancer and cigarette smoking. *New Engl J Med* 1984;310:92–94.
129. Hiatt RA, Fireman BH. Smoking, menopause and breast cancer. *J Natl Cancer Inst* 1986;76:833–838.
130. Adami HO, Bergstroem R, Hansen I. Age at first primary as a determinant of the incidence of bilateral breast cancer. Cumulative and relative risks in a population-based case-control study. *Cancer* 1985;55:643–647.
131. Chaudary MA, Millis RR, Hoskins EO. Bilateral primary breast cancer: a prospective study of disease incidence. *Br J Surg* 1984;71:711–714.
132. Horn PL, Thompson WD, Schwartz SM. Factors associated with the risk of second primary breast cancer: an analysis of data from the Connecticut Tumor Registry. 1987; *J Chron Dis* 40:1003–1011.
133. Chleboun JO, Gray BN. The profile of breast cancer in Western Australia. *Med J Austr* 1987;147:331–334.
134. Cohen P, Wax Y, Modan B. Seasonality in the occurrence of breast cancer. *Cancer Res* 1983;43:892–896.
135. Kirkham N, Machin D, Cotton DW, Pike JM. Seasonality and breast cancer. *Eur J Surg Oncol* 1985;11:143–146.
136. Mason BH, Holdaway JM, Skinner SJ, et al. Association between season of first detection of breast cancer and disease progression. *Breast Cancer Res Treat* 1987;9:227–232.
137. Nakao H. Birth seasonality of breast cancer patients and its variation according to menopausal status and histologic type in Japan. *Eur J Cancer Clin Oncol* 1986;22:1105–1110.
138. Vassilaros S, Tsiliakos S, Adamopoulos D, et al. Seasonal variations in the frequency distribution of breast cancer in Greek women according to the months of their birth. *J Cancer Res Clin Oncol* 1985;110:79–81.
139. Evans JS, Wennberg JE, McNeil BJ. The influence of diagnostic radiography on the incidence of breast cancer and leukemia. *New Engl J Med* 1988;315:810–815.
140. Harada T, Ishida M. Neoplasms among A-bomb-survivors in Hiroshima: first report of the research committee on tumor statistics. Hiroshima City Medical Association. Hiroshima, Japan. *J Natl Cancer Inst* 1960;25:1253–1264.
141. Tokunaga M, Norman JE, Asano M. Malignant breast tumors among atomic bomb survivors. Hiroshima and Nagasaki 1950–1974. *J Natl Cancer Inst* 1979;62:1347–1360.
142. Watanabe S. Cancer and leukemia developing among atom-bomb-survivors. In: E Grundmann, ed. *Handbuch Allg Pathologie VI Bd 5 Teil* Springer, Berlin Heidelberg New York, 1974; 461, 578.
143. Tokunaga M, Land CE, Yamamoto T, et al. Incidence of female breast cancer among atomic bomb survivors. Hiroshima and Nagasaki 1950-1980. *Radiat Res* 1987;112:243–272.
144. Shore RE, Hempelmann LH, Kowaluk E. Breast neoplasms in women treated with X-rays for acute post-partum mastitis. *J Natl Cancer Inst* 1977;59:813–822.
145. Tulinius H, Day NE, Bjarnason O, et al. Familial breast cancer in Iceland. *Int J Cancer* 1982b;29:365–371.
146. Statistisches Amt des Saarlandes. Morbidität und Mortalität an bösartigen Neubildungen im Saarland. 1986. 143/88.

147. Segi M. Age-adjusted death rates for cancer for selected sites in 43 countries in 1977. Segi-Institute of Cancer Epidemiology, Nagoya, 1982.
148. Lyon JL, Gardner JW. The rising frequency of hysterectomy: its effect on uterine cancer rates. *Am J Epidemiol* 1977;105:439.
149. Knox EG. Cancer of the uterine cervix. In: Magnus K, ed. *Trends in cancer incidence*. New York: Hemisphere Publishing, 1982;271–278.
150. Kelsey JL, Hildreth NG. *Breast and gynecological cancer epidemiology*. Boca Raton, FL: CRC Press, Inc 1983.
151. Marrett L, Elwood JM, Meigs JW. Recent trends in the incidence and mortality of cancer of the uterine corpus in Connecticut. *Gynecol Oncol* 1978;6:183–195.
152. Weiss NS. Assessing the risks from menopausal estrogen use: What can we learn from trends in mortality from uterine cancer? *J Chron Dis* 1978;31:705–708.
153. Robboy SJ, Bradley R. Changing trends and prognostic features in endometrial cancer associated with exogenous estrogen therapy. *Obstet Gynecol* 1979;54:269.
154. Roush GC, Holford TR, Schymura MJ, White C. *Cancer risk and incidence trends. The Connecticut perspective*. Washington: Hemisphere Publishing, 1987.
155. Dallenbach-Hellweg G. Krebsvorstadien und-frühstadien im Endometrium. *Verh Dtsch Ges Pathol* 1979;63:613–628.
156. Hendrickson MR, Kempson RL. Surgical pathology of the uterine corpus. Philadelphia: Saunders, 1980.
157. Horwitz RJ, Feinstein AR, Horwitz SM, Robboy SJ. Necropsy diagnosis of endometrial cancer and detection-bias in case-control studies. *Lancet* 1981;2:66.
158. Merletti F, Cole P. Detection bias and endometrial cancer. Lancet 1981;2:579.
159. Marrett LD. Estimates of the true population at risk of uterine disease and an application to incidence data for cancer of the uterine corpus in Connecticut. *Am J Epidemiol* 1980;111:373.
160. Pollack ES, Horm JW. Trends in cancer incidence and mortality in the United States 1969–1976. *J Natl Cancer Inst* 1980;64:1091.
161. Weiss NS, Szekely DR, Austin DF. Increasing incidence of endometrial cancer in the United States. *New Engl J Med* 1976;294:1259–1262.
162. Austin DF, Roe KM. The decreasing incidence of endometrial cancer. Public Health implications. *Am J Publ Health* 1982;72:65–68.
163. Ewertz M, Jensen OM. Trends in the incidence of the corpus uteri in Denmark 1943–1980. *Am J Epidemiol* 1984;119:725–732.
164. Hakulinen T, Andersen AA, Malker B, Pukkala E, Schou G, Tulinius H. *Trends in cancer incidence in the Nordic countries*. Copenhagen: Munksgard, 1986.
165. Kemp J, Boyle P. Atlas of cancer in Scotland. *IARC Scientific Pub* 72, Lyon, 1985.
166. Becker N, Frentzel-Beyme R, Wagner G. *Krebsatlas der bundesrepublik deutschland 2 Aufl* Berlin: Springer, 1984.
167. Wynder EL, Escher GC, Mantel N. An epidemiological investigation of cancer of the endometrium. *Cancer* 1966;29:489–520.
168. Berrino F, Panico S, Muti P. Dietary fat, nutritional status and endocrine associated cancers. In: Miller AB, ed. *Diet and the aetiology of cancer*. Berlin: Springer, 1989;3–12.
169. Lew EA, Garfinkel L. Variations in mortality by weight among 750,000 men and women. *J Chron Dis* 1979;32:563–576.
170. Kelsey JL, Livolsi VA, Holford TR. A case-control study of cancer of the endometrium. *Am J Epidemiol* 1982;116:333–343.
171. Henderson BE, Casagrande JT, Pike MC, Mak T, Rosario J, Duke A. The epidemiology of endometrial cancer in young women. *Br J Cancer* 1983;47:749–756.
172. Jensen H. Endometrial carcinoma. A retrospective, epidemiological study. *Dan Med Bull* 1985;32:219–228.
173. MacDonald PC, Edman CD, Hemsell DL, Porter JC, Siiteri PK. Effect of obesity on conversion of plasma androstenedione to estrone in postmenopausal women with and without endometrial cancer. *Am J Obstet Gynecol* 1978;130:448.
174. Rizkallah TH, Tovell NMM, Kelly WG. Production of estrone and fractional conversion of circulating androstenedione to estrone in women with endometrial carcinoma. *J Clin Endocrinol Metabol* 1975;40:1045.
175. La Vecchia C, Decarli A, Fasoli M, Gentile A. Nutrition and diet in the etiology of endometrial cancer. *Cancer* 1986;57:1248–1253.

176. Thomas DB, Chu J. Nutritional and endocrine factors in reproductive organ cancers: opportunities for primary prevention. *J Chron Dis* 1986;12:1031–1050.
177. Phillips RL. Role of lifestyle and dietary habits in risk of cancer among Seventh-Day Adventists. *Cancer Res* 1975;35:3513–3522.
178. Kolonel LN, Hankin JH, Lee J, Chu SY, Nomura AMY, Hinds MW. Nutrient intakes in relation to cancer incidence in Hawaii. *Br J Cancer* 1981;44:332–339.
179. MacDonald PC, Siiteri PK. The relationship between the extraglandular production of estrone and the occurrence of endometrial neoplasia. *Gynecol Oncol* 1974;2:259.
180. MacMahon B. Risk factors for endometrial cancer. *Gynecol Oncol* 1974;2:122.
181. Weiss NS, Szekely DR, English DR, Schweid AJ. Endometrial cancer in relation to patterns of menopausal estrogen use. *JAMA* 1979;242:261.
182. Jick H, Watkins RN, Hunter JR. Replacement estrogens and endometrial cancer. *New Engl J Med* 1979;300:218–222.
183. Mack TM, Pike MC, Henderson BE, et al. Estrogens and endometrial cancer in a retirement community. *New Engl J Med* 1976;294:1262.
184. Shapiro S, Kaufman DW, Slone D, et al. Recent and past use of conjugated estrogens in relation to adenocarcinoma of the endometrium. *New Engl J Med* 1980;303:485.
185. Salmi T. Endometrial cancer risk factors, with special reference to the use of oestrogens. *Acta Endocrinol (Suppl)* 1980;233:37.
186. Weiss NS, Sayvetz TA. Incidence of endometrial cancer in relation to the use of oral contraceptives. *New Engl J Med* 1980;302:551.
187. Schenker JG, Levinsky R, Ohel G. Multiple primary malignant neoplasms in breast cancer patients in Israel. *Cancer* 1984;54:145–150.
188. Vongtama V, Kurohara SS, Badib AO, Webster JH. Second primary cancers of endometrial carcinoma. *Cancer* 1970;26:842.
189. Doberneck RC, Garcia JE. Primary breast cancer in patients with previous endometrial or ovarian cancer. *J Surg Oncol* 1988;37:100–103.
190. MacMahon B, Austin JH. Association of carcinomas of the breast and corpus uteri. *Cancer* 1969;23:275.
191. Mansell H, Hertig AT. Granulosa-theca-cell tumors and endometrial cancer. *Obstet Gynecol* 1955;6:385.
192. Salerno LJ. Feminizing mesenchymomas of the ovary—an analysis of 28 granulosa-theca-cell tumors and their relationship to coexistent carcinoma. *Am J Obstet Gynecol* 1962;84:731.
193. Lesko SM, Rosenberg L, Kaufman DW, et al. Cigarette smoking and the risk of endometrial cancer. *New Engl J Med* 1985;313:593–596.

Endocrine Dependent Tumors, edited by
Klaus-Dieter Voigt and Cornelius Knabbe.
Raven Press, Ltd., New York © 1991.

2

Molecular Probes of the Structures and Functions of Androgen Receptors

Richard A. Hiipakka, Tehming Liang, Susumu Seino,
and Shutsung Liao

*The Ben May Institute, Departments of Biochemistry and Molecular Biology and
Medicine/Dermatology, The University of Chicago, Chicago, Illinois 60637*

Many steroid hormones enter target cells and bind to receptors without metabolic conversion. However, in the prostate and many other target organs of androgens, testosterone, the major testicular androgen circulating in blood, acts mainly after its conversion to 5α-dihydrotestosterone (DHT) by a 3-keto-5α-steroid reductase (5α-reductase) (Fig. 1). DHT then forms a complex with a specific receptor that binds tightly to nuclear acceptor sites that presumably contain DNA with an androgen response element (ARE). Specific inhibitors of 5α-reductase and antiandrogens that interfere with androgen binding to receptors can be used to analyze the roles of the reductase and receptors, as well as the active forms of androgens, in eliciting androgenic responses in target cells.

Recent success in cloning and sequencing of cDNA and determination of the deduced amino acid sequences of androgen receptors (ARs) have made it possible to analyze the roles of different AR domains in eliciting androgenic responses. Sequence analysis of AR-mRNA and AR-genes from individuals with androgen insensitivity has identified mutations that might be responsible for producing the abnormal androgenic response. Polyclonal and monoclonal anti-AR antibodies also are available now for immunocytolocalization and quantitation of ARs in target cells. Appropriate nucleotide probes can be constructed and used for qualitative and quantitative assays of AR-mRNA by *in situ* hybridization and other molecular hybridization methods.

In target cells ARs can go through a dynamic process of activation/inactivation, transformation and recycling. Many factors, either intracellular or external, are capable of interfering with individual steps involved in this dynamic process. Investigation of the these factors is important for the elucidation of the mechanism of action of androgen receptors. For example, recent studies in this area support the concept that AR and other steroid receptors (SR) might act not only at a transcriptional site but also at the level of RNA processing and protection. Understanding the

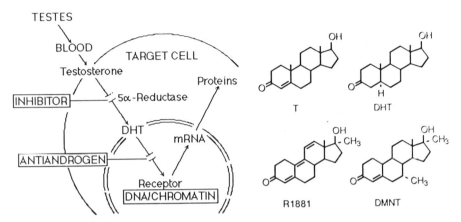

FIG. 1. Two points of control of androgen action in target cells using 5α-reductase inhibitors and androgen receptor-binding antiandrogens. The structures of testosterone (T), 5α-dihydrotestosterone (DHT), R1881 (17α-methyl-17β-hydroxyestra-4,9,11-trien-3-one or methyltrienolone), and DMNT (7α, 17α-dimethyl-19-nortestosterone or mibolerone) also are shown.

structure and function of ARs and their regulation also is useful for the design of new compounds that might have chemotherapeutic value in the control of the abnormal growth of prostates and androgen-sensitive tumors. This chapter will focus on recent progress in many of the aforementioned areas.

5α-REDUCTASE AND ITS INHIBITORS

Biological Importance of 5α-Reductase

DHT is formed from testosterone (T) by a NADPH-dependent 5α-reductase. In the rat prostate, most of the reductase in homogenates is associated with the microsomal and nuclear fractions (1). Because DHT binds more tightly than testosterone to AR and DHT-R associates more firmly than T-R to DNA/chromatin (2–5), the reductase plays an important role in amplifying the potency of the circulating hormone. It appears that the T-R might not be active in many target cells; therefore, a 5α-reductase deficiency can lead to a selective absence of an androgenic response in some organs. In fact, some forms of male pseudohermaphroditism (testicular feminization) are attributed to a 5α-reductase deficiency (6,7). In some tissues sensitive to androgen, including those deficient in 5α-reductase, T appears to act by binding to AR. Embryonic male urogenital tract differentiation, growth of kidney, muscle, phallus and scrotum and certain testicular functions, as well as voice change and sexual behavior in humans and some species of animals appear to be T-dependent (7–9).

Excessive DHT is implicated in certain androgen-dependent pathological conditions including benign prostatic hyperplasia (BPH), acne, male-pattern baldness, and female idiopathic hirsutism. Some investigators have shown that, in the benign hyperplastic prostate, 5α-reductase activity and the DHT level are higher than that of normal prostate (10,11). 5α-Reductase activity is reported to be higher in hair follicles from the scalp of balding men than that of nonbalding men (12) and in a given individual 5α-reductase activity is found to be higher in balding skin than from hairy skin (13). Some idiopathic hirsute women have a normal circulating level of testosterone, but their affected skin has a higher 5α-reductase activity than that of nonhirsute women (14). An increased 5α-reductase activity also has been reported for skin with acne (15). Genetic evidence also supports the suggestion that DHT plays an important role in the development of BPH and the skin conditions just mentioned. In men with hereditary 5α-reductase deficiency, their prostates remain small or nonpalpable after puberty. They do not develop acne, temporal hairline recession, or baldness. Compared to their fathers and brothers, they have scanty beards and reduced body hair.

5α-Reductase Inhibitors

In vivo inhibition of 5α-reductase would effectively limit the availability of DHT to AR and would suppress DHT-dependent androgen actions. Therefore, 5α-reductase inhibitors would be useful for analyzing whether T or one of its metabolites, such as DHT, is the active androgen in target organs. These inhibitors also should be useful in selective treatment of DHT-dependent abnormalities that are associated with the growth and functions of prostate, hair (hirsutism and baldness), skin, and sebaceous glands. Other hormonal therapies using GnRH analogs, estrogens, receptor binding antiandrogens (flutamide, cyproterone acetate, spironolactone), and orchiectomy, which impede all androgenic activities in the individual, can cause side effects, such as impotence, gynecomastia, and alteration of sexual behavior in males.

Among the inhibitors (Fig. 2) of 5α-reductase, the 4-azasteroidal compounds reported by Liang and coworkers are the most extensively studied to date (16–20). These inhibitors are 3-oxo-4-aza-5α-steroids with a bulky functional group at the 17β-position. The A-ring conformation of these compounds is thought to be similar to the presumed 3-enol transition state of the 5α-reduction of 3-oxo-Δ^4 -steroids. A prototype for 5α-reductase inhibitors is 4-MA, which behaves as an inhibitor of 5α-reductase *in vivo*, decreasing the prostatic concentration of DHT in intact male rats or in castrated male rats given testosterone proprionate. 4-MA attenuated the growth of the prostate of castrated rats induced by T, but had much less of an effect in rats given DHT (21). When dogs are treated with 4-MA, the prostate size decreases (22,23). Topical applications of 4-MA to the scalp of the stumptail macaque, a primate model of human male pattern baldness, also prevented the baldness that normally occurs at puberty in these monkeys (24). These results also suggest that the growth of the prostate in rats and dogs, and baldness in the stumptail macaque depend on DHT. On the other hand, studies in rat pituitary

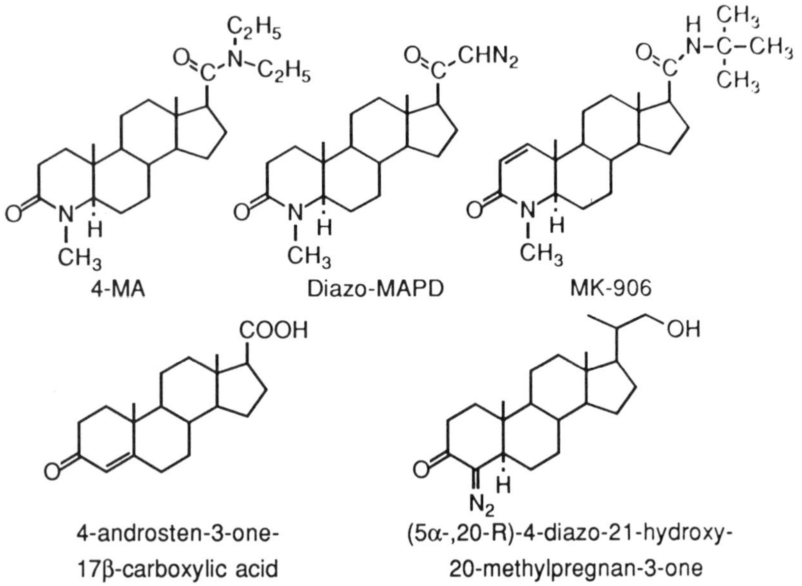

FIG. 2. Representative 5α-reductase inhibitors. Abbreviations are: 4-MA, 17β-N,N-diethylcarbamoyl-4-methyl-4-aza-5α-androstan-3-one; Diazo-MAPD, 21-diazo-4-methyl-4-aza-5α-pregnane-3,20-dione; MK-906, N-(2-methyl-2-propyl)-3-oxo-4-aza-5α-androst-1-ene-17β-carboxamide.

cultures showed that complete inhibition of T conversion to DHT by 4-MA did not affect T inhibition of LH release indicating direct action of T in this system (25).

MK-906 is a very potent inhibitor of 5α-reductase (Ki = 26 nM) in humans and is more potent than 4-MA in inhibiting the growth of the prostate. The inhibitor has no significant affinity for the rat prostate androgen receptor. A single oral dose of 0.5 mg of MD-906 decreases the plasma level of DHT to 50% 24 hours after administration (26). This compound is now under clinical testing for the treatment of BPH. Another potent inhibitor, diazo-MAPD (27), has been used in specific photolabeling of 5α-reductase. Other reported 5α-reductase inhibitors are 4-androsten-3-one-17β-carboxylic acid (28) and 4-diazo-21-hydroxy-methylpregnanone (29) (Fig. 2).

The primary structure of 5α-reductases, elucidated from cDNA sequences, should provide new information essential in analyzing reductase gene regulation, mutations, and intracellular membrane localization, and dynamics of the reductase at the molecular level. Polyclonal and monoclonal antibodies as well as various nucleotide (DNA and RNA) probes will be useful in basic studies, as well as in diagnostic analysis of 5α-reductase-linked abnormalities.

ANTI-ANDROGENS THAT BIND ANDROGEN RECEPTORS

Bioassays of various androgenic steroids (1,5,30) and studies of the structural requirements for binding of steroids to the AR suggested that multiple sites of an androgenic steroid are bound by the AR as though the steroid molecule was being enveloped. This is in marked contrast to steroid-metabolizing enzymes, antisteroid antibodies or blood steroid-binding proteins, which generally recognize only a portion of the steroid molecule. In fact, antisteroid antibodies can effectively remove steroids peripherally attached to these nonreceptor steroid-binding proteins, but not those bound to their SRs (30,31). The concept of steroid "enveloping" implies that it is chiefly the receptor protein, rather than the steroid, which interacts with other cellular components to produce the events leading to hormone action, and that the main function of the steroid is to transform the receptor protein to a form that can be recognized by acceptor sites in nuclear chromatin.

The action of classical steroidal antiandrogens (Fig. 3), such as cyproterone and its 17 α-acetate, have been attributed to their ability to compete with androgens for binding to AR (32,33). These antagonists act *in vivo* and during organ incubations by reducing the amount of DHT-AR complexes that are tightly associated with nuclear chromatin. Flutamide, a nonsteroidal antiandrogen, was found to act *in vivo* by the same mechanism apparently after a conversion to hydroxyflutamide (33,34), whereas Anandron appeared to act directly by binding to AR. Although these antiandrogens bind to AR with a low affinity (usually much less than 1/50th of natural androgens), they are useful as chemotherapeutic agents because they do not show significant side effects or toxicity.

Small compounds that easily can enter the androgen-binding cavity of AR (a high rate of association) and are trapped inside the binding cavity (a low rate of dissociation) should show a high affinity binding to AR. These compounds can act as antiandrogens. Several phenanthrene-related compounds have been studied to determine their ability to bind to AR and affect the androgenic response. Phenanthrene, a conjugated flat molecule that could presumably associate rapidly with AR, had a low affinity toward AR. In contrast, 9,10-dihydrophenanthrene, a compound hav-

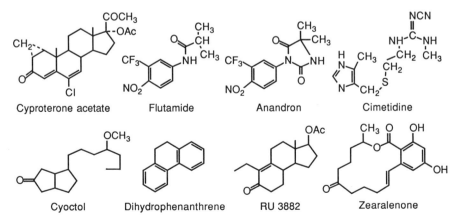

FIG. 3. Representative antiandrogens that apparently act by competing with androgens for binding to androgen receptors. Flutamide appears to act after conversion to a hydroxylated metabolite.

ing greater structural flexibility, which might allow the two end rings to conform to a structure compatible with the binding cavity of AR, was 80-fold more active than phenanthrene toward AR (35,36). The difference in the AR binding affinity for the two compounds is biologically significant. In castrated rats injected with testosterone, 9,10-dihydrophenanthrene reduced the androgen-dependent growth of the ventral prostate, seminal vesicle, and coagulating gland, whereas phenanthrene was far less active as an antiandrogen.

Studies with antiandrogens have clearly indicated that antagonistic activity is associated with a physical blockage of receptor binding to androgens and binding of these antiandrogens does not require the presence of specific functional groups. However, the hormonal action of a steroid or its agonists might be dependent on the interaction of AR with a precisely located functional group (17β-hydroxyl or 3-keto). The dependence of agonist activity on a specific functional group might be the reason that construction of a nonsteroidal androgen has not been successful, whereas many antiandrogenic compounds with very dissimilar structures have been synthesized. A more detailed study of the structural requirements for antagonists to interact with ARs in various organs *in vivo* might lead to the construction of compounds that can modulate AR function in an organ-specific manner. These antagonists will be useful as probes in the study of AR functions and also as chemotherapeutic agents in treating androgenic abnormalities.

ISOLATION OF THE cDNA AND STRUCTURAL ANALYSIS OF ANDROGEN RECEPTORS

Screening cDNA Libraries for Androgen Receptors and New Nuclear Receptors

For many steroid receptors, cDNAs have been cloned using specific antibodies to screen cDNA expression libraries. Because stable production of specific high-titer anti-AR antibodies has been very difficult, we employed an alternative approach (Fig. 4) based on the assumption that the DNA-binding domains of many members of the steroid receptor family may be very similar in their amino acid and DNA sequence. For this purpose, we prepared a radioactive oligonucleotide probe that was highly homologous to the nucleotide sequence encoding the DNA-binding domain of glucocorticoids receptors (GR). This probe was used to screen λGT11 cDNA libraries constructed from poly(A$^+$)RNA of human (h) prostate and testis or rat (r) ventral prostate. The selected clones were then screened again with oligonucleotide probes that were specific for individual receptors to eliminate clones that contained cDNAs for receptors previously cloned (37–39). The remaining clones were separated by molecular hybridization analysis into X-chromosome-linked and unrelated groups, because the AR gene had been shown to be linked to the X-chromosome (40,41). The cDNAs in the X-chromosome-linked clones were

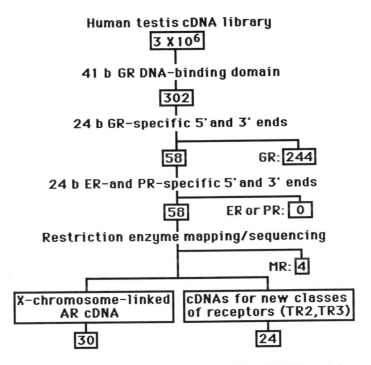

FIG. 4. Strategy used in the identification of clones containing AR cDNAs and clones containing other steroid receptors and new classes of nuclear receptors. A human testis cDNA library was screened with a 41-base oligonucleotide that was highly homologous to the nucleotide sequence of the DNA-binding domain of many steroid/thyroid receptors. The selected 302 clones were then screened with 24 base oligonucleotide probes that were specific to GR, ER, and PR. Restriction enzyme mapping and sequencing were used to identify and eliminate clones containing sequences for known receptors. The remaining clones were divided into two groups based on their ability to hybridizing to clones in an X-chromosome library. An AR-cDNA encoding a putative full-length AR was constructed from clones hybridizing to clones in the X-chromosome library. Other clones that were unrelated to X-chromosome DNA sequences were used to construct TR2- and TR3-cDNA that coded for new receptors.

analyzed by restriction mapping and sequencing, and full-length clones were constructed from overlapping DNAs by ligating appropriate restriction fragments and inserting the construct into the expression vector pGEM-3Z (37,42). The same approach was used to clone AR-cDNA by other investigators (43–45).

Some of the human cDNA clones that were identified and that contained steroid receptor-like DNA-binding domain sequences were not related to AR or other known receptors. From this group we isolated cDNAs for two new groups of nuclear receptors, which we designated TR2 and TR3 receptors (37,46), although the ligands for these receptors have not been identified. The TR3 receptor appears to be the human counterpart of the Nur/77 gene product originally identified in mouse fibroblasts stimulated by growth factors (47). This procedure (selection of receptor cDNAs for DNA-binding proteins and elimination of known receptor cDNAs) should be useful in finding cDNAs for novel receptors in many organs or tumors.

Characterization of Androgen Receptors Encoded by cDNAs

For the determination of the steroid-binding properties of the protein encoded by the constructed cDNAs, the pGEM-3Z vectors containing the cDNAs were linearized and transcribed by T7-RNA polymerase and the RNA produced was translated in a rabbit reticulocyte lysate. The receptor proteins produced were analyzed for their steroid-binding specificities and affinities by a hydroxylapatite-filter assay (36), sedimentation properties, and immuno-reactivities with human autoanti-AR antibodies (48).

The *in vitro* synthesized hAR and rAR firmly bound synthetic androgens, such as ^{3}H-R1881(Kd = 0.3–0.5 nM) and this binding was completed very well by DHT and the synthetic androgen, mibolerone (37,42) (Fig. 1). The ARs sedimented as 4 S forms either in low or high salt (0.4M KCl) media and in the absence or presence of androgen. In contrast, A-R complexes prepared from target organs such as the rat ventral prostate sediment as 3-5 S and 7-12 S or other heavier forms (30) in low salt media and as a 4 S form in high salt media. These observations suggested that the heavier forms of ARs are formed by association of ARs with other cellular components (RNA and/or other proteins) in the target organs. SRs have been shown to associate with 90 kDa heat shock proteins (49). By mixing experiments, we found that the ARs newly synthesized in the reticulocyte system, do not appear to interact with reticulocyte or prostate heat shock proteins to form 8-10 S components. It is not known whether AR binds a specific heat shock protein only after a chemical modification or interaction with specific factors in prostate cells.

cDNA-Nucleotide and Amino Acid Sequences of Androgen Receptors

Overall Structure

Analysis of the nucleotide sequence of AR cDNAs revealed open reading frames in hAR and rAR cDNAs that encode proteins with 918 and 902 amino acids. The molecular mass of these ARs is about 98 kDa. Because the site of translation initiation is not known for ARs, other possible translation products are proteins with 734 (hAR) and 753 (rAR) amino acids and molecular masses of 80kDa (translation initiation at the next ATG). The protein products obtained by translation of transcripts synthesized *in vitro* from AR-cDNAs included 98, 80, 70, 55, 46, 32, and 30-kDa proteins that bind to calf-thymus DNA and are immunoprecipitated by auto-immune-anti-AR antibodies (37,42). The 98 and 80kDa as well as some of the other proteins might be the products of translation at the first and other internal ATG codons, while other small peptides might be generated by proteolysis of larger forms. Preliminary studies, using an immunoblotting technique, indicated that some target organs of androgens had mostly the 98 kDa form, whereas other target organs had an 80 kDa AR and essentially no 98 kDa form. It is unknown if these tissue differences are biologically important or are the result of artifactual proteolysis.

Among the hAR sequences reported by us and four other groups (Fig. 5), there were two nucleotide differences in the N-terminal domain that changed two deduced amino acids. There are also differences in the number of amino acids in the two long Gln and Gly stretches in the N-terminal domain. For the rAR sequence there is only one nucleotide difference between our results and that of the North Carolina group, which changes the sequence by one amino acid. There is no disagreement in the reported cDNA nucleotide and deduced amino acid sequences in the C-terminal half (including DNA- and androgen-binding domains) of hAR or rAR.

Amino-terminal Domain

The various SRs do not have a uniform structure in the N-terminal domain, either in their amino acid sequence or in their length. In the N-terminal domain, 116 of 555 amino acids of hAR are not identical in the corresponding sequence of rAR. The most striking feature of hAR and rAR is the presence of many oligo- or poly(amino acid) sequences in this domain (Fig. 5). A long stretch of 27 consecutive Gly and another one with 17 Gln are present in hAR, whereas rAR has a stretch with 22 consecutive Gln. There are 11 oligo amino acid sequences in hAR, whereas rAR has 9. There are no oligo- or poly(amino acid) sequences in the DNA-binding domain, but there is one trimer of Leu in the androgen-binding domain of both hAR and rAR at equivalent positions. SRs including ARs are rich in Pro residues in the N-terminal region. In SRs, Pro residues might play a key role in structural conformations that are recognized by regulatory factors.

Repetitive nucleotide sequences that encode poly(amino acid) sequences have been found in some regulatory genes. For example, a GGN repeat that encodes poly(Gly) and a CAG repeat that encodes poly(Gln) have been found in several homeotic genes (50–52). A poly (Gln) sequence is also present in rGR (53), but no other SRs appear to have long stretches of poly(amino acids). It is possible that these oligo- or poly(amino acid) sequences are important in the regulation of AR function.

DNA-binding Domain

Although there are 14 nucleotide changes, hAR and rAR have an identical amino acid sequence in the DNA-binding domain. The 68-amino acids in this domain can fold into two 'zinc coordinated finger' structures (38,39) that bind to a hormone-response element as do other SRs (54). In estrogen receptor (ER) and GR (55), the first 'zinc finger' (nearest to the N-terminal) might be involved in recognition of the hormone responsive element (HRE) and this interaction then is stabilized by the

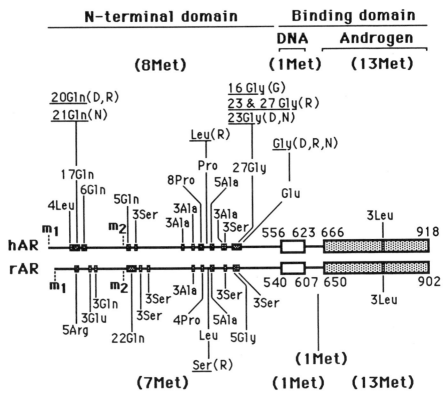

FIG. 5. The amino acid sequences of hAR and rAR deduced from the nucleotide sequences of cDNAs. The position and the number of amino acids in each oligo- or poly(amino acid) are shown based on our own data (37,42). The first and second methionines in the N-terminal domains are indicated by m_1 and m_2. The total number of methionines in each domain is shown in parentheses. The amino acid positions of the DNA- and androgen-binding domains are indicated by amino acid numbers started from m_1. The sequences that were reported by other research groups [N: North Carolina (43,56); D: Dallas (44); R: Rotterdam (45,57)] to be different from ours are underlined. The genomic (G) sequence reported by the Rotterdam group showed 16 Gly at the polyglycine stretch in hAR.

second 'zinc finger'. All 10 cysteines of rAR, hAR, progesterone receptor (hPR), and hGR as well as 9 of 10 cysteines in hER are conserved. There is a high homology (75% to 80%) among ARs and hPR, hGR, mineralocorticoid receptor (hMR) in this domain and they appeared to recognize the same SRE, possibly with different degrees of affinity. The homology in this domain among ARs and ER, or receptors for thyroid hormones, retinoic acids, or vitamin D is only 40% to 56%.

Androgen-binding Domain

The 253 amino acid sequence of the hormone-binding domain at the C-terminal end of hAR and rAR are identical, although there are 54 nucleotide differences in the

DNA coding for this region. The homology in this domain among ARs, GR, PR, and MR is only 50% to 54%. However, four short regions within this domain have 65% to 100% sequence similarity among these receptors. Another interesting feature is that the androgen-binding domain has a high methionine content (13 residues). The hormone-binding domains in other SRs also have a high methionine content. These amino acids can be part of unique structures that might have a role in structural recognition of hormonal ligands or factors that regulate the function of this domain.

Structure and Mutations of Androgen Receptor Genes

The gene for AR has been localized to the q11–q12 region of the human X-chromosome (58) using a cloned cDNA for AR. Structural organization of the human AR gene also has been analyzed recently (57). The total length of the hAR gene appears to be more than 90 kb and the AR coding region was separated over eight exons (57) (Fig. 6). There are striking similarities in the intron-exon organization among the SR genes analyzed so far (53,60–62). AR and other SRs are each encoded by one single-copy gene located on separate chromosomes (retinoic acid and thyroid hormone receptors seemed to have at least two genes on different chromosomes). Most of the N-terminal domain of a SR is coded by one large exon. The second exon codes for the first 'zinc finger' and the third exon codes for the second 'zinc finger'. All exon-intron junctions in hAR, hER, and cPR are located at similar positions, although the lengths of the introns are quite different.

AR Gene Mutations

Insensitivity of target organs and tumors to androgens has been observed in man and other animals. This abnormality might be caused by a mutation or altered ex-

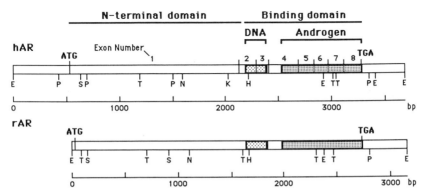

FIG. 6. Exon structure and restriction map of genes for hAR and rAR. Exon termini for hAR are taken from Kuiper and associates (128). Abbreviations for the restriction enzymes are: E, Eco RI; H, Hind III; K, Kpn I; N, Nru I; P, Pst I; S, SMa I; T, Taq I.

A. Receptor positive (low affinity androgen binding).

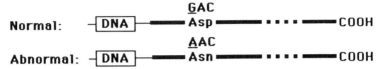

B. Receptor negative (no androgen binding).

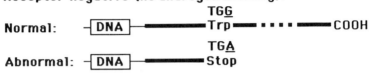

FIG. 7. Examples of G to A mutations in the androgen-binding domain of ARs. The bases changed are underlined. Example A shows a change in one amino acid (from Asp to Asn) might result in a lower androgen-binding affinity, whereas example B shows that a base change can result in the formation of a stop codon and production of a truncated receptor that does not bind androgen.

pression of the genes for the AR or 5α-reductase, as well as by defects in other cellular components that are needed for normal androgen responses in AR- and 5α-reductase-positive cells. A deficiency in 5α-reductase has been related to abnormal male sexual differentiation in men. A defect in the X-chromosome-linked AR also is considered to be responsible for syndromes of androgen resistance, such as testicular feminization (Tfm) (8,63). With the elucidation of the sequence of the AR, it is now possible to analyze whether mutations in the AR gene are responsible for abnormalities in androgen responsiveness. Brown and associates (64) have found a partial deletion in the DNA coding for the androgen-binding domain of the AR in one family and a possible point mutation in another family. In the Tfm Stanley-Gumbreck rat, a point mutation (CGG for arginine to CAG for glutamine) was found in the androgen-binding domain (127). A similar G to A transition (and change in amino acid sequence from valine to methionine) also has been found in an hAR gene from an androgen-insensitive individual (65). We also found that a reduction in the androgen-binding affinity of AR in an androgen-insensitive cell line was apparently because of a point mutation (G to A) in the androgen-binding domain of the AR, which changes the encoded amino acid from aspartic acid to asparagine. Another receptor-negative cell line derived from an androgen-insensitive individual also had a G to A mutation in the androgen-binding domain that changed TGG (trp) to TGA, creating a stop codon possibly resulting in the production of a truncated AR (Fig. 7).

Isoforms and Their Functions

Differences in the AR-sequences summarized in Fig. 5 and discussed in the last section suggest that there might be AR isoforms in various target organs or tumors. Besides the possibility of having more than one AR-gene, multiple forms of AR-mRNA can be generated by alternate splicing of AR-mRNA precursors. Govindan (66) reported recently the isolation of two different forms of hAR cDNA. The A-form had an amino acid sequence that was similar to that reported by other groups, but the B-form differed in the amino acid sequence of the androgen-binding domain and bound androgen poorly. Unlike the A-form, the B-form of AR did not transactivate MMTV-CAT nor bind specifically to the GRE. Isoforms of other SRs have been described, especially in the case of ERs and thyroid hormone receptor (TR).

Deletion analysis performed on GR estrogen receptors, (ER) and PR has shown that the hormone-binding domains of SRs and therefore their respective hormonal ligand, are not essential for SR recognition of HREs (67–69). Therefore, mutated SRs that do not bind hormones (because of mutation of an amino acid residue or deletion of the C-terminus) can act as hormone-independent transcription regulators. Interestingly, TR, which in the presence of thyroid hormone stimulates the expression of a responsive gene, suppresses activity of a responsive promotor if the hormone is absent (70,71). The oncogenic derivatives of TR, v-erbA, and other isoforms of TR have been shown to interfere with the interaction of a TR, with its TRE, and act as repressors (72). Structural changes in the ligand binding domain of a receptor also might alter the ligand preference and affinity. In such cases, mutated receptors that do not bind the natural hormone still can be controlled by new ligands or antagonists and this can be important in the development of hormone-insensitive tumors. For P_{450} enzymes, it has been shown that a one amino acid change in the enzyme can alter the substrate specificity (73). Considering the possible combination of multiple controls already discussed, it is plausible to suggest that the ratios of the cellular levels of AR isoforms and related receptors play an important role in determining the organ specificity and differential effectiveness of hormonal ligands and their receptors. Further studies of the isoforms of AR also can provide better understanding of positive and negative gene regulation by ARs.

Nucleotide Probes and Other Considerations

Based on the nucleotide sequence of cDNAs and genes for ARs it is possible to construct many useful primers for selection and amplification of particular nucleotide regions (by polymerase chain reaction methods) of ARs and to prepare probes for the analysis of potential defects in the AR gene and its expression. Sequences in the intron/exon junction will be especially useful in identifying affected regions of the gene. A point mutation might abolish a restriction enzyme site and provide a very simple analytical method for analyzing abnormalities by Southern blotting. AR-specific ribo- or deoxyribo-oligomers (20–30 bases) can be selected not only from the N-terminal and ligand-binding domains that have low homology among SRs, but also from the highly homologous DNA-binding domain as probes for blotting and *in situ* hybridization experiments.

Studies with several cell lines derived from androgen-insensitive individuals have shown that abnormalities in the androgen response often might be because of point mutations rather than gross structural alterations of the AR gene. To avoid misinformation because of cloning or sequencing errors, as well as errors because of mismatch during the polymerase chain reaction, it is important to confirm structural changes by analyzing both genomic DNA and AR-cDNA and to study androgen-binding activity and functionality in cells transfected with the DNA for these mutant ARs. Methylation of cytosine in DNA plays an important role in the regulation of gene exression. If 5'-methylcytosine undergoes deamination spontaneously in the cell to produce thymine, a GT-mistach can occur in DNA. This can lead to a G to A mutation during DNA replication. It has been suggested that a GT-mismatch can be corrected by a repair pathway involving a GT-binding protein (74). Therefore, a defect in GT-binding protein and its repair process can play a key role in altering hormone sensitive cells to insensitive tumor cells. Some point mutations or other small alterations in the AR gene might not be the molecular basis of functional AR abnormalities. Changes in the interaction of a receptor regulatory factor (RRF) with receptor domains or defects in the RRF itself can affect binding of androgens to ARs and binding of ARs to their HRE or chromatin, and affect AR functions. Because AR, GR, and PR appear to recognize similar HRE (75–78), differential expression of various SR in target cells or organs can determine the relative responsiveness of different hormones (79). Down regulation of the expression of SR genes by their respective hormones (80,81) including androgens (42,56) also can have a role in determining tissue responsiveness.

Steroid insensitivity also can occur irrespective of the presence of functional steroid receptors. For example, it has been shown that certain steroid-insensitive breast tumor cells contained functional receptors for glucocorticoids and androgens and so a defect existed at some other level of transcriptional control. It is also possible that an epigenetic mechanism can be involved in the switching off of certain genes after prolonged steroid withdrawal (82).

ANTI-ANDROGEN RECEPTOR ANTIBODIES

Human Autoantibodies

Autoantibodies to ARs are present in high titer in the sera of some patients with prostate diseases (48). These autoanti-AR antibodies were shown to be AR-specific and did not interact with GR, PR, or ER. Because of their specificity, these autoantibodies were important in analyzing whether ARs made in cell-free systems from cDNA constructs were immunoreactive and thus provided essential evidence that the cDNAs we constructed coded for ARs. So far high titer anti-AR antibodies have been found only in serum from males who had prostate cancer or who were older than 66 years (5 of 400 men from all age groups). Many prostate cancer patients, however, do not have high titer anti-AR antibodies. There is no apparent relationship between the presence of these autoantibodies and male infertility, gynecomastia, and liver cancer.

Monoclonal Antibodies and Immunocytolocalization

For the production of monoclonal antibodies, initially, we used Epstein-Barr virus to transform B-lymphocytes of prostate cancer patients who had higher titer auto-anti-AR antibodies. The transformed B-cells were fused with myeloma cells to obtain monoclonal antibody producing cells. Young and coworkers (83) also used this method successfully to obtain anti-AR antibodies and carefully characterized their properties. Unfortunately, the cloned human hybridomas were unstable and lost their ability to produce monoclonal antibodies.

A molecular fusion technique has been used to obtain large quantities of specific AR peptides linked to a E. coli protein, trpE. Polyclonal anti-AR antibodies were obtained from rabbits or rats immunized with fusion proteins that represent mainly the amino terminal portion, the DNA-binding domain, or the androgen-binding domain of rAR and hAR. Spleen cells from immunized rats were fused with mouse myeloma cells to produce hybridomas-secreting antibodies to AR. Based on immunoprecipitation assay and gradient centrifugation studies, the monoclonal anti-AR antibodies produced from cloned hybridomas were specific for AR (84).

Using these monoclonal antibodies ARs have been localized in epithelial cell nuclei of rat and human prostates as well as monkey seminal vesicles (85,86). These observations appear to confirm earlier findings based on autoradiographic localization of radioactive androgens in prostate cell nuclei (87,88). Because ARs have been found in the cytoplasmic compartment of target cells, such as the prostate, further studies are needed to define the role of ARs in different cellular compartments. Demura and associates (89) have immunized mice with partially purified ARs from human prostates and fused the mouse lymphocytes with myeloma cells to produce monoclonal antibodies to ARs. Although the receptor specificity of the monoclonal antibody was not described, the monoclonal antibody immunohistochemically stained the cytoplasm and nuclei of cells in benign prostatic hyperplastic tissues and mainly the nuclei of prostate cancer cells. Prostate cells in androgen-independent cancer tissue did not show immunoreactive staining, indicating the absence of AR. Because the antigenic site on AR for this monoclonal antibody was not clear, it was not possible to exclude the possibility that a truncated AR was present in the insensitive cells.

INTRACELLULAR DYNAMICS OF ANDROGEN RECEPTORS AND POSTTRANSCRIPTIONAL CONTROL

Dynamic Status of Prostate Androgen Receptors

The dynamic status of AR in prostate cells has been studied by incubation of rat ventral prostate with radioactive androgens in the presence and absence of respiratory poisons or inhibitors of protein and RNA synthesis, and also by isotope chasing of the radioactive A-R complexes (90). In the presence of 2,4-dinitro-

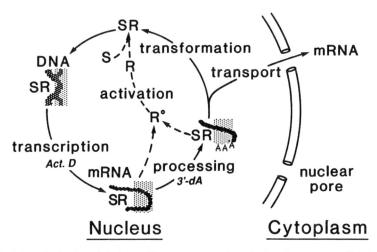

FIG. 8. A hypothetical model of steroid receptor recycling. An inactive receptor (R°) that does not bind steroid hormones goes through an energy-dependent activation process to become a steroid (S)-binding receptor (R). The complex then binds to the transcription site to regulate new RNA synthesis. The receptor complex then binds to RNA and is released from the chromatin. RNA is then processed and transported out of nucleus. The receptor (R) can be inactivated to R° again. Shaded areas represent the possible participation of other factors in the recycling process. Proposed points of inhibition of receptor recycling by actinmycin D (Act.D) and 3'-deoxyadenosine (3'-dA) are indicated.

phenol, AR is rapidly deactivated (half life, 2 min) to an inactive form (R°) that does not bind androgen unless it is reactivated by an energy-dependent process to an androgen-binding form (R) (Fig. 8). A majority of the A-R complexes formed might not bind to DNA/chromatin unless they are 'transformed' by a temperature-dependent process. It is not clear whether this is because of the need for a chemical modification of the newly formed A-R complexes or to the association/dissociation of other cellular factors. Isotope-chasing experiments with labeled androgen indicate that the steps involved in AR recycling between chromatin-bound and cytosolic forms are slow compared to other steps in the recycling process and the A-R complex has a half life of more than 50 min (91,92) in this part of the cycle. This slow process might reflect the participation of A-R in a time-consuming mechanism that is essential for hormone responses.

Steroid Hormone Regulation of Post-Transcriptional Processes

In addition to their effects on transcription of specific genes, steroid hormones also appear to be involved in post-transcriptional regulation of specific gene expression (93). In chick oviduct, for example, the level of a mRNA for a heat shock protein increases 20- to 50-fold with estrogen or progestin treatment, while the rate of transcription of the gene is increased only 2- to 4-fold (94). Androgens also enhance the transcription of genes for a steroid-binding secretory protein about 2- to 3-fold, but the level of the mRNA for this protein increases about 30-fold (95). Growth hormone gene transcription in pituitary cells is enhanced by glucocorticoids and thyroid hormones 5-fold, but the level of the mRNA increases about 50-fold (96). Many other examples have been described (97,98). Steroid hormones, therefore, appear to alter the stability of induced mRNA in their target cells. The possibility that E-R complexes might be involved in RNA transport in rat uterine nuclei also has been presented (99). Autoradiographic studies by Carmo-Fonseca also have suggested that, in the rat ventral prostate, androgens can stimulate intranuclear RNA transport and migration of RNA through the nuclear envelope (100).

RNA Binding of Steroid Receptors

To explain how SR recycling can be involved in the regulation of gene transcription and posttranscriptional processes, we suggested many years ago that S-R complexes not only can bind DNA to promote specific gene transcription, but can also bind RNA and regulate processing, transport, stabilization, and/or utilization of RNA (4,101,102). This hypothetical model (Fig. 8) was essentially identical with that proposed more recently for the action of *Xenopus* transcription factor IIIA, which binds to the 5S RNA gene to promote 5S RNA synthesis but can then bind and stabilize 5S RNA (103). In line with this view, it has been shown that both A-R and E-R complexes bind RNA or ribonucleoprotein in the rat ventral prostate (104) or uterus (105). In cell-free systems, certain single-stranded uridine(U)-rich poly-ribonucleotides (but not poly(A) or poly(C) can bind A-R, E-R, and G-R complexes and promote the release of these receptor complexes from DNA, and this effect is dependent on the nucleotide sequence of the polyribonucleotides (91,106). Because U-rich sequences are found in small nuclear RNAs that are essential in the function of the splicesome and stabilization of mRNA, SR might specifically recognize sequences in these RNAs.

In recent years, other investigators also have found that S-R complexes can bind to various types of RNA including small nuclear RNAs (107–113). Based on a computer analysis, Baker also pointed out that *Escherichia coli* tyrosyl-tRNA synthetase has a sequence similarity to a segment of human ER (114).

Probe of a Hypothetical Model

In our model, an S-R complex binds to the transcriptional complex on a responsive gene and promotes RNA synthesis. The S-R complex then binds to the RNA product, and the ternary complex formed is released from the target gene. This process allows the gene to participate in further RNA synthesis. Removal of RNA from the receptor complex is required for the S-R complex to recycle back to chromatin. To test the model, we used actinomycin D and 3'-dA, which selectively inhibit transcription and processing of newly synthesized RNA.

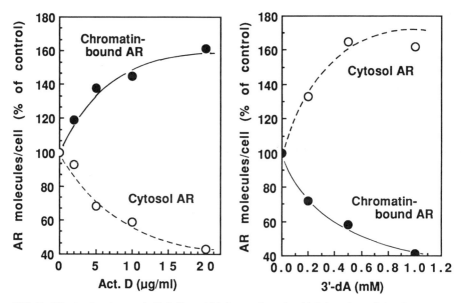

FIG. 9. Effects of actinomycin D (left) and 3'-deoxyadenosine (right) on the cellular distribution of AR in prostate cells. Minced ventral prostate from castrated rats was incubated with actinomycin D or 3'-deoxyadenosine at the concentration shown for 30 min and then with a radioactive androgen. The amount of the chromatin-bound and cytosolic A-R complexes were determined. The results are expressed as a percent of the value from a control, which was incubated without the inhibitors (92,119).

As shown in Fig. 9, A-R complexes appeared to be trapped at the site of transcription as a chromatin-bound form when minced rat ventral prostate was incubated with actinomycin D. If prostate tissue was incubated with 3'-dA instead of actinomycin D, the level of cytosolic A-R complex increased while the level of chromatin-bound A-R complex slowly decreased and reached a minimum. These results suggested that 3'-dA, a selective inhibitor of RNA polyadenylation (115, 116), splicing, and nucleo-cytoplasmic RNA transport (117,118) at the low concentration employed, was able to prevent recycling of the A-R complex back to the chromatin. The total level of A-R complexes in the prostate cell during this incubation did not change significantly.

Androgen-Receptor Complexes Formed in the Presence of 3'-dA

We found that 3'-dA actually increased the proportion of A-R complexes in the cytosol A-R fraction that does not bind to DNA-cellulose. The non-DNA-binding complexes had a sedimentation coefficient of 8-9 S. In comparison, the majority of A-R complexes in the cytosolic fraction of prostate incubated in the absence of 3'-

dA could bind to DNA-cellulose and had a sedimentation coefficient of 5 S (119). The non-DNA-binding A-R in the prostate incubated with 3'-dA were very similar to that of cytosolic A-R complexes prepared from the prostate homogenized in the presence of sodium molybdate. Molybdate has been shown to stabilize A-R complexes in an untransformed (non-DNA-binding) state (120). Whether the 3'-dA-induced A-R complexes contain U-rich or other type of RNA has not been clearly shown. Association of other factors also can be important in determining the nucleic acid-binding activity of A-R complexes.

3'-dA can exert its effect on the transformation and recycling of A-R complexes through mechanisms other than inhibition of polyadenylation and splicing of mRNA. 3'-dA has been shown to affect nuclear RNA methylation (121), and chromosomal protein phosphorylation (122). Phosphorylation of certain SRs and associated proteins have been studied (123–126), although the precise role of protein phosphorylation and other structural changes during receptor transformation remains uncertain.

CONCLUDING REMARKS

Recent progress in the analysis of the sequence of steroid receptors and their genes have provided many new methods to analyze the mechanisms of actions of steroid receptors and the causes of hormone insensitivity in various individuals and tumors. However, the precise molecular steps and factors involved in the function of SR in the target cells is far from clear. Further studies of the involvement of various isoforms of receptors in the positive and negative control of gene expression can lead to new understanding of the control of receptor mechanisms. It is now apparent that transcriptional regulation by a S-R complex requires the interaction of the zinc finger domain of a SR and the HRE of the affected genes. However, the actual event involved in specific hormonal regulation in the target cells is obviously much more complex. An intracellular receptor recycling process and RNA processing and stabilization also are important in hormonal regulation and require more indepth studies. In addition, various receptor regulatory factors can act in conjunction with SR to alter local chromatin structures and determine the genes that are available for positive or negative regulation. Several new androgen-sensitive and androgen-repressed gene products have been found recently. Some of these protein markers can be useful in analyzing androgen receptor functions. Better understanding of the mechanism involved in the mutation of androgen-sensitive cells to insensitive cells might lead to new therapeutic approaches in the treatment of hormone-insensitive tumors.

Acknowledgment

The work described in this article was supported by Grants DK37694, and DK41670 from U.S. National Institutes of Health

REFERENCES

1. Liao S. Cellular receptors for steroid hormone actions. *Intl Rev Cytology* 1975;41:87–172.
2. Fang S, Anderson KM, Liao S. Receptor proteins for androgens: on the role of specific proteins in selective retention of 17β-hydroxy-5α-androstan-3-one by rat ventral prostate *in vivo* and *in vitro*. *J Biol Chem* 1969;244:6584–6595.
3. Fang S, Liao S. Androgen receptor: steroid- and tissue-specific retention of a 17β-hydroxy-5α-androstan-3-one protein complex by cell nuclei of ventral prostate. *J Biol Chem* 1971;246:16–24.
4. Liao S, Fang S. Receptor proteins for androgens and the mode of action of androgens on gene transcription in ventral prostate. *Vitam Horm* 1969;27:17–90.
5. Liao S, Liang T, Fang S, Castaneda E, Shao TC. Steroid structure and androgenic activity: specificities involved in the receptor binding and nuclear retention of various androgens. *J Biol Chem* 1973;248:6154–6162.
6. Bardin CW, Bullock LP, Sherins RJ, Mowszowicz I, Blackburn WR. Androgen metabolism and mechanism of action in male pseudohermaphroditism: a study of testicular feminization. *Rec Progr Hormone Research* 1973;29:65–109.
7. Peterson RE, Imperato-McGinley J, Gautier, Teofilo A, Sturia E. Male pseudohermaphroditism due to steroid 5α-reductase deficiency. *Amer J Med* 1977;63:170–191.
8. Bardin CW, Catterall JF. Testosterone: a major determinant of extra genital sexual dimorphism. *Science* 1981;211:1285–1294.
9. Williams-Ashman HG (1988): Perspective in the male sexual physiology of eutherian mammals. In: Knobil E, Neill J, eds. *The Physiology of Reproduction*, New York: Raven Press, pp 727–751.
10. Isaacs JT, Brendler CB, Walsh PC. Changes in the metabolism of dihydrotestosterone in the hyperplastic human prostate. *J Clin Endocrinol Metab* 1983;56:139–146.
11. Siiteri PK and Wilson JD. Dihydrotestosterone in prostatic hypertrophy. *J Clinical Invest* 1970;49:1737–1745.
12. Schweikert, HU and Wilson JD. Regulation of human hair growth by steroid hormones. I. Testosterone metabolism in isolated hairs. *J Clin Endocrinol Metab* 1974;38:811–819.
13. Bingham KD, Shaw DA. The metabolism of testosterone by human male scalp skin. *J Endocr* 1973;57:111–112.
14. Serafini, P. and Lobo, RA. Increased 5α-reductase activity in idiopathic hirsutism. *Fert Steril* 1985;43;74–87.
15. Sansone G, and Reisner RM. Differential rates of conversion of testosterone to dihydrotestosterone in acne and in normal human skin—a possible pathogenic factor in acne. *J Invest Dermat* 1971;56:366–372.
16. Liang T, Cascieri MA, Cheung AH, Reynolds GF, Rasmusson GH. Species differences in prostatic steroid 5α-reductase of rat, dog, and human. *Endocrinology* 1985;115:571–579.
17. Liang T, Heiss CE. Inhibition of 5α-reductase, receptor binding, and nuclear uptake of androgens in the prostate by a 4-methyl-4-aza-steriod. *J Biol Chem* 1981;256:7998–8005.
18. Liang T, Heiss CE, Cheung A, H, Reynolds GF, Rasmusson GH. 4-Azasteroid 5α-reductase inhibitors without affinity for the androgen receptor. *J Biol Chem* 1984;259:734–739.
19. Liang T, Rasmusson G, Brooks JR. Biochemical and biological studies with 4-aza-steroidal 5α-reductase inhibitors. *J Steroid Biochem* 1983;19:385–390.
20. Rasmusson, GH, Reynolds G, Steinberg N, Walton E, Patel GF, Liang T, Cascieri MA, Cheung AH, Brooks, Berman C. Azasteroid: structure-activity relationships for inhibition of 5α-reductase and of androgen receptor binding. *J Med Chem* 1986;29:2298–2315.
21. Brooks JR, Baptista EM, Berman C, et al. Response of rat ventral prostate to a new and novel 5α-reductase inhibitor. *Endocrinology* 1981;109:830–836.
22. Brooks JR, Berman C, Glitzer MS, et al. Effect of a new 5α-reductase inhibitor on size, histologic characteristic and androgen concentrations of the canine prostate. *Prostate*, 1982;3:35–44.
23. Wenderoth UK, George FW. The effects of a 5α-reductase inhibitor on androgen mediated growth of the dog prostate. *Endocrinology*, 1983;113:569–573.
24. Rittmaster RS, Uno H, Povar ML, Mellin TN, Loriaux DL. The effects of N,N-diethyl-4-methyl-3-oxo-4-aza-5α-reductase inhibitor and antiandrogen, on the development of baldness in the stumptail macaque. *J Clin Endocrinol Metab* 1987;65:188–193.
25. Liang T, Brady EJ, Chung A, Saperstein R. Inhibition of luteinizing hormone (LH)-releasing

hormone-induced secretion of LH in rat anterior pituitary cell culture by testosterone without conversion to 5α-dihydrotestosterone. *Endocrinology* 1984;115:2311–2317.

26. Vermeulen A, Giagulli VA, De Schepper P, Buntinx A, and Stoner E. Hormonal effects of an orally active 4-azasteroid inhibitor of 5α-reductase in humans. *Prostate* 1989;14:45–53.

27. Liang T, Cheung AH, Reynolds GF, Rasmusson GH. Photoaffinity labeling of steroid 5α-reductase of rat liver and prostate microsomes. *J Biol Chem* 1985;260:4890–4895.

28. Voigt W, Fernandez EP, and Hsia SL. Transformation of testosterone into 17β-hydroxy-5α-androstan-3-one by microsomal preparations of human skin. *J Biol Chem* 1970;245:5594–5599.

29. Blohm TR, Metcalf BW, Laughlin ME, Sjoerdsma A, Schatzman GL. Inhibition of testosterone 5α-reductase by a proposed enzyme-activated, active site-directed inhibitor. *Biochem Biophy Res Commun* 1989;95:273–280.

30. Liao S. Molecular actions of androgens. In: Litwack G, ed. *Biochemical Actions of Hormones,* New York: Academic Press 1977; Vol. 4, 351–406.

31. Castaneda E, Liao S. The use of anti-steroid antibodies in the characterization of steriod receptors. *J Biol Chem* 1975;250:883–888.

32. Fang S, Liao S. Antagonistic action of anti-androgens on the formation of a specific dihydrotestosterone-receptor protein complex in rat ventral prostate. *Molecular Pharmacol* 1969;5:428–431.

33. Liao S, Howell DK, Chang TM. Action of a non-steroidal anti-androgen, flutamide, on the receptor binding and nuclear retention of 5α-dihydrotestosterone in rat ventral prostate. *Endocrinology* 1974;94:1205–1209.

34. Neri RO. Studies of the biology and mechanism of action of nonsteroidal antiandrogens. In: Matini L, Motta M, eds. *Androgens and Antiandrogens,* New York: Raven Press, 1977; 179–189.

35. Chang C, Liao S. Topographic recognition of cyclic hydrocarbons and related compounds by receptors for androgens, estrogens, and glucocorticoids. *J Steroid Biochem* 1987;27:123–131.

36. Liao S, Witte D, Schilling K, Chang C. The use of hydroxylapatite-filter steroid assay method in the study of the modulation of androgen receptor interactions. *J Steroid Biochem* 1984;20:11–17.

37. Chang C, Kokontis J, Liao S. Molecular cloning of human and rat complementary DNA encoding androgen receptors. *Science* 1988;2:324–326.

38. Liao S, Chang C, Kokontis J, Popovich T, Hiipakka RA. Structure and intracellular dynamics of androgen receptors. In: Carlstedt-Duke J, Eriksson J, Gustafsson J-A, eds. *The Steroid/Thyroid Hormone Receptor Family and Gene Regulation,* Basel: Birkhauser Verlag, 1988; 83–92.

39. Liao S, Kokontis J, Sai T, Hiipakka RA. Androgen receptors: structures, mutations, antibodies, and cellular dynamics. *J Steroid Biochem* 1989;34:41–51.

40. Lyon M, Hawkes, SG. X-linked gene for testicular feminization in the mouse. *Nature (Lond),* 1970;227:1217–1219.

41. Meyer WJ III, Migeon BR, Migeon CJ. Locus on human X-chromosome for dihydrotestosterone receptor and androgen insensitivity. *Proc Natl Acad Sci U S A* 1975;72:1469–1472.

42. Chang C, Kokontis J, Liao S. Structural analysis of complementary DNA and amino acid sequences of human and rat androgen receptors. *Proc Natl Acad Sci U S A* 1988;85:7211–7215.

43. Lubahn DB, Joseph DR, Sar M, Tan J, Higgs HN, Larson RE, French FS, Wilson EM. The human androgen receptor: Complementary deoxyribonucleic acid cloning, sequence analysis and gene expression in prostate. *Mol Endocrinol* 1988;2:1265–1275.

44. Tilley WD, Marcell M, Wilson JD, McPhaul MJ. Characterization and expression of a cDNA encoding the human androgen receptor. *Proc Natl Acad Sci U S A* 1989;86:327–331.

45. Trapman J, Klaassen P, Kuiper GGJM, et al. Cloning, structure and expression of a cDNA encoding the human androgen receptor. *Biochem Biophys Res Commun* 1988;153:241–248.

46. Chang C, Kokontis J. Identification of a new member of the steroid receptor super-family by cloning and sequence analysis. *Biochem Biophys Res Commun* 1988;155:971–977.

47. Hazel TG, Nathans D, Lau LF. A gene inducible by serum growth factors encodes a member of the steroid and thyroid hormone receptor superfamily. *Proc Natl Acad Sci U S A* 1988;85:8444–8448.

48. Liao S, Witte D. Autoimmune anti-androgen receptor antibodies in human serum. *Proc Natl Acad Sci U S A* 1985;82:8345–8349.

49. Howard KJ, Distelhorst CW. Evidence for intracellular association of the glucocorticoid receptor with the 90-kDa heat shock protein. *J Biol Chem* 1988;263:3474–3481.

50. Beachy PA, Helfand SL, Hogness DS. Segmental distribution of bithorax complex proteins during Drosophila development. *Nature (Lond)* 1985;313:545–551.

51. McGinnis W, Garber RL, Eirz J, Kuroiwa A, Gehring WJ. A homologous protein-coding se-

quence in Drosophila homoeotic genes and its conservation in other metazoans. *Cell* 1984;37:403–408.

52. Scott MP, Carroll SB. The segmentation and homeotic gene network in early Drosophila development. *Cell* 1987;51:689–698.
53. Miesfeld R, Rusconi S, Godowski PJ, et al. Genetic complementation of a glucocorticoid receptor deficiency by expression of cloned receptor cDNA. *Cell* 1986;46:389–399.
54. Evans R. The steroid and thyroid hormone receptor superfamily. *Science* 1988;240:889–895.
55. Green S, Kumar V, Theulaz I, Wahli W, Chambon P. The N-terminal DNA-binding 'zinc finger' of the oestrogen and glucocorticoid receptors determines target gene specificity. *EMBO J* 1988; 7:3037–3044.
56. Tan J, Joseph DR, Quarmby VE, Lubahn DB, Sar M, French FS Wilson EM. The rat androgen receptor: primary structure, autoregulation of its messenger ribonucleic acid, and immunocytolocalization of the receptor protein. *Mol Endocrinol* 1988;2:1276–1285.
57. Faber PM, Kuiper GGJM, van Rooij HCJ, van der Korput JAGM, Brinkmann AO, Trapman J. The N-terminal domain of the human androgen receptor is encoded by one large exon. *Mol Cell Endocrinol* 1989;61:257–262.
58. Brown CJ, Goss SJ, Lubahn DB, et al. Androgen receptor locus on the human X-chromosome: regional localization to Xq11-12 and description of a DNA polymorphism. *Am J Hum Genet* 1989;44:264–269.
59. Kuttenn F, Mowszowicz I, Schaison G, Mauvais-Jarvis PC. Androgen production and skin metabolism in hirsutism. *J Endocrinol* 1977;75:83–91.
60. Green S, Chambon P. Nuclear receptors enhance our understanding of transcription regulation. *Trends in Genetics* 1988;4:309–314.
61. Huckaby CS, Conneely OM, Beattie WG, Dobson ADW, Tsai M, O'Malley BW. Structure of the chromosomal chicken progesterone receptor gene. *Proc Natl Acad Sci U S A* 1987;84:8380–8384.
62. Ponglikitmongkol M, Green S, Chambon P. Genomic organization of the human estrogen receptor gene. *EMBO J* 1988;7:3385–3388.
63. Pinsky L, Kaufman M. Genetics of steroid receptors and their disorders. *Adv Human Genetics* 1987;16:299–472.
64. Brown TR, Lubahn DB, Wilson EM, Joseph DR, French FS, Migeon CJ. Deletion of the steroid-binding domain of the human androgen receptor gene in one family with complete androgen insensitivity syndrome: evidence for further genetic heterogeneity in this syndrome. *Proc Natl Acad Sci U S A* 1988;85:8151–8155.
65. Lubahn DB, Brown TR, Simental JA, Higgs HN, Migeon CJ, French FS. Cloning, sequencing and amplification by the polymerase chain reaction of coding exons in the human androgen receptor gene in normal and androgen insensitive genetic males. *Endocrinology, 1989; 71st Ann Meeting Abst.*: No. 621.
66. Govindan MV. Evidence for two androgen receptors. Molecular cloning, expression and functional analysis of the two androgen receptors. *Endocrinology 1989; 71st Ann Meeting Abst.*: No. 184.
67. Godowski PJ, Rusconi S, Miesfeld R, Yamamoto KR. Glucocorticoid receptor mutants that are constitutive activators of transcriptional enhancement. *Nature* 1987;325,365–368.
68. Gronemeyer H, Turcotte B, Quirin-Striker C, et al. The chicken progesterone receptor: sequence, expression and functional analysis. *EMBO J* 1987;6:3985–3994.
69. Hollenberg SM, Evans RM. Multiple and cooperative trans-activation domains of the human glucocorticoid receptor. *Cell* 1988;55:899–906.
70. Damm K, Thompson CC, Evans RM. Protein encoded by v-erbA functions as a thyroid-hormone receptor antagonist. *Nature (Lond)* 1989;339:593–597.
71. Graupner G, Wills KN, Tzukerman M, Zhang X, Pfahl M. Dual regulatory role for thyroid-hormone receptors allows control of retinoic-acid receptor activity. *Nature (Lond)* 1989;340:653–656.
72. Koenig RJ, Lazar MA, Hodin RA, et al. Inhibition of thyroid hormone action by a non-hormone binding c-erbA protein generated by alternative mRNA splicing. *Nature (Lond)* 1989;337:659–661.
73. Lindberg RLP, Negishi M. Alteration of mouse cytochrome P450$_{coh}$ substrate specificity by mutation of a single amino-acid residue. *Nature (Lond)* 1989;339:632–634.
74. Jiricny J, Hughes M, Corman N, Rudkin BB. A human 200-kDa protein binds selectively to DNA fragments containing GT mismatches. *Proc Natl Acad Sci U S A* 1988;85:8860–8864.

75. Denison SH, Snads A, Tindall DJ. A tyrosine aminotransferase glucocorticoid response element also mediates androgen enhancement of gene expression. *Endocrinology* 1989;124:1091–1093.

76. Ham J, Thomson A, Needham M, Webb P, Parker M. Characterization of response elements for androgens, glucocorticoids and progestins in mouse mammary tumour virus. *Nucleic Acids Res* 1988;16:5263–5276.

77. Matuskik RJ, Cattini PA, Lecco KJ, et al. In: Kar J, ed. *Molecular and Cellular Biology of Prostate Cancer*. Bethesda, NIH, in press.

78. Tsai SY, Carletsdt-Duke J, Weigel, NL, Dahlman K, Gustafsson J-A, Tsai, M-J, O'Malley BW. Molecular interactions of steroid hormones receptor with its enhancer element: evidence for receptor dimer formation. *Cell* 1988;55:361–369.

79. Strahle U, Boshart M, Klock G, Stewart F, Schat G. Glucocorticoid- and progesterone-specific effects are determined by differential expression of the respective hormone receptors. *Nature* 1989;339:629–632.

80. Okret S, Poellinger L, Dong YU, Gustafsson JA. Down-regulation of glucocorticoid receptor RNA by glucocorticoid hormones and recognition by the receptor. *Proc Natl Acad Sci U S A* 1986;83:5899–5903.

81. Rosewicz S, McDonald AR, Maddux BA, Goldfine ID, Miesfeld RL, Logsdon CD. Mechanism of glucocorticoid receptor down-regulation by glucocorticoids. *J Biol Chem* 1988;263:2581–2584.

82. Darbre PD, King RJB. Progression to steroid insensitivity can occur irrespective of the presence of functional steroid receptors. *Cell* 1987;51:521–528.

83. Young CYF, Murthy LR, Prescott JL, et al. Monoclonal antibodies against the androgen receptor: recognition of human and other mammalian androgen receptors. *Endocrinology* 1989; 123:601–610.

84. Chang C, Whelan CT, Popovich TC, Kokontis J, Liao S. Fusion proteins containing androgen receptor sequences and their use in the production of poly-and monoclonal anti-androgen receptor antibodies. *Endocrinology* 1989;123:1097–1099.

85. Brenner RM, West NB, Chang C, Liao S. Immunocytochemical localization of the androgen, estrogen and progestin receptors in the seminal vesicle of the Rhesus monkey. *Endocrinology, 71st Ann Meeting abstract* No. 190; 1989.

86. Chang C, Chodak G, Sarac E, Takeda H, Liao S. Androgen receptor: Immunolocalization and mRNA characterization. *J Steroid Biochem* 1989;34:311–313.

87. Peters CA, Barrack ER. A new method for labeling and autoradiographic localization of androgen receptors. *J Histochem Cytochem* 1987;35:755–762.

88. Sar M, Liao S, Stumpf WE. Nuclear concentration of androgens in rat seminal vesicles and prostate demonstrated by dry-mount autoradiography. *Endocrinology* 1970;86:1008–1011.

89. Demura T, Kuzumaki N, Oda A, et al. Establishment of monoclonal antibody to human androgen receptor and its clinical application for prostatic cancers. *Am J Clin Oncol* 1988; 11 (suppl): S23–S26.

90. Liao S, Rossini GP, Hiipakka RA, Chen C. Factors that can control the interaction of the androgen-receptor complex with the genomic structure in the rat prostate. In: Bresciani F, ed. *Perspectives in Steroid Receptor Research*, New York: Raven Press, 1980; pp. 99–112.

91. Hiipakka RA, Liao S. Modulation of androgen receptor activity in the rat ventral prostate. *Ann New York Acad Sci* 1984;43:54–60.

92. Rossini GP, Liao, S. Intracellular inactivation, reactivation and dynamic status of prostate androgen receptors. *Biochem J* 1982;208:383–392.

93. Liao S, Hiipakka RA. Mechanism of action of steroid hormones at the subcellular level. In: Makin HLJ, ed. *Biochemistry of Steroid Hormones*, Oxford: Blackwell Scientific Publications, 1984; pp. 630–680.

94. Baez M, Sargan DR, Elbrecht A, et al. Steroid hormone regulation of the gene encoding the chicken heat shock protein Hsp 108, *J Biol Chem* 1987;262:6582–6588.

95. Page MJ, Parker MG. Effect of androgens on the transcription of rat prostatic binding protein genes. *Mol Cell Endocrinol* 1982;27:343–355.

96. Diamond DJ, Goodman HM. Regulation of growth hormone messenger RNA synthesis by dexamethasone and triiodothyronine. *J Mol Biol* 1985;181:41–62.

97. Shapiro DJ, Blume JE, Nielsen DA. Regulation of messenger RNA stability in eucaryotic cells. *BioEssays* 1987;6:221–226.

98. Shapiro DJ, Brock ML. Messenger RNA stabilization and gene transcription in the estrogen induction of vitellogenin mRNA. In: Litwack G, ed. *Biochemical Actions of Hormones*, New York: Academic Press, 1985; Vol. 12, pp. 39–172.

99. Thampan RV. Estradiol-stimulated nuclear ribonucleoprotein transport in the rat uterus: a molecular basis. *Biochemistry* 1988;27:5019–5026.
100. Carmo-Fonseca M. Quantitative ultrastructural autoradiographic study of RNA transport in rat ventral prostate. *J Ultrastruct Res* 1986;94:63–76.
101. Hiipakka RA, Liao S. Steroid receptor recycling and interaction with RNA. *Am J Clin Oncol* 1988;2:518–522.
102. Liao S, Tymoczko JL, Howell DK, Lin AH, Shao TC, Liang T. Interaction of ribonucleoprotein particles and sex-steroid-receptor complexes: a model for receptor recycling and possible function. *Excerpta Medica Int Congr Ser* 1972;273:404–407.
103. Miller J, McLachlan AD, Klug A. Repetitive zinc-binding domains in the protein transcription factor IIIA from *Xenopus* oocytes. *EMBO J* 1985;4:1609–1614.
104. Liao S, Liang T, Tymoczko JL. Ribonucleoprotein binding of steroid receptor complexes. *Nature (Lond)* 1973;241:211–213.
105. Liang T, Liao S. Association of the uterine 17β-estradiol-receptor complex with ribonucleoprotein *in vitro* and *in vivo*. *J Biol Chem* 1974;249:4671–4678.
106. Liao S, Smythe S, Tymoczko JL, Rossini GP, Chen C, Hiipakka RA. RNA-dependent release of androgen and other steroid-receptor complexes from DNA. *J Biol Chem* 1980;245:5545–5551.
107. Ali M, Vedeckis WV. Interaction of RNA with transformed glucocorticoid receptor. *J Biol Chem* 1987;262:6778–6784.
108. Anderson EE, Tymoczko JL. Stabilization of glucocorticoid receptor association with RNA by a low molecular weight factor from rat liver cytosol. *J Steroid Biochem* 1985;23:299–306.
109. Chong MT, Lipmann ME. Effects of RNA and ribonuclease on binding of estrogen and glucocorticoid receptors from MCF-7 cells to DNA-cellulose. *J Biol Chem* 1982;257:2996–3002.
110. Feldman M, Kallos J, Hollander VP. RNA inhibits estrogen receptor binding to DNA. *J Biol Chem* 1981;256:1145–1148.
111. Rossini GP, Wikstrom A-C, Gustafsson J-A. Glucocorticoid-receptor complexes are associated with small RNA *in vitro*. *J Steroid Biochem* 1989;32:633–642.
112. Rowley DR, Premont RT, Johnson MP, Young CYF, Tindall DJ. Properties of an intermediate-sized androgen receptor: association with RNA. *Biochemistry* 1986;25:6988–6995.
113. Webb ML, Litwack G. Association of RNA with the glucocorticoid receptor and possible role in activation. In: Litwack G, ed. *Biochemical Actions of Hormones*, New York: Academic Press, 1986; Vol. 13, pp. 379–403.
114. Baker ME. Similarity between tyrosyl-tRNA synthetase and the estrogen receptor. *FASEB J* 1989;3:2086–2088.
115. Darnell JE, Philipson L, Wall R, Adesnik M. Polyadenylic acid sequences: role in conversion of nuclear RNA into messenger RNA. *Science* 1971;174:507–510.
116. Penman S, Rosbach M, Penman M. Messenger and heterogeneous nuclear RNA in HeLa cells: Differential inhibition by cordycepin. *Proc Natl Acad Sci U S A* 1970;67:1878–1885.
117. Agutter PS, McCaldin B. Inhibition of ribonucleic acid efflux from isolated SV-40 3T3 cell nuclei by 3′deoxyadenosine (cordycepin). *Biochem J* 1979;180:371–378.
118. Kletzein RF. Nucleocytoplasmic transport of RNA: the effect of 3′-deoxyadenosinetriphosphate on RNA release from isolated nuclei. *Biochem J* 1980;192:753–759.
119. Hiipakka RA, Liao S. Intracellular inhibition of chromatin binding and transformation of androgen receptor by 3′-deoxyadenosine. *J Biol Chem* 1988;263:17590–17595.
120. Traish AM, Muller RE, Wotiz HH. Resolution of non-activated androgen receptors based on differences in their hydrodynamic properties. *J Steroid Biochem* 1985;22:601–609.
121. Glazer RI, Peale AL. Cordycepin and xylosyladenine: inhibitors of methylation of nuclear RNA. *Biochem Biophys Res Commun* 1978;81:521–526.
122. Legraverend M, Glazer RI. Inhibition of the phosphorylation of non-histone chromosomal proteins of rat liver by cordycepin and cordycepin triphosphate. *Cancer Res* 1978;38:1142–1146.
123. Auricchio F, Migliaccio A, Rotondi A. Inactivation of estrogen receptor *in vitro* by nuclear dephosphorylation. *Biochem J* 1981;194:569–574.
124. Logeat F, Le Cunff M, Pamphile R, Milgrom E. The nuclear bound form of the progesterone receptor is generated through a hormone-dependent phosphorylation. *Biochem Biophys Res Commun* 1985;131:421–427.
125. Orti E, Mendel DB, Munck A. Phosphorylation of glucocorticoid receptor-associated and free forms of the 90-kDa heat shock protein before and after receptor activation. *J Biol Chem* 1989;264:231–237.

126. Pike JW, Sleator NM. Hormone-dependent phosphorylation of the 1,25-dihydroxyvitamine D_3 receptor in mouse fibroblasts. Biochem Biophys Res Commun 1985;131:378–385.
127. Yarbrough WG, Quarmby VE, Simental JA, Olsen KL, French FS Molecular basis of androgen insensitivity in the Tfm rat. *Endocrinology, 71st Ann Meeting abstract*: No. 620.
128. Kuiper GGJM, Faber PW, van Rooij HCJ, et al. Structural organization of the human androgen receptor gene. *J Mol Endocrinol* 1989;2:R1–R4.

Endocrine Dependent Tumors, edited by
Klaus-Dieter Voigt and Cornelius Knabbe.
Raven Press, Ltd., New York © 1991.

3

Programmed Cell Death of Normal and Malignant Prostatic Cells

Natasha Kyprianou, Paula Martikainen, and John T. Issacs

*James Buchanan Brady Urological Institute and The Johns Hopkins Oncology Center,
The Johns Hopkins Medical Institutions, Baltimore, Maryland, 21205*

Most prostatic cancers retain an androgen responsiveness for stimulation of their growth. Prostatic cancer thus is often highly responsive to androgen ablation therapy. Nearly all men with metastatic prostatic cancer treated with androgen ablation therapy have an initial, often dramatic, beneficial response to such androgen withdrawal therapy (1). Although this initial response is of substantial palliative value, essentially all treated patients eventually relapse to an androgen-insensitive state in which additional forms of antiandrogen therapy are ineffective no matter how aggressively given (1–4). Because of this nearly universal relapse phenomenon, the annual death rate from prostatic cancer has not decreased at all over the subsequent 40 years since androgen withdrawal has become standard therapy (5). Over the last 40 years, the superficially benign nature of androgen withdrawal therapy has tended to disguise the fact that metastatic prostatic cancer is still a fatal disease for which no therapy is available that effectively increases survival (6,7).

THERAPEUTIC IMPORTANCE OF ANDROGEN-INDEPENDENT PROSTATIC CANCER CELLS

Studies by a series of laboratories have demonstrated that a major reason for this universal relapse of metastatic prostatic cancer to androgen ablation is that prostatic cancer within an individual patient is heterogeneously composed of clones of both androgen-dependent and -independent cancer cells even before hormone therapy is begun (8–11). Development of such tumor cell heterogeneity can occur by a variety of mechanisms [e.g., multifocal origin of the tumor, adaptation, or genetic instability (12)]. Regardless of the mechanism of development of such cellular heterogeneity, once androgen-independent cancer cells are present within individual prostatic cancer patients, the patient is no longer curable by androgen withdrawal therapy alone, no matter how complete, because this therapy kills only the androgen-dependent cells without eliminating pre-existing androgen-independent

prostatic cancer cells. To effect all the heterogenous prostatic cancer cell populations within an individual cancer, effective chemotherapy, specifically targeted
against the pre-existing androgen-independent cancer cell, must be simultaneously
combined with androgen ablation to effect the androgen-dependent cells. The val-
idity of each of these points has been demonstrated by a series of animal (11,13–16)
and human studies (17). The animal studies demonstrated that only by giving such a
combined chemohormonal treatment, is it possible to produce any reproducible
level of cures in animals bearing prostatic cancers (18). To produce cures however,
treatment must be started early in the course of the disease, the chemotherapy must
have definitive efficiency against androgen-independent cells, it must be given for a
crucial period, and it must be begun simultaneously with not sequential to androgen
ablation. The cure rate, even under these ideal conditions, in animals is not high,
that is, 25% (18). Although the concept of early combinational chemohormonal
therapy for prostatic cancer is valid, for such an approach to be therapeutically
effective in humans, a chemotherapeutic agent that can effectively control the
growth of the preexisting androgen-independent prostatic cancer cells must be available. There are presently no highly effective chemotherapeutic agents that can control the growth of androgen-independent prostatic cancer cells (7).

NEW APPROACHES TO CONTROL THE GROWTH OF ANDROGEN-INDEPENDENT PROSTATIC CANCER CELLS

The inability to control androgen-independent prostate cancer cells in human and
rodent tumors by standard chemotherapeutic methods has lead to a search for new
approaches. Growth of a cancer is determined by the relationship between the rate
of cell proliferation and the rate of cell death. Only when the rate of cell proliferation is greater than cell death does tumor growth continue. If the rate of cell proliferation is lower than the rate of cell death, then involution of the cancer occurs.
Therefore, a successful treatment of a cancer can be obtained by either lowering the
rate of proliferation and/or by raising the rate of cell death so that the rate of cell
proliferation is lower than the rate of cell death.

Most of the presently available chemotherapeutic agents are targeted at proliferating cancer cells. It is not surprising that there is a good correlation in a large variety
of cancers between the effectiveness of these agents and the respective cancer's rate
of cell proliferation (19,20). These previous studies have demonstrated that in cancers with high cell proliferation rates, chemotherapy can disturb the relationship
between cell proliferation and death such that the rate of cancer cell death is now
greater than production and involution of the cancer is induced, thus producing
complete clinical responses. In contrast, in cancers with a low cell proliferation
rate, similar chemotherapy is unable to shift the relationship between proliferation
and death into a negative balance thus producing, at best, only partial responses. In
order for chemotherapy to be effective, not only the rate of cell proliferation, but
also the rate of cell death, must be high (20).

If the daily cell death rate of a cancer is high enough, then antiproliferative
chemotherapy that induces even a small reduction in the daily cell proliferation rate

can produce tumor regression resulting in a high rate of complete durable response. In contrast, if the daily cell death rate is too low (e.g. slow growing cancers), then antiproliferative chemotherapy must induce a much larger reduction in the daily cell proliferation rate. Unfortunately, the reduction in cell proliferation achievable at the maximum tolerated therapeutic intensity using presently available agents in slow growing cancers are not high enough to produce high complete response rates or durable complete responses (19).

Thus, a sufficient death rate is crucially important in allowing even small differences in cell proliferation rates induced by chemotherapy to be clinically useful. Although the exact magnitude of either the cell proliferation rate or cell death rate has not been determined precisely for many human prostatic cancers, available data on the thymidine labelling index suggest that it has both a low cell proliferation rate and a low cell death rate (21,22). Successful treatment of slow growing prostatic cancers probably will require simultaneous antiproliferative chemotherapy targeted at the small number of dividing cancer cells and some type of additional therapy targeted at increasing the low cell death rate of the majority of androgen-independent cancer cells not proliferating within the prostatic cancer.

There is a large variety of effective antiproliferative chemotherapy presently available that can lower the rate of cell proliferation without increasing the rate of cell death (i.e., cytostatic agents) or agents that lower the rate of cell proliferation and also increase the rate of cell death (i.e., cytotoxic agents). Unfortunately, the cytotoxic agent presently available only lead to death of cancer cells if they subsequently undergo cell proliferation. Therefore, cancer cells not in cycle (i.e., cell in G_0 of the cell cycle) at the time of exposure or not undergoing cell division soon enough after exposure to the cytotoxic chemotherapeutic agent can repair the damage induced by cytotoxic agent and are not killed by the therapy. What is needed is some type of cytotoxic therapy that leads to the death of cancer cells, not requiring the cell to undergo proliferation to be killed.

Is it possible to induce the death of cells without requiring them to attempt to divide? The answer to this question is yes, as demonstrated by the rapid involution of the normal prostate following androgen ablation. Only about 2% of the cells in the normal adult prostate of intact male rats are undergoing cell proliferation on any day (23). Androgen ablation (i.e., castration) of the male rat leads to a decrease in cell proliferation and to an increase in the rate of cell death such that 20% of the cells present per day die within the prostate between 2 to 7 days following castration (23). By 7 days following castration more than 70% of the total number of cells in the rat prostate have died (23). Thus the vast majority of prostatic cells that die following castration did not undergo cell proliferation (i.e., the cells are in G_0 when they die).

RESPONSE OF THE NORMAL RAT PROSTATE TO ANDROGEN ABLATION

Androgen has the dual ability to stimulate cell proliferation and inhibit cell death of normal rat prostatic glandular epithelial cells (23). Androgen ablation induces a series of discrete biochemical events that lead to a cessation of cell proliferation and the activation of programmed death of these androgen-dependent prostatic cells ultimately resulting in the involution of the gland (24–37). Within 12 hours after castration of adult male rats, serum testosterone concentration decreases to below 2% of the value present in intact hosts (24). This rapid decline in serum androgen results in the ventral prostatic DHT concentration decreasing within the first 24 hours following castration to below a critical threshold value that results in cessation of proliferation and the death of the androgen-dependent ventral prostatic glandular epithelial cells (24,26,27).

Because it has been demonstrated that transforming growth factor-β (TGF-β) is a potent inhibitor of cell proliferation of both normal and malignant prostatic epithelial cells (38), the expression of TGF-β in the rat ventral prostate was studied following castration (36). Steady state levels of TGF-βmRNA were determined by Northern blot analysis and compared with mRNA levels for prostatein C_3, (39) the major androgen-dependent secretory protein of ventral prostate. Within the first day following castration there is a dramatic increase in the levels of TGF-β mRNA in the ventral prostate (approx. 10-fold) and by 4 days postcastration (36), TGF-β mRNA is maximally expressed (approx. 40-fold increase), by which time the androgen-dependent C_3 secretory protein mRNA transcripts diminish to undetectable levels. Androgen administration to 4-day castrated rats leads to a marked decrease in TGF-β mRNA to a level comparable to its constitutive expression obtained in the intact control animals, indicating that expression of TGF-β in the rat ventral prostate is under negative androgenic regulation (36). Scatchard analyses of the binding of TGF-β to membranes from rat ventral prostate reveals the presence of high affinity ($K_d = 140$ pM) saturable binding sites for [^{125}I] TGF-β to prostatic membranes, which are displaced in the presence of excess unlabeled TGF-β, but are unaffected by epidermal growth factor, nerve growth factor, fibroblast growth factor, or insulin, indicating the specificity of binding (40). Castration results in a significant increase in the total [^{125}I] TGF-β binding per total prostate, with no apparent change in the affinity of membrane receptors for TGF-β. These studies demonstrate that additional TGF-β receptors are synthesized during the first 4 days following castration because the total number of receptors per gland increases 2 to 3 fold even though the total number of cells per gland decreases $1/3$ during this time period (40). The elevated TGF-β receptor and mRNA expression might be a major mechanism for the inhibition of cell proliferation observed following castration.

The mechanism of prostatic glandular cell death induced following castration has been studied by a variety of investigators (24–37). These studies have demonstrated that the death of a cell can occur via one of two major pathways (41). The first type of cell death is termed necrotic cell death. Necrotic death is a response to pathological changes initiated outside of the cell and can be elicited by any of a large series of rather nonspecific factors that produce a hostile microenvironment for the cells (i.e., freezing and thawing, osmotic stock, ischemia, solubilizing agents, membrane ATPase inhibition, etc.). In necrotic cell death, the cell has a passive role in initiating the process of cell death (i.e, the cell is "murdered" by its hostile microenvironment). In addition to the necrotic cell death, there is a second type of cell death termed programmed cell death. In contrast to necrotic cell death, which is a pathological process, programmed cell death is a physiological process whereby a cell is activated by specific signals to undergo an energy-dependent process of cell death (i.e., the cell is induced to commit suicide by specific signals in an otherwise normal microenvironment) (41,42). Programmed cell death is a widespread phenomenon occurring normally at different stages of morphogenesis, growth, and development of metazoans (43). It also occurs in adult tissues (43). Programmed cell death is initiated in specific cell types by tissue specific extra cellular agents, generally hormones or locally diffusing chemicals. The activation of this programmed cell death can occur either because of the positive presence of a tissue specific inducer (e.g., glucocorticoid induce death of small thymocytes (44)) or because of the negative lack of a tissue specific repressor (e.g., decrease in serum ACTH results in cell death in the zona reticularis of the adrenal (45)). Once initiated, either by the positive presence of inducer or the negative lack of a repressor, programmed cell death leads to a cascade of biochemical and morphological events that results in the irreversible degradation of the genomic DNA and fragmentation of the cell (44,46–49). The morphological pathway for programmed cell death is rather stereotypic and has been given the name apoptosis to distinguish this process from necrotic cell death.

Apoptosis originally was defined by Kerr and associates (42) as the orderly and characteristic sequence of structured changes resulting in the programmed death of the cell. The temporal sequences of events of apoptosis comprise chromatin aggregation, the nuclear and cytoplasmic condensation, and the eventual fragmentation of the dying cell into a cluster of membrane-bound segments (apoptotic bodies), which often contain morphological intact organelles. For example, in apoptosis (as opposed to necrotic death), mitochondria do not swell and lose their function as an early event in the process. Instead, functionally active mitochondria often are contained in apoptotic bodies. These apoptotic bodies are rapidly recognized, phagocytosed, and digested by either macrophages or adjacent epithelial cells.

In an intact adult male, the supply of androgen is normally sufficient to maintain a balance between prostatic cell death and proliferation such that neither involution nor overgrowth of the gland occurs (23). Biochemical and morphological studies have demonstrated that the involution of the normal prostate following castration is not the result of necrotic cell death, but is an active process brought about by the initiation of a series of specific biochemical steps that lead to the program death (apoptosis) of the androgen-dependent glandular epithelial cells within the prostate (23–37). In the androgen-maintained ventral prostate of an intact adult male rat, the rate of cell death is very low, approximately 2% per day, and this low rate is balanced by an equally low rate of cell proliferation, also 2% per day (23). If animals are castrated, the serum testosterone levels drop to less than 10% of the intact control value within two hours (24). By 6 hours postcastration the serum testosterone level is only 1.2% of intact control (24). By 12 to 24 hours following castration, the prostatic DHT levels (i.e., the active intracellular androgen in prostatic cells) are only 5% of intact control values (24). This lowering of prostatic DHT leads to changes in nuclear androgen receptor function (i.e., by 12 hours after castration, androgen receptors are no longer retained in biochemically isolated ventral prostatic nuclei) (24). These nuclear receptor changes results in the synthesis of a series of proteins normally not present in the intact prostate (32,33), because of the novel expression of genes normally repressed in the intact prostate. The most notable of these are the TRPM 2 gene (i.e., testosterone repressed prostate message-2) (34), the Ca^{+2} responsive *c-fos* gene (35), heat shock 70 kilodalton gene (35) and the TGF-β gene (36).

The exact function of any of these epigenetic changes, activated following androgen ablation, is not entirely clear. It is known, however, that as with other systems in which programmed cell death occurs (44,46–49), this type of cell death initially involves fragmentation of genomic DNA. This fragmentation involves enzymatic degradation of the genomic DNA into nucleosomal oligomers (i.e., multiples of a 180 nucleotide base pair subunit) lacking intranucleosomal breaks in the DNA. This fragmentation of prostatic DNA is a result of activation of a Ca^{2+} $-Mg^{2+}$-dependent endonuclease present within the nucleus induced by elevation of intracellular free Ca^{2+} occurring following androgen ablation (24,25,36,37). This Ca^{2+}-Mg^{2+}-dependent nuclease selectively hydrolyzes prostatic DNA at sites located between nucleosomal units, resulting in the sterotypic ladder of DNA fragments (24). This DNA fragmentation is subsequently followed by irreversible morphological changes, histologically characteristic of apoptosis (i.e., chromatic condensation, nuclear disintegration, cell surface blebbing, and eventually cellular fragmentation into a cluster of membrane-bound apoptotic bodies (39).

Although the process of DNA fragmentation is completed in a portion of the androgen-dependent glandular epithelial cells in the prostate as early as 1 day following castration, the first morphological signs of apototic bodies formation occurs during the second day following castration (25–27,30). This demonstrates that the fragmentation of the genomic DNA does not occur after the cells are dead but instead occurs as an irreversible commitment step for viable cells to die. During the next several days (i.e., days 2 to 7 following castration), the level of the Ca^{+2}-Mg^{+2}-dependent endonuclease (24–26), TRPM 2 gene expression (34) TGF-β (36), and series of other proteins (32) continues to increase with the maximal levels obtained on day 4 postcastration. The fragmentation of the genomic DNA of the androgen-dependent glandular epithelial cells likewise continues, as does the production of apoptotic bodies (25,26) and the decrease in m-RNA for the secretory proteins (39). By day 10 following castration, the androgen-dependent glandular epithelial cells all have died and there is no longer any indication of either DNA fragmentation, TRPM-2 expression, or apoptotic bodies.

These temporal studies demonstrate that DNA fragmentation is an important irreversible commitment step in the process of the programmed cell death of the androgen-dependent glandular epithelial cells in the prostate following castration (37,39). The DNA fragmentation observed in the rat ventral prostate following castration is not because of a change in the chromatin conformation increasing its sensitivity/accessibility to endogenous nucleases (25). The fact that castration induces a 2 to 4-fold increase in the prostatic nuclear Ca^{2+}-Mg^{2+}-dependent endonuclease raises the possibility that the enzyme might be inactive or highly suppressed in the ventral prostate of intact rats, because of a limited intranuclear concentration of free Ca^{2+}. To investigate the relationship between perturbation of intracellular calcium homeostasis and prostatic cell death, ventral prostates of intact rats were implanted locally with pellets of the calcium ionophore, A23187. Unfortunately, these studies were severely hindered by the fact that local administration of the calcium ionophore in the ventral prostate consistently resulted in a dramatic enlargement (i.e., >5-fold) of the gland within 1 week because of nonbacterial prostatitis (25). This effect is because of the ionophores ability to act as a chemotactic factor for lymphocytes.

The involvement of an increase in intracellular free calcium in castration-induced prostatic cell death was demonstrated; however, from studies in which rats were castrated and immediately implanted in the prostate with either a placebo or a time-release pellet containing the calcium channel blocker, nifedipine. The temporal pattern of castration-induced prostatic involution is significantly slowed in the nifedipine-treated group, compared to the placebo-treated castrated group. This nifedipine-induced delay in prostatic cell death is evident between days 3 and 7 postcastration (25,37). Histological examination of ventral prostates from intact rats revealed the characteristic pattern of tall columnar glandular epithelium and highly dilated lumen. By 3 days following castration, the columnar glandular epithelium is no longer maintained, the glandular cells are now cuboidal, and numerous apoptotic bodies are evident either singly or in small groups. In contrast, prostates of rats 3 days postcastration treated with nifedipine pellets demonstrated involuted cuboidal glandular epithelial cells, but the incidence of apoptotic bodies was distinctively reduced compared to the castrated placebo group (25,37). In ventral prostates from rats castrated and given nifedipine, the degree of DNA fragmentation also is significantly decreased as compared to castrated-placebo group and this inhibition correlates well with the degree of inhibition obtained in prostatic weight and DNA loss by nifedipine (25).

Additional studies have demonstrated that it is possible to use prostatic organ culture to study the effects of increased Ca^{+2} levels on prostatic cell death *in vitro* under conditions in which neither drug toxicity to the host nor lymphocytic infiltration into the gland is a problem. Using this organ culture system, it has been demonstrated that ventral prostatic glandular epithelial cells can be maintained in G_o organ culture for a period of up to 14 days with a low rate of cell death (i.e., ~5% per day) if androgen is included in the media. If androgen is not included in the media, the rate of glandular cell death increases to approximately 12% per day. Using this organ culture system, it has been demonstrated that rate of programmed death of the glandular epithelial cells can be shifted from 5% to approximately 12% of the cells dying per day when testosterone plus 10 μM of the Ca^{2+} ionophore, A23187 are both in the media. Thus, in the presence of the ionophore, the rate of cell death in the presence of testosterone is identical to that induced when testosterone is not present. Additional studies have demonstrated that if the organ cultures are maintained in media lacking testosterone, but containing 10 μM of the Ca^{+2} channel blocks, nifedipine, the rise in the rate of cell death from 5% to 12% of the cells dying per day usually induced can be totally prevented (i.e., in the presence of nifedipine the rate is also 5%). These results suggest that increases in intracellular free Ca^{+2} probably derived from extracellular Ca^{+2} pools, are a crucial early event involved in triggering the subsequent process of programmed cell death (i.e., specifically DNA fragmentation) in the rat ventral prostate following androgen ablation.

Regardless of the specific mechanism, once a prostate cell fragments its genomic DNA into such small pieces, the DNA is no longer functional for cell replication or gene expression, as evidenced by the fact that the m-RNA levels for the major secretory proteins decrease abruptly (30) and thus the cell is terminally committed to death. The terminal process of prostatic cell death following castration is not known with certainty. Based upon data in other systems in which programmed cell death has been studied (50–53) particular glucocorticoid induced programmed cell death of thymocytes (53), this might involve activation of the poly (ADP-ribose) synthetase pathway within the nucleus of the prostatic cells. In these other cell death systems, this nuclear enzyme is specifically activated by the fragmentation of the DNA (50–53) and its chronic activation results in the enzymatic depletion of the nucleotide co-factor NAD^+. Because of the unique role of NAD^+ in both glycolysis and oxidative phosphorylation, depletion of NAD^+ results in the eventual depletion of ATP. It is this rapid depletion of NAD^+ and ATP induced by increased poly ADP-ribosylation that is believed to be the actual cause of the rapid demise of the cell (50–53).

PROGRAMMED CELL DEATH OF HUMAN PROSTATIC CANCER CELL FOLLOWING ANDROGEN ABLATION

Recent completed studies have demonstrated that not only normal rat prostatic cells, but also human androgen-responsive prostatic cancer cells activate the pathway of programmed cell death following androgen ablation. The PC-82 human prostatic cancer is highly androgen-responsive when grown as a xenograft in nude mice (59). If intact male nude mice are inoculated with human PC-82 prostatic cancer, continuously growing tumors are produced. If the host mice are castrated when the PC-82 tumor is approximately 0.5 cc in size the rate of cell proliferation decrease about 7-fold from 3.5% of the cells proliferating per day to 0.5% of the cells proliferating per day and the rate of cell death increases approximately 11-fold from 0.5% of the cell dying per day to 4.7% of the cells dying per day. Because of these changes, the tumor involutes rapidly following castration reaching approximately $1/2$ of its starting size within three weeks of castration. Biochemical analysis during this involution period has demonstrated that both TGF-β and TRPM-2 m-RNA levels as well as DNA fragmentation into nucleosomal size pieces are detectably increased within the first day following castration. The levels of all of these parameters increase to a maximum on day 3 following castration. In addition, if exogenous androgen is given back to the castrated host, DNA fragmentation ceases, TGF-β, mRNA and TRPM-2 mRNA levels drop, involution stops, and growth of the tumor resumes.

PROGRAMMED CELL DEATH IN ANDROGEN-INDEPENDENT PROSTATIC CANCER CELLS

Although androgen-independent prostatic cancer cells do not activate the program of cell death following androgen ablation, these cells still retain the major portion of the program cell death pathway. This has been demonstrated using a series of Dunning R-3327 androgen-independent prostatic cancers established as continuously growing *in vitro* cell lines. For example, the Duning AT-3 androgen-independent, highly metastatic, anaplastic prostatic cancer cells have been treated *in vitro* with a variety of nonandrogen ablative agents that induce "thymine-less death" of the cells (e.g. cells treated with 5-fluorodeoxyuridine (5-Fdur) or trifluorothymidine (TFT)). Analysis has revealed that "thymine-less death" results in an increase in the expression of the TRPM-2 gene and an increase in the nuclear $Ca^{+2}Mg^{+2}$ dependent endonuclease with the resultant fragmentation of the genomic DNA of the AT-3 cells into a similar nucleosomal ladder, as seen in the death of androgen-dependent prostate cells following castration (55). This cascade of events requires 6 to 12 hours before fragmentation of the DNA is complete. The AT-3 cells are not "dead," as defined by their ability to metabolize a mitochondrial vital dye, until 24 hours of treatment. This demonstrates that the fragmentation of the genomic DNA is an early, irreversible, commitment step in programmed cell death of even androgen-independent prostatic cancer cells (55). If the AT-3 cells are treated with osmotic shock induced by exposure to distilled water or agents that inhibit the plasma membrane ATPase activity (i.e., ouabain or iodoacetate), the cells rapidly lyze in less than 3 hours after treatment and do not metabolize the vital dye (i.e., they are dead) even though they do not fragment their DNA into nucleosomal size pieces nor do they elevate TRPM-2 mRNA levels (55). This data demonstrates that agents that induce necrotic death of the AT-3 cells (i.e., osmotic effects) do not lead to the activation of the programmed cell death of these cells. Programmed cell death can be activated, however, even in androgen-independent prostatic cancers, by specific agents (e.g., those able to induce a "thymine-less" state).

The problem with agents of this latter type, however, is that cell proliferation is required for the "thymine-less" state to activate the program of cell death in these AT-3 cells. Therefore some type of agent that can likewise activate this death program in androgen-independent prostatic cancer cells not in the cell cycle and not requiring the cell to attempt to proliferate, still must be identified. The effect of TGFβ on AT-3 cells *in vitro* also have been studied (38). At a concentration of 0.1 ng/ml, TGFβ has a profound inhibitors effect upon the growth of AT-3 cells in culture (i.e., >80% reduction in growth rate). TGFβ, even at a concentration of 20 ng/ml, however, does not induce death of the AT-3 (i.e., TGFβ is cytostatic not cytotoxic to these cells).

If AT-3 cells are treated *in vitro* with 10 μM of either the calcium ionophores, A23187, or ionomycin, cell death can be induced. Using microfluorescence image analysis (56) on AT-3 cells loaded with the fluorescent dye "fura-2" to measure intracellular free Ca^{+2} level such ionomycin treatment has been demonstrated to elevate the intracellular free Ca^{+2} levels from <30 nM to >200nM within the first minute of treatment. After the first few minutes, the intracellular free Ca^{+2} returned to ~ 50–100 nM. Such sustained elevations in intracellular free Ca^{+2} results in cell proliferation stopping within hours of treatment; then the cells begin to die after ~ 48 to 72 hours. Biochemical analysis during this time course demonstrated that DNA fragmentation into nucleosomal oligomers begins as early as 6 hours after Ca^{+2} ionophores treatment. Interesting, there is no elevation of the TRPM-2 mRNA levels during the chronic elevation of intracellular free Ca^{+2} induced by ionophore. This might be significant because such chronic elevation in free Ca^{+2} levels does activate the DNA fragmentation suggesting that TRPM-2 elevation is not required for this step in the process of cell death. These results suggest that TRPM-2's site of action in the cell death might be involved in inducing an increase in intracellular free Ca^{+2}, which the ionophores are fully capable of doing without any TRPM-2 involvement. This possibility is further strengthened by the recent clarification that TRPM-2 is highly related—if not identical to—the previously identified sulfated glycoprotein 2 normally secreted by rat sertoli cells (57). This SGP2 protein has been demonstrated to be secreted by Sertoli cells and to bind to the acrosomal membrane of sperm (58). This might be significant because for sperm to undergo the capitation reaction it must proceed through an acrosomal reaction step that involves the breakdown of the acrosomal membrane, a process that is known to involve Ca^{+2}.

CONCLUSIONS

To increase survival for men with metastatic prostatic cancer what is desperately needed is a modality that can effectively eliminate the clones of androgen-independent cancer cells already present, even before therapy is begun within individual heterogeneous prostate cancers. By combining such an effective modality with any of the various types of androgen ablation presently available, all of the populations of tumor cells within individual heterogeneous prostatic cancer can be affected, thus optimizing the possibility for cure. Unfortunately, such an effective form of therapy for the androgen-independent prostatic cancer cell is not presently available. Effective chemotherapy for the androgen-independent prostatic cancer cell will probably require two types of agents; one having antiproliferative activity affecting the small number of dividing androgen-independent cells, and the other able to increase the low rate of cell death among the majority of nonproliferating androgen-independent prostatic cancer cells present. Androgen-dependent prostatic epithelial cells can be made to undergo programmed death, even if the cells are not in the cell cycle (i.e., G_0 cells), simply by means of androgen ablation. Androgen-independent prostatic cancer cells retain the major portion of this programmed cell death pathway, only there is a defect in the pathway such that it is no longer activated by androgen ablation. The long-term goal, therefore, is to develop some type of nonandrogen ablative method to activate this programmed cell death cascade in androgen-independent prostatic cancer cells distal to the point of the defect.

REFERENCES

1. Scott WW, Menon M, Walsh PC. Hormonal therapy of prostatic cancer. *Cancer* 1980;45:1929–1936.
2. Schulze H, Isaacs JT, Coffey DS. A critical review of the concept of total androgen ablation in the treatment of prostatic cancer. In: Murphy GP, Khoury S, Kuss R, Chatelain C, Denis L eds. Prostate Cancer Part A: Research Endocrine Treatment, and Histopathology *Progress in Clinical and Biological Research*, vol. 243A. New York: Alan R. Liss, 1987;1–19.
3. Smith JA, Eyse HJ, Roberts TS, Middleton RG. Transphenoidal hypophysectomy in the management of carcinoma of the prostate. *Cancer* 1984;53:2385–2387.
4. Menon M, Walsh PC. Hormonal therapy for prostatic cancer. In: Murphy GP ed. Prostatic Cancer, Littleton, MA: PSG Publ. Co., pp 175–200, 1979.
5. Devese SS, Silverman DT. Cancer incidence and morbidity trends in the United States: 1935–1974. *J Natl Cancer Inst* 1978;60:545–571.
6. Lepor H, Ross A, Walsh PC. The influence of hormonal therapy on survival of men with advanced prostatic cancer. *J Urol* 1982;128:335–340.
7. Raghavan D. Non-hormone chemotherapy for prostate cancer: principles of treatment and application to the testing of new drugs. Semin Oncol 1988;15:371–389.
8. Prout GR, Leiman B, Daly JJ, MacLoughlin RA, Griffin PP, Young HH. Endocrine changes after diethylstilbestrol therapy. *Urology* 1976;7:148–155.
9. Sinha AA, Blackard CE, Seal US. A critical analysis of tumor morphology and hormone treatment in the untreated and estrogen treated responsive and refractory human prostatic carcinoma. *Cancer* 1977;40:2836–2850.
10. Smolev JK, Heston WDW, Scott WW, Coffey DS. An appropriate animal model for prostatic cancer. *Cancer Treat Rep* 1977;61:273–287.
11. Isaacs JT, Coffey DS. Adaptation vs selection as the mechanism responsible for the relapse of prostatic cancer to androgen ablation as studied in the Dunning R-3327 H adenocarcinoma. *Cancer Res* 1981;41:5070–5075.
12. Isaacs JT. Cellular factors in the development of resistance to hormonal therapy. In: Bruchovsky N, Goldie J eds. Drug and Hormone Resistance in Neoplasia, vol. 1. Boca Raton: CRC Press, 1982; 139–156.
13. Ellis WJ, Isaacs JT. Effectiveness of complete vs partial androgen withdrawal therapy for the treatment of prostatic cancer as studied in the Dunning R-3327 system of rat prostatic carcinomas. *Cancer Res* 1985;45:6041–6050.
14. Redding TW, Schally AV. Investigation of the combination of the agonist D-Trp-6-LHRH and the antiandrogen flutamide on the treatment of Dunning R-3327 H prostatic cancer model. *Prostate* 1985;6:219–232.
15. Kung TT, Mingo GG, Siegel MI, Watnick AS. Effect of adrenalectomy, flutamide and leuprolide on the growth of the Dunning R-3327 prostatic carcinomas. *Prostate* 1988;12:357–364.
16. Isaacs JT. The timing of androgen ablation therapy and/or chemotherapy in the treatment of prostatic cancer. *Prostate* 1984;5:1–18.
17. Schulze H, Isaacs J, Senge T. Inability of complete androgen blockade to increase survival of patients with advanced prostatic cancer as compared to standard hormone therapy. *J Urol* 1987;137:909–914.
18. Isaacs JT. Relationship between tumor size and curability of prostate cancer by combined chemohormonal therapy. *Cancer Res* 1989;49:6290–6294.
19. Schackney SE, McCormack GW, Curhural GJ. Growth rate patterns of solid tumours and their relation to responsiveness to therapy. *Ann Intern Med* 1978;89:107–113.
20. Tubiana M, Malaise EP. Growth rate and cell kinetics in human tumours: some prognostic and

therapeutic implications. In: Symington R, Carter RL eds. *Scientific Foundations of Oncology*, Chicago: Year Book Med Publishers, 1975;126–136.

21. Helpap B, Steins R, Bruhl P. Autoradiographic in vitro investigations of prostatic tissue with C-14 and H-3 thymidine double labelling method. *Beitr Pathol Anta Allgem Path* 1974;151:65–72.

22. Meyer JS, Sufrin G, Martin SAS. Proliferative activity of benign human prostate, prostatic adenocarcinoma and seminal vesicle evaluated by thymidine labeling. *J Urol* 1982;128:1353–1356.

23. Isaacs JT. Antagonistic effect of androgen on prostatic cell death. *Prostate* 1984;5:545–558.

24. Kyprianou N, Isaacs JT. Activation of programmed cell death in the rat ventral prostate after castration. *Endocrinology* 1988;122:552–562.

25. Kyprianou N, English HF, Isaacs JT. Activation of a Ca^{2+}-Mg^{2+}-dependent endonuclease as an early event in castration-induced prostatic cell death. *Prostate* 1988;13:103–118.

26. English HF, Kyprianou N, Isaacs, JT. Relationship between DNA fragmentation and apoptosis in the programmed cell death in the rat prostate following castration. *Prostate 15* 1989;(in press).

27. Kerr JFR, Searle J. Deletion of cells by apoptosis during castration-induced involution of the rat prostate. *Virchows Archiv B* 1973;13:87–102.

28. Lesser B, Bruchovsky N. The effects of testosterone, 5α-dihydrotestosterone and adenosine 3',5'-monophosphate on cell proliferation and differentiation in rat prostate. *Biochem Biophys Acta* 308:426–437, 1973.

29. Lee C. Physiology of castration-induced regression of the rat prostate. *Prog Clin Biol Res* 1982;75A:145–159.

30. Sanford ML, Searle JW, Kerr JFR. Successive waves of apoptosis in the rat prostate after repeated withdrawal of testosterone stimulation. *Pathology* 1984;16:406–410.

31. Stanisic T, Sadlowski R, Lee C, Grayhack JT. Partial inhibition of castration-induced ventral prostate regression with actinomycin D and cycloheximide. *Invest Urol* 1978;16:19–22.

32. Lee C, Sensibar JA. Protein of the rat prostate: synthesis of new proteins in the ventral lobe during castration-induced regression. *J Urol* 1985;138:903–908.

33. Saltzman AG, Hiipakka RA, Chang C, Liao S. Androgen repression of the production of a 29 kilodalton protein and its mRNA in the rat ventral prostate. *J Biol Chem* 1987;262:432–437.

34. Montpetit ML, Lawless KR, Tenniswood M. Androgen repressed messages in the rat ventral prostate. *Prostate* 1986;8:25–36.

35. Buttyan R, Zaker Z, Lockshin R, Wolgemuth D. Cascade induction of c-*fos*, c-*myc* and heat shock 70K transcripts during regression of the rat ventral prostate gland. *Mol Endocrinol* 1988;2:650–657.

36. Kyprianou N, Isaacs JT. Expression of transforming growth factor-β in the rat ventral prostate during castration-induced programmed cell death. *Mol Endocrinol* 1989;3:1515–1522.

37. Connor J, Sawdzuk IS, Benson MC, et al. Calcium channel antagonists delay regression of androgen-dependent tissues and suppress gene activity associated with cell death. *Prostate* 1988;13:119–130.

38. McKeehan WL, Adams PS. Heparin-binding growth factor/prostatropin attenuates inhibition of rat prostate tumor epithelial cell growth by transforming growth factor type β. *In Vitro Cell Dev Biol* 1988;24:243–246.

39. Viskochil DH, Perry ST, Lea DA, Stafford DW, Wilson EM, French FS. Isolation of two genomic sequences encoding the mr ~ 1400 subunit of rat prostatein *J Biol Chem* 1983;258:8861–8866.

40. Kyprianou N, Isaacs JT. Identification of a cellular receptor for transforming growth factor-β in rat ventral prostate and its negative regulation by androgens. Endocrinology 1988;123:2124–2131.

41. Wyllie AH, Kerr JFR, Currie AR. Cell death: the significance of apoptosis. *Int Rev Cytol* 1986;68:251–306.

42. Kerr JFR, Wyllie AH, Currie AR. Apoptosis: a basic biological phenomenon with wide ranging implications in tissue kinetics. *Brit J Cancer* 1972;26:239–257.

43. Bowen ID, Lockshin RA. Cell Death in Biology and Pathology. London: Chapman and Hill, 1981.

44. Wyllie AH. Glucocorticoid induces in thymocytes a nuclease-like activity associated with the chromatin condensation of apoptosis. *Nature* 1980;284:555–556.

45. Wyllie AH, Kerr JFR, Macaskill IAM, Currie AR. Adrenocortical cell deletion: the role of ACTH. *J Pathol* 1973;111:85–94.

46. Umansky SR, Korol BA, Nelipovich PA. *In vivo* DNA degradation in thymocytes of γ-irradiated or hydrocortisone-treated rats. *Biochem Biophys Acta* 1981;655:9–17.

47. Cohen JJ, Duke RC. Glucocorticoid activation of a calcium-dependent endonuclease in thymocyte nuclei leads to cell death. *J Immunol* 1984;132:38–42.

48. Wyllie AH, Morris RG, Smith AL, Dunlop D. Chromatin cleavage in apoptosis: association with

condensed chromatin morphology and dependence on macromolecular synthesis. *J Pathol* 1984;142:67–77.

49. Compton MM, Cidlowski JA. Rapid *in vivo* effects of glucocorticoids on the integrity of rat lymphocyte genomic deoxyribonucleic acid. *Endocrinology* 1986;118:38–45.

50. Seto S, Carrera CJ, Kubota M, Wasson DB, Carson DA. Mechanism of deoxyadenosine and 2-chlorodeoxyadenosine toxicity to nondividing human lymphocytes. *J Clin Invest* 1985;75:377–383.

51. Carson DA, Seto S, Wasson DB, Carrera, CJ. DNA strand breaks, NAD metabolism, and programmed cell death. *Exp Cell Res* 1986;164:273–281.

52. Berger NA. Poly(ADP-ribose) in the cellular response to DNA damage. *Radiation Res* 1985;101:4–15.

53. Berger NA, Berger SJ, Sudar DC, Distelhorst CW. Role of nicotinamide adenine dinucleotide and adenosine triphosphate in glucocorticoid-induced cytotoxicity in susceptible lymphoid cells. *J Clin Invest* 1987;79:1558–1563.

54. van Steenbrugge GJ, Groen M, Romijn JC, Schroder F. Biological effects of hormonal treatment regimens on a transplantable human prostate tumor line (PC-82). *J Urol* 1984;131:812–817.

55. Kyprianou N, Isaacs JT. Thymine-less death in androgen-independent prostatic cancer cells. *Biochem Biophys Res Comm* 1989;165:73–81.

56. Tucker RW, Meade-Cobun K, Loats H. Measurement of free intracellular calcium (Ca_i) in fibroblasts. Digital image analysis of Fura 2 fluorescence. In: Fiskum G ed. New York: Plenum Publ Corp, 1989;239–248.

57. Bettuzzi S, Hiipakka RA, Gilna P, Liao S. Identification of an androgen-repressed mRNA in rat ventral prostate as coding for sulphated glycoprotein 2 by cDNA cloning and sequence analysis. *Biochem J* 1989;257:293–296.

58. Sylvester SR, Skinner MK, Griswold MD. A sulfated glycoprotein synthesized by Sertoli cells and by epididymal cells is a component of the sperm membrane. *Biol Reproduc* 1984;31:1087–1101.

Endocrine Dependent Tumors, edited by
Klaus-Dieter Voigt and Cornelius Knabbe.
Raven Press, Ltd., New York © 1991.

4

Endocrine Factors in the Initiation, Diagnosis, and Treatment of Prostatic Cancer

*K. Griffiths, *P. Davies, *C.L. Eaton, *M.E. Harper,
*A. Turkes, and †W.B. Peeling

*Tenovus Institute for Cancer Research, University of Wales College of Medicine,
Heath Park, Cardiff CF4 4xx, United Kingdom, and †Department of Urology,
St Woolos' Hospital, Newport, Gwent, United Kingdom*

Prostatic carcinoma and benign prostatic hypertrophy (BPH) are conditions that rarely present in men under the age of 50. Indeed, prostatic disease with its associated difficulties with micturition is generally considered by many men to be merely a feature of the aging process to be borne with some degree of stoicism. It is, however, becoming very evident, especially with life expectancy increasing throughout the world, that prostatic disease, both BPH and carcinoma of the prostate, must now be recognized as serious clinical problems. In the United Kingdom, carcinoma of the prostate is the fourth most common cause of death from malignant disease in men and results in approximately 4,000 deaths each year (1,2). Nearly 100,000 new cases of prostatic cancer will present and be treated during this year in the United States with an estimated 26,000 deaths. Such statistics reveal a dramatically rising incidence (3,4) and a mortality rate for the black population that is nearly double that of the white community. Moreover, the proportion of the male population over the age of 65 years continues to increase (3) in both North America and the countries of Western Europe.

A possible etiological relationship between carcinoma of the prostate and BPH has been a subject of controversy for many years. The frequency with which nodular hyperplasia, found at autopsy, was associated with prostatic cancer (5) led Armenian and his colleagues (6) to reassess the possibility that patients with BPH might be at risk of subsequently developing malignant disease. The consensus among urologists is that prostatic carcinoma and BPH do not have a common etiology, BPH does not represent a premalignant condition, and there is general support for the concept that benign and malignant diseases of the prostate are independent clinical conditions arising in different regions of the gland, probably with distinct etiologies. BPH appears to develop from the prostatic periurethral glands opening into the upper segment of the urethra exclusively above the verumontanum (7–11),

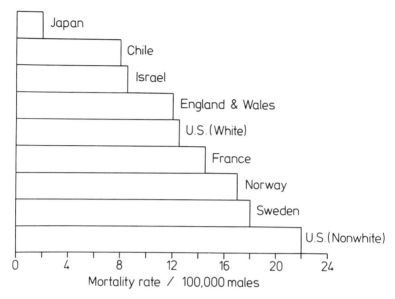

FIG. 1. Mortality rates for cancer of the prostate, age-standardized to world population, 1964–1965 (13).

whereas prostatic cancer originates in the peripheral zone of the true prostate (10) and could become relatively large and possibly metastasize before clinical symptoms of urinary obstruction become manifest (12).

Both diseases are features of advancing years and it might be expected that both nodular hyperplasia and cancer would be found together in the same prostate. More than 50% of the approximately 34.5 million men in the United States over the age of 45 are considered to have some degree of BPH (3). Of particular interest, however, is that the incidence of prostatic disease is influenced not only by age but also by race (Fig 1) (13). The incidence of prostatic cancer is high in both North Americans and Northern Europeans, but not in the people of Japan, China, and the Philippines. The age-adjusted incidence rate in various parts of the United States is 10 to 30 times that in Osaka, Japan and up to 125 times that in Shanghai, China (13,14). The disease is more prevalent in the North American black community, whereas it is comparatively rare in West Africa, although prostatic cancer is not often diagnosed in men below the age of 50 (15) and the mean life expectancy in many black African countries is little beyond 40 years (16). Of particular interest, however, is that the incidence of carcinoma of the prostate is low in Japanese men whose mean life expectancy and socioeconomic standards are eminently comparable with those in North America and Western Europe.

Environmental or dietary factors must clearly influence the etiology of the disease and the study of migrating populations indicates that the mortality rate for carcinoma of the prostate, although low in Japan, increases to half that of the indigenous American people for those Japanese migrants who become domiciled in the United States (17,18). Of equal interest, however, in relation to these studies, is that the classic investigations of Rich (19) indicated that by the age of 50, 30% of Western men have latent carcinoma, intraprostatic microscopic foci of cancer cells and, furthermore, latent carcinoma is just as common in Japanese males as in Caucasians of a similar age (20).

Estimates seem to indicate (3) that of the 34 million men over the age of 45 in the United States, and presumably of a similar number of men representing the population of Western Europe, 10 million on each continent, or 30% of the men, will have latent carcinoma of the prostate. Again the data indicate (3) that of these American men with latent carcinoma, nearly 1%, (74,000), present annually with clinically manifest disease. The hormones or growth factors and associated biological processes that are concerned in the promotion, growth, and development of latent carcinoma to the aggressive clinical manifestation of the cancer must be identified. It is of equal importance, however, to consider the possibility that particular growth-restraining factors might be involved in preventing the progression of latent cancer in the oriental man.

The hormone-related processes that are concerned with the maintenance of the prostate gland and the regulation of its growth have been extensively investigated through the past two or three decades (21,22). The prostate is regarded as a primarily androgen-dependent gland controlled essentially by the levels of plasma testosterone, of which 90% to 95% of a daily 6 to 7 mg production rate (Fig. 2) is synthesized and secreted by the testis (23,24). Androgens are indeed necessary for the development of the prostate and for the maintenance of morphology, cell number, and functional activity of the adult gland. Furthermore, androgens have been implicated in the pathogenesis of prostatic disease, and because prostatic carcinoma retains some degree of androgen dependence in the earlier phases of its growth, the treatment of the disease has been centered essentially on the removal of the source of testosterone, directed to either orchidectomy, estrogen therapy, or to the use of LH-RH analogues (25–28).

Because the clinical behavior of prostatic cancer reflects some degree of androgen dependence, it is of paramount importance that the fundamental biological processes concerned with the hormonal control of prostatic growth and function are understood. The adult normal prostate gland is maintained and functions within a "multihormonal environment" and has the capacity to respond to a range of growth regulatory factors. The role of the androgenic steroids in regulating the growth of the prostate therefore must be critically assessed relative to the influence of other growth factors on these molecular processes. A complete understanding of the fundamental endocrinology and biochemistry concerned with the initiation and progression of abnormal prostatic growth must inevitably lead to more rational therapeutic regimes for cancer control.

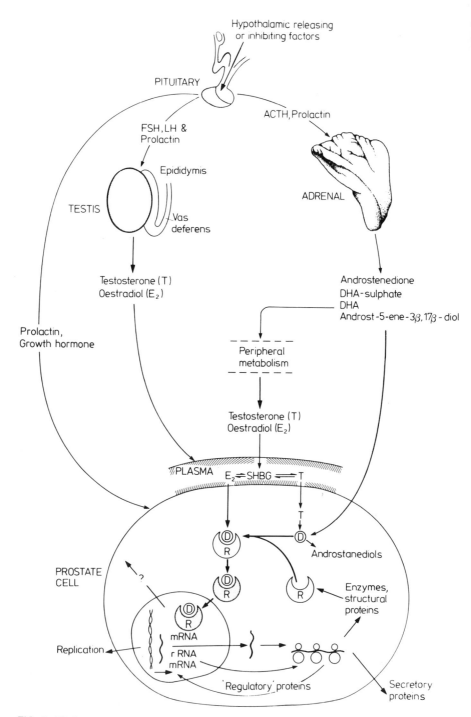

FIG. 2. Pituitary–testicular–adrenal–prostatic interrelationships. D = 5α-dihydrotestosterone; R = 5α-dihydrotestosterone receptor; DHA = dehydroepiandrosterone; SHBG = sex hormone-binding globulin; mRNA = messenger RNA; rRNA = ribosomal RNA.

MOLECULAR PROCESSES CONCERNED WITH ANDROGEN ACTION

Testosterone is metabolized, within the prostatic cell, to 5α-dihydrotestosterone (DHT), which has a greater affinity than testosterone for the intracellular androgen-receptor protein. Metabolism of DHT can abnegate, attenuate, or redirect the androgenic stimulus (21,22). The selective association of the androgen receptor with acceptor sites within the nucleus influences gene expression eliciting a tissue-specific biological response. Although fundamental detailed studies over the past several years have provided a greater understanding of these complex molecular processes, the basic features remain those originally outlined by Mainwaring (29). In particular, the localization of the 5α -reductase and the intracellular distribution of the steroid receptor protein in the absence of steroid now might be considered controversial (30) but this does not detract from the essential, well-established concept that the steroid-receptor complex is the modulator of gene expression (31), with the binding of DHT altering the intramolecular or intermolecular associations of the receptor protein to liberate a domain with high affinity for selective chromatin sites.

A considerable amount of information regarding androgenic modulation of gene expression has been derived from an extensive investigation of the principal secretory product of the rat ventral prostate, generally referred to as prostate binding protein (PBP) (32), but diversely by others as prostatein (33), prostate secretory protein (34) and estramustine-binding protein (35). It is a tissue-specific glycoprotein, comprising three polypeptides, C1, C2 and C3 (36–38) encoded by three highly homologous genes of probably similar ancestral derivation (39). Long-term castration reduces the proportion of these polypeptides, which normally constitute 30% to 50% of the protein synthesized by the rat prostate to less than 1% (40–44). Normal levels of protein secretion are restored by androgen administration (41,43). Androgenic control appears to be exercised through the availability of PBP mRNA (41,44–46) but not exclusively at the level of transcription (47,48).

Rapidly advancing technology in molecular biology has allowed the biochemical interaction of androgen-receptor complexes and genes to be examined in greater detail.

Androgen receptor (AR) belongs to the steroid receptor branch of a nuclear receptor multigene family comprising ligand-inducible *trans*-acting regulatory factors (30,49–53). The structure of the AR protein, as deduced from the sequences of cloned AR cDNA from rat (54–56) and human (54,55,57–59) prostate conforms with the functional segmentation previously described for other steroid receptors (49,50,54) with defined domains (Fig. 3) intuitively assigned both steroid- and DNA-binding functions. It is assumed that other regions, including the N-terminal region, constitutively and inducibly confer promoter-selective, *trans*-acting and transcriptional activation specifications (60–62).

The human AR is a 110 kDa protein (63) encoded by a single-copy gene (64) located on the X-chromosome (58,59) and extending over more than 90 kb. The coding sequence is divided into 8 exons (64) with introns positioned similarly to

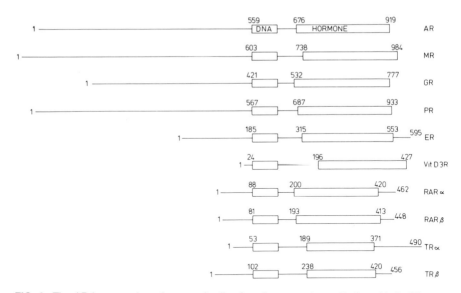

FIG. 3. The AR is a member of a superfamily of nuclear receptors with ligand-inducible transcriptional activation capability, which included receptors for mineralocorticoids (MR), glucocorticoids (GR), progestins (PR), estrogens (ER), vitamin D3 (Vit D3R), retinoic acid (RAR) and thyroid hormone (TR), as well as other DNA-binding proteins whose activating ligands have not been determined. The functional segmentation of the protein is shown with reference to the DNA and ligand-binding domains. Numbering is of amino acids from the aminoterminus (65). Structures are aligned on the first cysteine residue of the 66-amino acid DNA-binding domain. The DNA-binding domain of AR shares approximately 80% homology with those of PR, GR, and MR, approximately 20% with that of ER, and less with others. Conserved cysteines in the DNA-binding domains confer the capacity for formation of zinc fingers. Note that the major difference in receptor size is contributed by the aminoterminal domain, which might be responsible for fidelity and accuracy of transcriptional activation. Structures shown are of the human family of proteins.

other steroid hormone receptor genes (66,67). The sequence encoding the N-terminal region comprises one large exon (68): the two putative DNA-binding fingers (49,51) are encoded separately by two small exons and the information for the hormone-binding domain is split over 5 exons (64).

Defects in human AR have been directly correlated to several forms of the X-linked androgen insensitivity syndrome (69) and similar considerations cannot be excluded from those biological processes implicated in the progression of prostatic cancer from the androgen dependent to the independent state.

The inducible enhancer nucleotide sequences that are recognized by the DNA-binding domains of the steroid receptors are termed hormone response elements (HRE). These have been defined for glucocorticoids and estrogens (70–72). Because the DNA-binding domains of the GRs, MRs, PRs, and ARs are all highly homologous, it is not surprising that AR appears to function through the glucocorticoid response elements of the tyrosine aminotransferase (TAT) gene (73) and the mouse mammary tumor virus (MMTV) long terminal repeat (LTR) region (74,75).

High affinity binding of AR to restriction fragments of the MMTV LTR is in accord with these observations (76).

High affinity AR-binding regions of the PBP C3(1) gene (77,78) do not function effectively as androgen response elements (AREs) in transient transfection analyses (79). All PBP genes (C1, C2, and C3) do, however, have AR-binding sites both in the promoter region and in the first intron (80). This suggests therefore, a possible requirement for spatial juxtaposition in chromatin to exercise maximal effect (81). This concept is supported by their linear disposition in terms of nucleotides, which correlates with the oligomeric chromatin unit, the hexanucleosome preferentially released during cleavage by micrococcal nuclease (82,83). Such a relationship, frequently displayed by multiple HREs (84–86), might be a consistent feature of androgen action. Furthermore, HREs usually coexist with clusters of transcription factor binding sites with which they also might synergise (87–90). Binding of AR to HREs is ameliorated in the presence of NF-I or NF-III consensus sequences (91).

Putative androgen response elements in PBP genes resemble, both in structure (at least with regard to the TGTTCT motif at the right hand of the 15 bp imperfect palindrome) and binding properties (80,49,91), the HREs of the MMTV LTR and the TAT gene. A gradation of response to androgens has been shown through the four HREs of the LTR (75). Moreover, variations in the estrogen response elements appear to modify response quantitatively (92,71). Taken together with the fact that the estrogen and glucocorticoid response elements differ in only a few nucleotides (93,81), these observations suggest that a family of nucleotide sequences, coevolving with the receptor gene superfamily, also might have diverged to ensure the tissue and gene-specificity of the steroid hormone response.

It is very reasonable to expect that the biochemical processes concerned in the androgenic regulation of prostatic growth depend on chromosomal positioning, cooperative intragenic androgen response elements, tissue-specific transcription factors, and the extragenic regions responsible for the correct chromatin structure surrounding the "response information." These delicate regulatory systems require intensive study if we are to develop a greater understanding of the biochemistry of abnormal growth of the human prostate gland (94). Clearly, however, not all the actions of androgens can be accounted for by interaction between AR-complex and gene promoter regions. The intranuclear distribution of the complexes in relation to transcriptional activity and chromatin structure (82,83) and the logical necessity for the involvement of androgens in the stabilization of transcripts (47,48) suggest an organizational role. The diverse distribution of AR throughout transcriptionally active and inactive chromatin and amongst chromatin structures and the nuclear matrix (95,96), direct attention to the wide-ranging involvement of AR-complexes in cellular homeostasis.

Understanding the molecular mechanisms whereby androgens influence gene expression becomes truly relevant to prostatic disease through their involvement in regulating processes in the human prostate gland. This applies to the production of secretory proteins (97–101), the genes encoding the best known of which have now been cloned (102–111). Included are those most frequently used to monitor the course of prostatic disease, acid phosphatase, which has phosphotyrosine phosphatase activity, and the kallikrein-like prostate specific antigen (PSA). Also of paramount importance is the elucidation of the androgenic involvement with those entities frankly eliciting growth responses, growth factors, growth factor receptors, and the cellular protooncogenes, to which reference is made in greater depth later in this chapter.

ANDROGENS AND THE PROCESSES REGULATING CELL GROWTH

The molecular processes by which androgens influence prostatic growth are less well understood than those concerned with the regulation of the secretory protein genes. Androgens clearly are essential because the prostate gland cannot develop, differentiate, or maintain its size or function in their absence. The adult prostate does not, however, enlarge in response to exogenous androgens (112), but maintains its normal size through a balance between cell renewal and cell death in the presence of high concentrations of androgenic steroids (113).

Processes concerned with both the pre- and postnatal development of the prostate are androgen-dependent (114) and administration of testosterone to immature male rats accelerates prostatic growth to its normal maximal size (112). Both 5α-reductase activity and intracellular androgen receptors have been detected in the urogenital sinus (115,116) and an impairment of either results in a rudimentary prostate or, alternatively, in the complete absence of the gland (117,118).

Castration of the adult animal produces a remarkable reduction in prostate size. Studies on rat ventral prostate have shown that after an initial lag period with no cell loss, there is a rapid decrease in cell number and DNA content to less than 10% of the normal levels by 10 days postcastration (113,119). Because this rate of cell loss was vastly in excess of normal cell turnover, Bruchovsky and his colleagues (119) suggested that prostatic involution is an active process.

Although prostatic regression is characterized by a net decrease in synthetic processes (120,121), the rapid rate of cell death is dependent upon the synthesis of specific macromolecules, a process that can be blocked by inhibitors of RNA and protein synthesis (122).

Specific proteins and RNAs have been observed after androgen withdrawal (123–125) for which a role in prostatic involution has not been defined. At least one androgen-repressed gene in the rat ventral prostate, testosterone-repressed prostate message -2, (TRPM-2) which appears involved in the processes of cell regression and programmed cell death, can be induced with antiandrogens (126–128). TRPM-2, the most abundant mRNA species, appeared 2 days after castration, and after 4 days, peaked at a level 400-fold higher than in intact animals. The mRNA for the protooncogene c-myc increases 6-fold in the involuting prostate (129), apparently as part of a sequential pattern of gene expression involving c-fos, c-myc, and heat shock protein (hsp)70 (130).

Hydrolytic enzymes, not surprisingly, have been considered relevant to prostatic cellular autolysis (131–133) including a Ca/Mg-dependent endonuclease (134) and the proteolytic plasminogen activators (135). Interestingly, administration *in vivo* of inhibitors of plasminogen activators caused a decrease in their activity and also in prostatic involution (136). Equally noteworthy are the observations that the suppression of Ca/Mg-dependent endonuclease (134), the activity of c-fos and TRPM-2 and prostate regression (137), can be achieved by inhibitors of calcium ion influx. These results offer intriguing insights into the cellular phenomena programmed by androgens and the means whereby they could be exploited.

The repression of these catabolic processes within the normal gland has been defined by Isaacs (113) as an antagonistic action of androgens on cell death, an effect that can be functionally dissociated from an androgenic action on cell proliferation on the basis of differential dose requirements. This phenomenon is exemplified by the Dunning R-3327-G rat prostatic adenocarcinoma that has retained

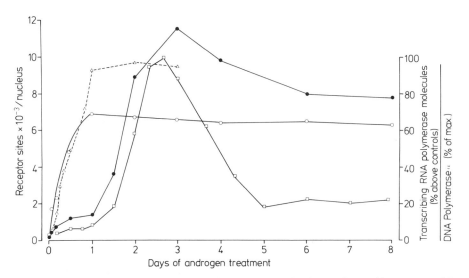

FIG. 4. Nuclear deployment of ARs in relation to macromolecular syntheses. Rats castrated 7 days previously were administered daily injections of 5α-dihydrotestosterone (DHT: 400 μg/100 g body weight) intramuscularly, as shown, and accumulation of ventral prostate nuclear AR extractable by (○) and resistant to (●) micrococcal nuclease was assessed, with activity of RNA polymerase B (△) and nuclear matrix-associated DNA polymerase (□). Activation of RNA polymerase was rapid; the basal level of 5,100 molecules engaged in transcription increased to 7,600 12 hours after administration of DHT, and reached a maximum of 10,100 36 hours later. Matrix-associated DNA polymerase was undetectable in prostates of 7-day castrated rats, and did not increase significantly until 36 to 48 hours after DHT injection. Maximum levels (820 pmol [³H]TMP incorporated/mg DNA) were attained 64 hours after DHT administration began and thereafter declined. The coreplenishment of nuclease-resistant AR and matrix-associated DNA polymerase probably results from nuclear restructuring in response to androgen and androgen-induced factors rather than direct correlation.

responsiveness to the antagonistic effect of androgens on cell death, but not the agonistic effect of androgens on cell proliferation (138).

The involuted rat ventral prostate has been the model of choice for studying the influence of androgens on cellular proliferation and differentiation but presents certain disadvantages when assessing such effects on different cellular populations (114,139). Administration of androgens to long-term castrated animals does influence the rate of DNA synthesis. After a lag period of 24–48 hours, the rate of DNA synthesis increases, peaking at 72 to 96 hours (119,121,140) but the effect is transitory, being sustained only until normal cell number is achieved, whereupon, basal levels of DNA synthesis are reestablished. Such changes in DNA synthesis are paralleled by the activity of enzymes involved in the process (121,141,142). Furthermore, androgen receptors are lost from the prostate of the castrated rat well before a net loss of cells can be determined and the appearance of receptors in the nucleus after androgen administration precedes DNA synthesis by several hours (119). Moreover, synthesis of nuclear receptors was not in synchrony (Fig. 4) with either the onset or shutdown of DNA synthesis (143), but dependent on cell division. Kyprianou and Isaacs (144) proposed that the androgen-induced increase in cell number was dependent upon a crucial, intracellular concentration of DHT. Above a threshold value of 600 receptors per nucleus, each increment in the number of androgen receptors was paralleled by an increase in the number of prostate cells recruited into the growth process (145).

Because a direct involvement of androgen receptors in the initiation of DNA synthesis has not yet been established, the inevitable conclusion must be drawn (119) that androgens are essential but not solely responsible for the initiation of prostatic cell proliferation and it would seem that the intercession of other associated controlling factors is probably mandatory.

THE INFLUENCE OF OTHER STEROID HORMONES ON THE PROSTATE GLAND

Estrogens influence the prostate indirectly through effects at the hypothalamic and pituitary level, reducing gonadotrophin secretion and hence the synthesis and secretion of testicular testosterone (21,22,146). Estrogens also might modulate adrenal synthesis of C_{19}-steroids such as dehydroepiandrosterone (DHA) sulphate, DHA, and androstenedione by promoting prolactin secretion, and also might act directly upon the testis (22). A large proportion of the estrogen in the male is directly secreted by the testis (see Fig. 2), although the adrenal gland contributes through the peripheral aromatisation of androstenedione and interestingly, aromatase activity also has been detected in the human prostate (147). In the aging male, an imbalance in the estradiol/testosterone ratio in plasma with a relatively higher estrogen concentration has often been cited as a possible cause of abnormal prostate growth (21,22,146). Certainly estrogens have been implicated in the development of BPH (148–151) but a role in the etiology of prostate carcinoma is more nebulous (146).

The antigonadotrophic effect of progestins also would modulate the androgenic influence on the prostate, but progestational steroids designed as antiandrogens also interact directly with the androgen receptor (152). A more direct involvement of both estrogens and progestins can be deduced from the presence of receptors for both classes of steroid in the prostate (153,154). Mobbs and Johnson (155,156) have observed a relationship between estrogen administration and the concentration of cytosolic progesterone receptor. More than one receptor binding site for estradiol has been observed (157–159) with the nuclear sites of lower affinity being assigned to the nuclear matrix (160).

It has been proposed (161) that both androgens and estrogens act upon the same cells, but that the observed effects of estrogen can be rationalized through the intra-prostatic distribution of their receptors, with the stromal elements of the prostate implicated as the primary site of action. Many investigators (162–165) have reported that there is a higher concentration of estrogen receptors in the stromal tissue and, moreover, the effects of antiestrogens also appear to be stromally biased (166–168). Immunocytochemical studies (169) identified a greater localization of estrogen receptor in the stroma and ductal epithelium of the periurethral region of the normal canine prostate, but not in the acinar epithelium. This observation is of particular interest because the periurethral region of the prostate in man has been implicated as the zone in which BPH develops (170), fostering further speculation on the role of estrogens in the etiology of BPH.

Estrogens certainly have a direct effect on fibromuscular stroma (114) and lack mitogenic activity on prostatic epithelium in culture (171). Estrogen administration can cause squamous metaplasia of prostate epithelium (172,173), but synergizes with androgens to elicit prostate growth in the dog (149,174). The estrogen-induced squamous metaplasia of the canine prostate was associated with a comparatively smaller gland, but with a high level of DNA synthesis, indicative of elevated rates of cell turnover. The level of DNA synthesis and rate of prostate cell turnover, however, was lower in dogs treated with estrogen and androgen together (161) than in those treated with androgen alone, suggesting that the growth promoting effect of estrogen could be because of a complementary inhibitory influence on cell death.

In considering the endocrine factors that might exercise a role in prostate carcinogenesis and cancer progression, the influence of the adrenocorticosteroids should not be neglected (22). Both rat and human prostate contain significant levels of glucocorticoid receptor (GR) mRNA (175) which, in the former, are induced by castration (176). Glucocorticoids stimulate prostatic epithelial cells in culture (139) and are able to maintain PBP secretion during the first 7 days of prostate organ culture at a level equivalent to that produced by testosterone (177). Cortisol treatment of castrated rats retarded cell and weight loss in the prostate and inhibited the castration-induced rise in plasminogen activators (135,136). Furthermore, cortisol substantially reduced the castration-induced increase in transcripts for TRPM-2, c-fos and hsp 70, but sustained PBP C1 mRNA at 50% of noncastrate levels (176). This circumstantial evidence, which in relation to reports of studies with the androgen/glucocorticoid-dependent Shionogi carcinoma (178,179) suggests that the

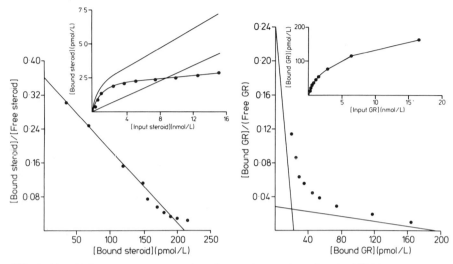

FIG. 5. (A, left) Scatchard representation of saturation analysis (inset) of [³H]dexamethasone binding in prostatic nuclei shows one class of high-affinity receptor sites with dissociation constant (K_d) of approx. 0.5 nmol/l. (B, right) Similar appraisal of [³H]dexamethasone-receptor binding to prostate chromatin reveals two classes of acceptor sites. The higher affinity sites have a K_d of approximately 90 pmol/l and the lower affinity sites a K_d of 6.5 nmol/l. These compare with the two affinity classes of acceptor sites previously described for androgen receptors (see ref. 83).

TABLE 1. *Androgen receptors and glucocorticoid receptors in rat ventral prostate*

| Days after castration | Receptor (molecules/cell) | | | | | |
| | Androgen | | | Glucocorticoid | | |
	Total	Nuclear	Cytosolic	Total	Nuclear	Cytosolic
0	17,300	15,900	1,400	1,500	1,150	1,350
1	16,900	4,800	12,100	6,970	2,680	4,290
3	2,200	700	1,500	10,850	5,200	5,200

Following castration, there is a rapid decline in those ARs with high affinity for DNA (nuclear) and over the first 24 hours, a stoichometric increase in those with lesser affinity for DNA (cytosolic). By 3 days after castration, total cellular receptors have decreased to basal values, and 'nuclear': cytosolic ratios are probably more indicative of an intracellular equilibrium than any meaningful activity. Over this period of time, however, there is a considerable increase in total cellular GRs evenly distributed between nuclear and cytosolic. It should be noted, however, that the nuclear complement of GR is insufficient to maintain priority of chromatin domains or gene transcriptional activity without administration of exogenous cortisol. Acceptor sites for GR are numerically similar to those for AR, and competition can be demonstrated *in vitro*. The relative cellular content of AR and GR can preclude a role at the nuclear level for the latter under normal conditions: under conditions of androgen withdrawal, GR effects would be dependent on circulating levels and relative efficacy of glucocorticoids. However, an extranuclear role for GR cannot be discounted. (Data have been adapted from refs. 83,142,180.)

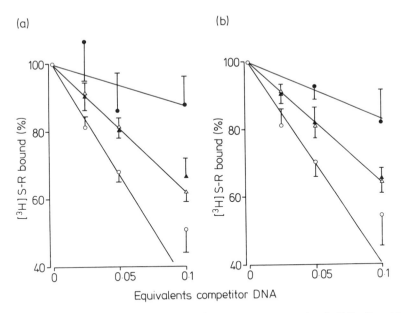

FIG. 6. A 300 bp HindII-BstEII restriction fragment (a) and a 500 bp BglII-PvuII restriction fragment (b), derived from the promoter region and the first intron, respectively, of the PBP C3(i) gene, both of which show comparative high affinity for androgen-receptor complexes (78), were tested for their ability to compete with immobilized calf-thymus DNA for [³H]estradiol-receptor complexes (●), [³H]ORG2058-receptor complexes (▲) and [³H]dexamethasone-receptor complexes (△). [³H]DHT-receptor complexes (○) were included in the experiments to confirm earlier results. The moderately high affinity for PRs and GRs is not surprising because ARs, PRs, GRs, and MRs are active through the GREs of the MMTV LTR, and AR can act through the GRE of the TAT gene. AREs presumably belong to the same family of nucleotide sequences as GREs. The promoter fragment contains the hexanucleotide TCTTGT and the intronic fragment contains TGTTCT. Single-point mutations in the latter destroy androgen-dependent enhancer activity in transfection assays (181). A comparison of the 15-mer GRE of the TAT gene (TGTACAGGATGTTCT), the four GREs of the MMTV LTR (GTTACAAACTGTTCT, AGCTCTTAGTGTTCT, GGTATCAAATGTTCT, ATTTTCCTATGTTCT, in order of their androgeninductive ability (75), and the putative ARE of the C3(1) intron (AGTACGTGATGTTCT) suggests that relative activity for GR and AR might be dependent on the affinity of the complex dimer for the left arm of the response element. However, it is worth noting that in the promoter and intronic sequence the perfect complements to the TCTTGT and TGTTCT motifs reside 40 bp and 60 bp upstream, respectively, and chromatin conformation and DNA structures *in vivo* play an important part.

role of glucocorticoids in this dual-hormonal action is mediated through the GR. Not surprisingly, in view of the previous comments, human prostate, rat prostate, and prostate cell lines that respond to glucocorticoids have been found to contain varying levels of GR (Fig. 5). In rat ventral prostate, nuclear GR levels rise significantly after castration (Table 1), attaining after 3 days, 30% of the "normal" AR level. The major proportion of this increase is directed toward nuclease/salt-extractable sites that are associated with oligomeric transcriptionally active chromatin. Interactions *in vitro*, with restriction fragments of PBP genes containing HREs (Fig. 6) emphasize the capacity of glucocorticoids to regulate these genes (49). Under normal circumstances, the relative levels of AR and GR militate against the latter, competing effectively for cooperative enhancer factors (182), but under conditions of AR loss or AR impairment, GR can assume a greater role, a concept opening up another interesting facet of prostatic growth regulation.

PROSTATIC CELL INTERACTIONS MODULATING STEROID-RESPONSIVENESS

Androgens are a necessary prerequisite for prostate cell proliferation, but proliferation is not an inevitable consequence of the presence of androgens nor of AR-complexes. Clearly other determinant factors must be involved. Bruchovsky and his colleagues (119) suggested that growth responsiveness to androgens was dependent upon cell number within the prostate. The concept was further extended by Cunha (114) who proposed that the relative proportion of different cell types within the gland could be the crucial controlling factor. Disproportionate losses of epithelial cells compared to stromal tissue are observed following castration (183). Both epithelial and stromal cells of the prostate are potential targets for androgen action. Both contain 5α-reductase activity (184–186) although whether the activity is higher in epithelium (187) or stroma (188,189) is an issue still to be resolved. Both types of cells contain ARs (189,190).

The impressive investigations of Cunha and his colleagues (114) have firmly established that the epithelium-mesenchyme "balance" plays a principal role in the regulation of prostatic growth and development. It seems that many of the biological processes of epithelial tissue are indirectly controlled by androgens through androgen-dependent mediators of stromal origin. In similar manner, estrogen receptors in the stroma could elicit an "estrogenic effect" on the epithelium by regulating the production of stimulatory or inhibitory factors by the stroma, thereby exercising a paracrine influence on the adjacent epithelial tissue.

The embryonic prostatic rudiment with massive growth potential as it develops into the adult organ has a large proportion of mesenchymal tissue. During development, epithelial tissue eventually predominates, but Chung and Cunha (191) suggest that the original amount of mesenchyme present could determine the final size of the adult organ. Prostatic growth *in situ* was observed when urogenital mesenchyme, or intact urogenital sinus, was directly grafted into the gland of intact adult male rats (192,193). Atrophy or loss of cells from the prostate is therefore not a prerequisite for the induction of proliferation if the proportion of the mesenchymal elements is experimentally increased. Such a concept could explain the lack of "overgrowth" of the prostate in the presence of high concentration of androgens but with a controlling limited amount of stroma.

Fundamental to the concepts of Cunha and his colleagues (114) is the fact that whereas androgens stimulate DNA synthesis in prostate epithelial tissue in organ culture when stroma is present (194–196), the evidence is equivocal that androgens have a mitogenic effect on cultured *isolated* epithelial cells. The evidence to date, in many respects, suggests a lack of effect (139,197) and should thereby direct attention to other growth regulatory factors of greater importance.

The existence of diffusible factors, or other agents capable of paracrine cell stimulation, most effectively explains the observed effects of androgens and estrogens on the prostate and considerable research activity is currently directed to the identity of such prostate-orientated growth factors.

After castration, two days elapse before cell loss occurs (119), the tissue presumably being maintained during this period by a balance between residual growth factors and gradual derepression of androgen-inhibited genes. An increase in matrix acceptor sites during this period (83) ensures that these sites are preferentially reoccupied (96,198) as the cells attempt to restore normality by reorganization of nuclear processes. Administration of androgens to long-term castrates results, however, in ARs being distributed more extensively in nuclease-sensitive regions (198) and associated with processes concerned with transcription (142). Cunha and associates (114) called into question the relevance of the epithelial cell ARs if stromal elements are the essential mediators of the androgenic response. Apart from a secretory function, ARs might have a role in preparing the epithelial cell response mechanisms that are influenced by the stromally secreted growth factors.

GROWTH FACTORS AND THE PROSTATE

The probability that diffusible trophic factors play an important role in the normal growth regulatory processes within the prostate provides a new, exciting research initiative and stimulates the quest for a greater understanding of these factors and their relationship to abnormal growth, both benign and malignant. An interest originally developed in this area from the fact that carcinoma of the prostate was frequently associated with osteogenic metastases and human prostate extracts stimulated the growth of rat calvarial osteoblasts and skin fibroblasts (199).

In the past decade, prostate-derived growth factors have been identified in BPH, prostatic cancer, prostatic secretions, and normal and cancerous rat prostatic tissue (200–212). Preliminary investigations (213) suggested that epidermal growth factor (EGF) was not the principal agent in human prostate extracts and with certain exceptions (200,204), subsequent studies have shown, on the basis of molecular mass and affinity for heparin, that this agent could be identified as a member of the endothelial cell growth factor family (bFGF), possibly an aminoterminally extended form (214,215).

Distinct mitogens for cells of the osteoblast phenotype have been found in prostate cancer extracts (199,216–218) and in one study (219), mRNA extracted from a human prostate cell line and micro-injected into Xenopus oocytes, directed the synthesis of mitogenic and stimulatory material for osteoblast-like cells.

Quantitative increases in the bFGF-like factor appear to be restricted to BPH (207) although this was not reflected in mRNA expression, which was similar in normal, hypertrophic, and cancerous human prostate samples (220). This does not preclude a role for bFGF in the etiology of prostatic disease because other factors probably are implicated, and at least circumstantial evidence exists to indicate a hormonal dependence for the production and action of prostate-derived growth factors (200,209,218).

In addition, constitutive production of platelet-derived growth factor-1 (PDGF-1) and PDGF-2/sis genes and concomitant production of PDGF-like proteins by the prostate carcinoma cell lines DU145 and PC3, neither of which contain PDGF receptors, have been reported (221). A transforming growth factor (TGF)-related substance also was induced in a prostate cancer cell line by tamoxifen (222).

Several regulatory peptides have been found in the prostate gland including endorphins (223), relaxin (224), vasopressin and oxytocin (225), inhibin (226), somatostatin (227), nerve growth factor (228), thyrotropin-releasing hormone (229), prolactin (230,231), growth hormone (230–232) and insulin or insulin-like peptides (233). A large proportion (47%) of the growth factor activity of the rat ventral prostate, however, can be attributed to EGF (234), a factor also identified in guinea pig (235) and human (236) prostate and a constituent of human prostatic fluid (237). Synthesis of EGF by the mouse (238) and rat ventral (239) prostate is reported to require androgens and its secretion into prostatic fluid is under both α-adenergic and cholinergic control (240).

The proliferative effects of a considerable number of peptide growth factors in various prostatic cells in culture have been demonstrated. They include EGF (139,197,241,242), TGFα (241), TGFβ (243), insulin (242,197), prolactin (197,244) and a neural tissue-derived "prostatropin" (197,245), which has 90% homology with acidic FGF (246). Such observations are in accord with reports of receptors in prostatic cells for EGF (241,247–249), insulin (250) and insulin-like growth factor (IGF-I) (251), prolactin (252) and TGFβ (253).

Production and secretion of EGF suggests that its target is extraprostatic. Rat ventral prostate EGF receptors are down-regulated by androgens (249,254) and it has been suggested (249) that androgen deprivation might promote EGF receptor induction and thereby prevent complete prostatic regression after castration. Aberrations in the biological control processes of the androgen-repressed genes concerned with programmed cell death and in androgen-mediated neuroendocrine-controlled secretory mechanisms could instigate androgen-independent growth in such an abnormal situation. Of interest, therefore, is that EGF receptors of LNCaP cells are reported to be up-regulated by androgen (248) an effect inhibited by TGFβ (255).

Data from the Tenovus Institute for Cancer Research from a comparative study of tissue from normal human prostate and from BPH and cancer biopsies (247) showed, in prostatic carcinoma, an inverse relationship in the concentration of EGF receptors and ARs (Fig. 7) together with a developing imbalance of high and low affinity sites associated with dedifferentiation. Contemporaneously, in addition to formal sites, cryptic binding sites appeared for IGF-I (247).

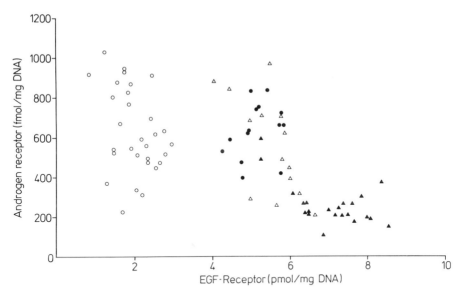

FIG. 7. Comparison of androgen receptor and EGF binding capacity in samples of BPH (○) and well (●), moderate (Δ) and poorly (▲) differentiated carcinomas. An inverse relationship was apparent between androgen and EGF binding capacity within carcinoma samples. BPH samples contained relatively elevated levels of androgen receptors and depressed levels of EGF binding.

The functional significance of heterogeneous arrays of high and low affinity EGF (TGFα) binding sites on the surfaces of epithelial cells is at present only partially understood. High affinity binding appears to be associated with receptor aggregation and the formation of dimers from dispersed monomers (M_R175kDa) with lower affinity for EGF (256–258). Aggregation is EGF-dependent and seems to greatly augment the autophosphorylative activity of the tyrosine kinase-bearing internal domain of the receptor, a process identified as an early event in the cellular response to EGF. Controversy still surrounds the relative functions of the monomeric and dimeric forms of the receptor in modulating the biological activities of EGF, but it has been suggested that initial activation and subsequent regulation of kinase activity might be independently controlled by aggregation/dissociation (259). With regard to this, noteworthy is the recent identification of truncated forms of the EGF receptor, lacking the internal domain, but with biological function, apparently down-regulating kinase activity by aggregation with intact receptors (259).

Ligand activation of EGF receptor and subsequent control of kinase activity is clearly a dynamic process involving aggregation, autophosphorylation, internalization and a high level of receptor recycling rather than *de novo* synthesis (260). It is interesting, therefore, that receptor-recycling in at least one system does not appear to require ligand dissociation, implying the possibility of continuous activation. Observed variations (Fig. 8) in EGF binding capacity and the relative expression of

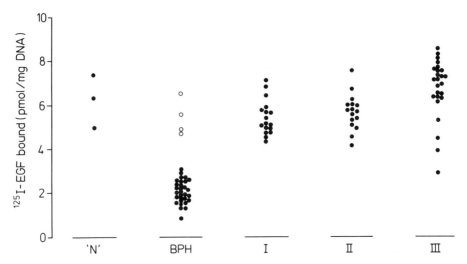

FIG. 8. Summary of total, saturable (^{125}I) EGF-binding concentrations in histologically normal prostatic tissue ('N') in BPH and in three grades of carcinoma of well (I), moderate (II), and poorly differentiated (III) histology. Values are for unfractionated tissue (○) and for separated epithelial fractions (●). Median values did not differ significantly between carcinoma samples of different grades, although there did appear to be a small increase in mean values (I: 5.45 ± 0.84, II: 5.62 ± 0.85, III: 6.74 ± 1.33 pmol/mg DNA SD) with increasing grade. Mean EGF binding was however significantly lower in BPH samples than either histologically normal or carcinoma samples.

high and low affinity receptors in human tissue samples from histologically normal, BPH and from various grades of carcinoma may reflect differences in these tissues in both the mechanism and capacity for response to EGF and related ligands. In poorly differentiated tumors, for example, the relatively increased EGF binding capacity is differentially expressed in favor of a greatly elevated proportion of high affinity binding sites and not simply of total receptor content. This is, therefore, suggestive of continually activated receptors, either as a result of constant or renewing ligand occupancy, or by some other mechanism related to aggregation. A clearer understanding of these processes is fundamental to any future consideration of rational anti-growth factor-based therapy, which, although an exciting concept, would be likely to affect many other tissues as well as the target tumor-cell population. This concept forms the basis from which some of the Institute's current research is developing using well-defined culture systems and cell lines derived from normal and neoplastic prostatic tissues. These cell lines contain both high and low affinity EGF binding sites, expressed at varying levels (Fig. 9) and are responsive to EGF and TGFα. Receptor expression is being studied in relation to population growth phase (Fig. 10), growth rate, and response to both EGF and other potentially interactive growth regulators.

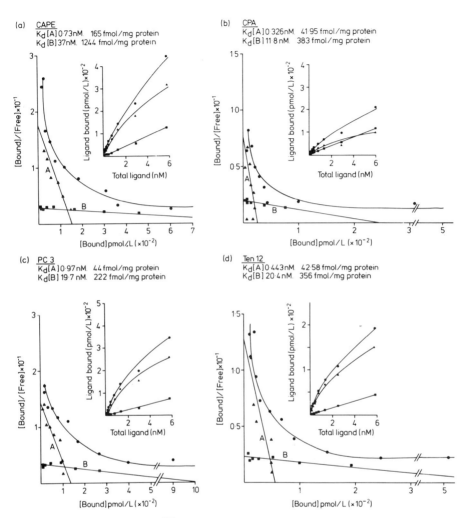

FIG. 9. Saturation analysis of (^{125}I) EGF binding in membrane preparations from four cell lines derived from normal (CAPE) and neoplastic (CPA) canine prostatic tissue and from human prostatic tumors (PC3, Ten 12). CAPE, CPA, and PC3 were grown as continuous cell cultures and Ten 12 was passaged as xenografts in athymic mice. Remarkably similar levels of high affinity binding were observed in the three tumor cell lines (41.95–44 fmol/mg membrane protein). Significantly higher concentrations of this binding component were present in membranes derived from the CAPE cell line (165 fmol/mg protein). Evaluations of Kds and site concentrations of lower affinity binding components were made difficult because of the presence of nonsaturating components; however, best estimates suggested that the levels of these components are 5- to 10-fold higher than high affinity binding present in each cell line.

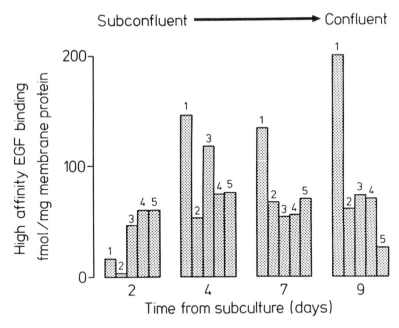

FIG. 10. Summary of the concentration of high-affinity EGF-binding components present in membrane preparations derived from five cell lines measured at various cell densities throughout a sigmoidal growth curve. Cell lines were derived from normal (1, CAPE) and neoplastic (2:CPA) canine tissue and from human prostatic tumors (3:LNCAP, 4:DU145, 5:PC3). After a short rise time, not exceeding 48 hours, high-affinity binding did not alter significantly with cell density within each cell line. Significantly higher levels of high-affinity binding were present in the cell line derived from normal tissue than in any of the tumor-derived populations. (Cf. Fig. 9). High-affinity EGF-binding data within each cell line remained constant with cell density, after the initial rise following subculture, and was not altered by challenge of sensitive cell cultures with androgens (not shown).

PREMALIGNANCY AND ENDOCRINE STATUS

The cornerstone of our understanding of prostatic cancer is the series of investigations of Dr. Charles Huggins and his colleagues (25,172,261), which established that prostate cancer cells retained some degree of hormone dependence. Although reference was made (262,263) in the latter part of the nineteenth-century to the use of orchidectomy for the treatment of enlarged prostates, it was the classic experimentation of Huggins that provided the scientific basis for the acceptance of anti-androgen therapy, orchidectomy, or estrogen administration, for the management of advanced carcinoma of the prostate. In the ensuing years, prostatic endocrinology has been dominated by the concept that the growth, maintenance, and functional

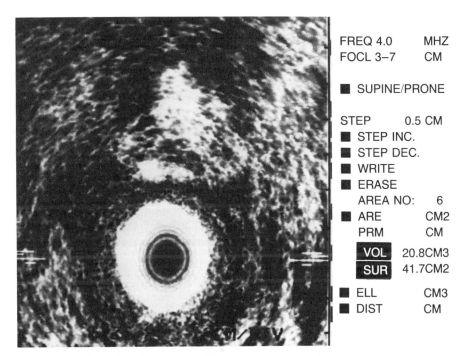

FIG. 11. Per-rectal ultrasound scan of a patient with a small hypoechoic prostatic carcinoma in the peripheral zone and a small benign adenoma anteriorly.

activity of the gland are largely dependent upon testosterone secreted by the testis. Furthermore, through these five decades, the treatment of disseminated prostatic cancer has centered on endocrine therapy, most effective in the short term, in that 70% to 80% of patients experienced symptomatic relief (264,265), although relapse occurs within 1 to 2 years (266,267) and median survival is then six months. Disease progression clearly expresses the inexorable growth of the clones of hormone-independent cancer cells.

It is now clear that although the influence of steroid hormones, particularly testosterone, has been extensively studied as modulators of prostatic growth and differentiation, there is now a whole range of factors, some derived from the organ's "microenvironment," that experimental evidence suggests also could play a principal role in the regulation of prostatic growth. The prostate, including both the epithelial cells and stromal elements, is the focus of a barrage of regulatory stimuli elicited by steroid hormones and peptide growth factors and a greater appreciation of the influence they exercise on intracelluar processes is a prerequisite to understanding the tumor biology of this gland. The prostate is an androgen-dependent gland, yet the precise details of the androgen involvement in growth regulation remain undetermined. The stroma has been implicated as the mediator of the androgenic, perhaps the estrogenic response. BPH can result from the reactivation of the embryonic inductive potential of the stroma in the adult prostate (114,170,268). Carcinoma of the prostate is a disease where epithelial proliferation escapes from androgenic control and stromal intervention, and because there is evidence to suggest that the growth factor requirements of tumor cells differ from those of normal cells (251), it is imperative that we increase our knowledge of these processes as quickly as possible.

In the programs of research directed to the search for endocrine or biochemical factors that could be implicated in carcinogenesis of the prostate gland, the determination of steroid and peptide hormone concentrations in plasma of patients with the disease has failed to identify any endocrine disturbance or any difference from the normal asymptomatic man that could lead to a greater understanding of disease etiology (21,22). Despite such relatively disappointing investigations, the search continues for evidence to incriminate excessive androgen stimulation as the cause of prostatic carcinoma, and certainly it is well recognized that the disease does not occur in the prepubertally castrated man.

The central and peripheral zones of the prostate atrophy with advancing years, although McNeal (10) described in certain glands an age-related increase in atypical hyperplasia, diffuse, or multifocal proliferation of ductal and epithelial tissue, changes that he considered related to premalignancy. Such changes normally would be associated with the glandular morphology present in the prostate of a younger man. Previous studies (269) have shown that these diffuse areas of hyperplasia occur more frequently in prostatic tissue from patients with cancer than from controls. The relationship of this atypical hyperplasia to the well-established (270) high incidence of small, clinically asymptomatic latent carcinoma seen at autopsy in the peripheral zone of the prostate, remains undetermined. The time course by which these small foci of carcinoma develop into the malignant, clinically manifest cancer is unknown, but the process could take at least 20 years (271). It would seem that despite a high incidence of latent carcinoma in men past the age of 50 years, only 1% annually present with clinical cancer (3), and the progression from latent to malignant cancer occurs only rarely in the oriental man. Extensive growth of the cancer in the peripheral region of the gland with capsular involvement and disease dissemination often occurs before local clinical symptoms are recognized. There is a certain propensity for prostatic cancer to metastasize from the primary site and data indicate that approximately 60% of those who present with prostatic cancer have advanced disease (3).

The essential problem of prostatic cancer is one of early diagnosis and it has to be recognized that the principal means of diagnosis is still the rectal examination. If men could be investigated during the period when preneoplasia or early malignancy was becoming established, it might be possible to understand better the biochemical or hormonal factors that influence the promotion of the disease. The possibility of screening populations for elevated PSA levels in plasma, or some such similar protein specifically associated with prostatic cancer, must be considered, especially in association with secondary investigation involving ultrasonography by rectal probe.

Such ultrasonic scanning procedures (272) are now capable of recognizing small, early cancers within the prostate (Fig. 11) and appropriate sampling techniques could allow tissue biopsy for biochemical examination. Measures would then have to be taken to identify the "high risk" cancer as distinct from that which urologists have long believed merely should be "watched." Recognition could then be given to the most effective means of managing the disease in these earlier stages, possibly using 5α -reductase inhibitors, LH-RH analogues, specific drug-targeting or even laser technology for the destruction of this small primary cancer rather than radical prostatectomy, which is currently in vogue.

TREATMENT OF ADVANCED CARCINOMA OF THE PROSTATE

The clinical behavior of prostatic cancer does reflect androgen stimulation and a large proportion of patients respond well to antiandrogenic therapy that effectively lowers plasma levels of testosterone. The treatment is palliative, and the disease inevitably recurs or progresses. The patients are not cured of cancer and the autonomous proliferation of the hormone-independent cancer cells eventually kills the patient. Those who fail to respond initially to primary endocrine therapy, the "high-risk," bad prognosis group, probably represent patients in whom a large proportion of cancer cells, if not all, are hormone independent. Those patients who initially respond, but quickly relapse, represent the same high risk group for which endocrine therapy has only limited value.

There is clearly an urgent need for new, innovative therapy for this high-risk group of patients to extend the time before relapse occurs and to improve survival time.

When Huggins and his colleagues (25,172,261) showed that the symptoms and general well-being of men with advanced prostatic cancer could be improved by orchidectomy or by treatment with diethylstilboestrol (DES), there was a new, real sense of hope among those concerned with the management of this previously untreatable disease. These new forms of therapy, particularly the orally active DES, based on scientific studies of the physiologic control of the prostate gland, must have evoked considerable optimism that even more efficacious procedures would follow.

Through these past 50 years, it has become universally accepted that orchidectomy is the simplest and most direct procedure to remove the major proportion (90% to 95%) of the testosterone in the human male. This surgical procedure resulted in an overall, symptomatic response of 70% to 80% in patients with disseminated disease. It also became well established that bilateral orchidectomy was the yardstick, the gold standard, against which other forms of primary endocrine therapy should be assessed and against this, DES was seen as an inexpensive but effective synthetic estrogen for the management of metastatic carcinoma of the prostate. After treatment with DES, the concentration of testosterone in plasma falls to "castration levels" of approximately 2 nmol/l. As with orchidectomy, 70% to 80% of patients experience a clinical response.

Bilateral orchidectomy or treatment with DES have been the mainstay of primary endocrine therapy for these past five decades. During later years, however, the use of DES was not without some degree of controversy and concern as the results of the Veterans Administration Cooperative Urological Research Group directed attention to the potential danger of the side effects of this therapy including cardiovascular problems, gynecomastia, nausea, and occasional allergies (273,274). Because total orchidectomy is seen by many as a permanent, mutilating, and generally distasteful form of therapy, in certain urological centers, particularly in the United Kingdom, there was a reversion to subcapsular orchidectomy as the principal first-line treatment. Data from various centers including our own (275,276) indicate that the procedure effectively removes all testicular tissue concerned with the synthesis and secretion of androgens and the operation is considered to be cosmetically more acceptable to the patient.

Initiatives were sought and these were dominated by either the need to remove the source of testicular testosterone or to inhibit its biological action on the prostatic cancer (28). Few drugs other than DES have gained universal acceptance. The long-acting intramuscular polyoestradiol phosphate (Estradurin) is popular in Scandinavia but only weakly suppresses LH secretion (277) and the use of Premarin (2.5 mg. t.d.s), a mixture of conjugated equine estrogens, or the synthetic ethinyloestradiol (0.15–1.0 mg./day) were not generally accepted and were more expensive than DES. Various progestational steroids have been used for primary therapy including medroxyprogesterone acetate (Provera), hydroxyprogesterone acetate (Delalutin), cyproterone acetate (Cyprostat), and chlormadinone acetate. Some have been reported to show clinical promise, but apart from cyproterone acetate and medroxyprogesterone acetate, their clinical effectiveness has not been critically established by rigorous, randomized trials. The past decade, however, has been dominated by the potential value of LH-RH analogues as the primary form of endocrine therapy.

Because the isolation and characterization of LH-RH in the early part of 1970, various analogues with marked physiological and pharmacological effects have been synthesized and studied (278–280). Physiologic doses of the analogues were shown to mimic the action of LH-RH whereas, paradoxically, long-term administration of pharmacologic doses produced antigonadal effects and regression of hormone-dependent mammary and prostatic tumors in experimental animals (281–283).

The early experimental work of the Institute (282,283) involved the LH-RH analogue, ICI 118630, (D-Ser(Bu^t)^{6}Azgly^{10}LH-RH: Zoladex, (ICI Pharmaceuticals, Macclesfield, Cheshire, U.K.). It was established from phase I and phase II clinical studies that the slow-release (depot) formulation with the analogue (3.6 mg) incorporated in a 50:50 lactide:glycolide copolymer in the form of a small cylindrical rod, injected every 28 days, effectively reduced serum testosterone concentrations to castrate levels by the 15th day (284–286). Patients responded well to the treatment that had few significant side effects. A phase III randomized clinical trial involving 18 urologic clinics of the British Prostate Study Group and coordinated by the Tenovus Institute (27,28,287) has indicated that the long-term administration of

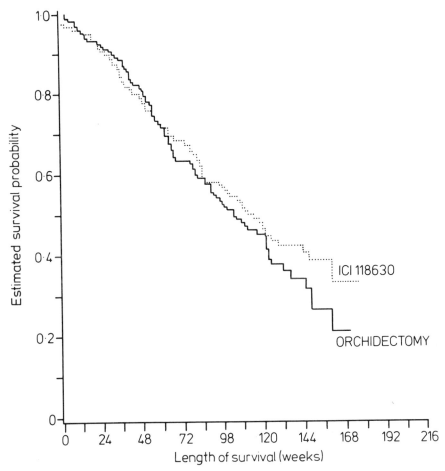

FIG. 12. Survival curves for patients with advanced prostatic cancer treated either by orchidectomy or administration of Depot-Zoladex: ICI trial 118630:1501.

depot-Zoladex, 3.6 mg. monthly, was equally as effective as orchidectomy for the treatment of advanced prostatic cancer.

Survival time was similar for patients in both groups (Fig. 12). Treatment with Zoladex produced minimal side effects (Table 2) and it is very clear that this depot preparation offers an innovative, effective, alternative form of primary endocrine therapy.

Current interest centers, however, on the clinical potential of a more aggressive approach to primary endocrine therapy, the "complete androgen blockade" (289), the simultaneous treatment with an LH-RH analogue and an antiandrogen. Although there is little doubt that the residual testosterone in the castrated or Zoladex-

TABLE 2. *Incidence of reported adverse reactions*

	Orchidectomy (n = 182)	Zoladex (n = 176)
Postoperative complications	14	n/a
Problems at the injection site	n/a	0
Transient increase in pain	0	6
Systems:		
Gastrointestinal	0	6
Cerebrovascular	0	2
Central nervous system	0	4
Respiratory	1	8
Musculoskeletal	0	1
Skin	0	5
Other	0	1

Phase III Trial orchidectomy vs. depot Zoladex in advanced prostatic cancer patients. n/a, not applicable; n = number of patients.

treated patient is of adrenal origin (21), relapse or disease progression is rarely associated with a secondary rise in testosterone levels (290). Adrenal C_{19}-steroids are metabolized peripherally to produce testosterone and can be utilized by prostatic tissue for the synthesis of DHT (290), although their role in maintaining the growth of prostatic cancer in patients who have been either medically or surgically castrated must remain in doubt. Complete androgen blockade, whereby the antiandrogen administered together with LH-RH analogue inhibits the action of these adrenal androgenic steroids at the target organ is currently being assessed with randomized clinical trials in Europe and the United States.

It is hoped that such treatment will extend the period of time to relapse, but the possibility that complete androgen blockade will increase survival time is awaited with some degree of scepticism. Early results reported from two of the European trials are shown in Fig. 13, where it appears that the combined therapy provides no further benefit than from LH-RH analogue treatment alone. Further detailed reports on the progress of these trials are awaited with considerable interest.

The concept of total androgen withdrawal is not new. Huggins and Bergenstal (291) removed the adrenals of patients who had suffered relapse in an attempt to restrain disease progression, although this was second-line endocrine therapy, after estrogen treatment or castration, and the patients were considerably more debilitated by this stage. Brendler (292) reported that neither adrenalectomy nor hypophysectomy offered effective therapy for the relapsed patient, a conclusion strongly supported by Coffey and his colleagues (293). Schroeder (294) has recently reviewed all the data from these earlier, classic studies. Geller and his associates (295) have long advocated the use of progestational agents, such as megestrol acetate, in a therapeutic regime to both remove the effects of testicular androgens by inhibiting pituitary secretion of LH and influence the effects of the adrenal androgens at the level of the target organ.

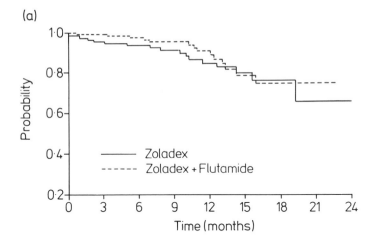

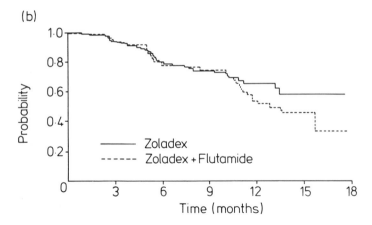

FIG. 13. (a) Preliminary data from the EORTC 30853 clinical trial, orchidectomy versus Zoladex and Flutamide combined, for the management of metastatic carcinoma of the prostate. Data show the relationship between the treatment and duration of survival. **(b)** Preliminary data from the ICI 118630:1509 clinical trial Zoladex versus Zoladex and Flutamide combined, showing time to progression in the two groups of patients.

The possibility of total androgen withdrawal as primary endocrine therapy was in many respects innovative and much credit is due to Fernand Labrie and his colleagues for introducing such a concept. Controversy has, however, surrounded this work, since Labrie originally described (289,296–298) the preliminary clinical data on the treatment of patients by such means. Substantial, 100% remission rates were reported for patients who were followed for 18 months, with less disease progression and fewer deaths. More conservative assessments have subsequently been reported, but the "Labrie concept" stimulated particular excitement and controversy and thereby provoked the urologic community into establishing most effectively designed, prospective randomized trials to determine the clinical value of total androgen withdrawal therapy. The results from these worldwide studies are currently being assessed by the various groups, but as illustrated (see Fig. 13), combination therapy might not ultimately furnish the much hoped for success.

Essentially, therefore, Zoladex or indeed any other similar LH-RH analogue, offers a new, safe form of medical castration with 70% to 80% of patients showing clinical improvement. The treatment, however, is palliative and progression occurs through the growth of the androgen-independent tumor cells. Proliferative processes then access other, as yet poorly defined, growth regulatory pathways and only a complete understanding of these systems provides the rational means of designing new therapeutic regimes. Treatment with LH-RH analogues offers a new form of fine tuning to the endocrine approach to primary therapy, but 50 years after the classical experiments of Charles Huggins, there are many who believe that orchidectomy still provides the simplest and cheapest treatment and a cure for this most common type of cancer remains a dream.

SOME CURRENT TRENDS IN THE FIELD OF PROSTATE CANCER

It is important that we continue to search for innovative, but rational, approaches to therapy. Many patients presenting with metastatic prostate cancer fail to respond to endocrine therapy, or respond, but quickly relapse. Identification of this "bad prognostic" group of patients is necessary and data from the British Prostate Study Group (21,299) and from Adlercreutz and his colleagues (300) suggest that a prognostic index could be used to select patients for a more aggressive combination cytotoxic–hormonal therapy regimen. These investigations have revealed that lower plasma concentrations of testosterone and estradiol-17β, together with elevated plasma growth hormone levels relate to the high risk patients. The results might reflect the inhibitory effects of cortisol on the testis of the more stressed, severely ill patient. Other analytical procedures (301) will soon provide additional capacity in the search for prognostic indices to identify individual tumor characteristics.

If the high risk patients can be identified either by analysis of plasma hormone concentrations or by the recognition of particular characteristics of the tumor tissue, than research is necessary to establish the most appropriate, but acceptable, chemotherapeutic approach for first-line treatment of at least the younger element of this group of patients. Certainly with the potential of the androgen receptor analysis for the identification of androgen responsive cancer still to be realized (21), such an approach would allow progress to be made. In the United States, (302) patients with advanced disease are entering trials where combination chemotherapy and hormonal therapy is being assessed; these studies will provide valuable data. The difficulties in determining the most effective and best tolerated chemotherapeutic agents for patients with prostate cancer are appreciated by all in this field of medicine.

The treatment of the relapsed patient with chemotherapy has always been limited by the toxicity of the agents and there had always been an interest in the possibility of specific targeting of such agents to the site of the cancer to effect a response with reasonably acceptable side effects. The concept of drug targeting was incorporated into the research program of the Tenovus Institute in the late 1960s with an attempt to localize the action of cytotoxic agents within the tumor. In association with the late Dr. Arthur Walpole (I.C.I. Pharmaceuticals, Alderley Park, Macclesfield, U.K.) nitrogen mustard derivatives of diethylstilboestrol (I.C.I. 85966) and of tamoxifen (I.C.I. 79792) were prepared and their biological effects studied (303). The introduction of estramustine phosphate [Estracyt] with the alkylating agent, nor-nitrogen mustard attached as a carbamate *via* C-3 of estradiol-17β was equally of interest. Despite being estrogenic and cytotoxic, Estracyt has never been as universally accepted as might have been expected. As primary endocrine therapy, Estracyt is only as effective as conventional estrogen treatment (304–307), although it was reported (308) that approximately 40% of patients refractory to orchidectomy or estrogen treatment responded to the drug. These results should be substantiated by appropriately coordinated randomized clinical trials, possibly comparing the effects of Estracyt with mitomycin C. Whatever its chemotherapeutic effect, part of Estracyt's clinical action will be endocrine-directed because plasma estradiol-17β concentrations are significantly elevated in patients treated with Estracyt (244).

Antibodies have long been considered potentially valuable as the carrier of cytotoxic drugs (309) and evaluating some of the Tenovus Institute data gives little doubt that this approach deserves further consideration and support (310,311). In these studies, methotrexate (MTX) was linked to a purified IgG fraction of a rabbit polyclonal antiserum raised against cell membranes prepared from the human prostatic cell line PC3. The ability of the MTX-antibody conjugate to bind to cell membranes was substantially retained as assessed by immunocytochemical techniques and a solid-phase competition assay, and there was only a small loss in the capacity of the MTX-antibody complex to inhibit dihydrofolate reductase compared to an equimolar amount of free drug. The cytotoxic effects of the MTX-antibody conjugate were evaluated *in vitro* using cultured PC3 cells by measuring the release of ^{51}Cr from preloaded cells, the number of cells remaining in culture after treatment and the distribution of cell volume. At a dose of 4μg MTX/ml, the MTX-antibody conjugate significantly reduced the number of cells remaining in the culture and significantly increased ^{51}Cr-release when compared to similar conjugates prepared from nonimmune IgG (Fig. 14).

Studies *in vivo*, using athymic nude mice bearing PC3 tumors, demonstrated a significant retardation of tumor growth (Fig. 15) when animals receiving anti-membrane MTX-antibody conjugates were compared to those receiving MTX, anti-

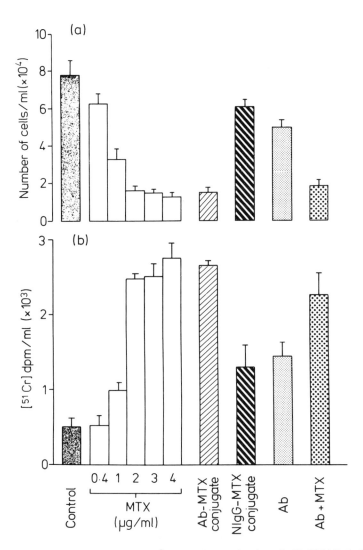

FIG. 14. PC3 cells at a density of 5 × 10³ cells/well were incubated with MTX (0.4–4 μg/ml), antimembrane immunoglobulin-MTX conjugates (4 μg MTX/ml; 90 μg IgG/ml), nonimmune IgG-MTX conjugates (4 μg MTX/ml; 83 μg IgG/ml), antimembrane immunoglobulin alone (90 μg IgG/ml), antimembrane immunoglobulin plus MTX (4 μg MTX/ml; 90 μg IgG/ml) or media only for 2 hours at 37°C. Following washing (5 × 2 ml PBS) the monolayers were incubated in fresh media at 37°C. (a) The number of cells remaining in each well was measured 72 hours after treatment. Data represent the mean + SD of quadruplicate cultures. (b) Cells were pre-loaded with [51Cr], (20 μCi × 10⁶ cells) for 30 minutes at 37° and washed (6 × 2 ml PBS before incubation with antibody-drug conjugates and controls. The amount of [51Cr] released into the media was measured 24 hours later and the data represented as the mean + SD from eight wells per experimental group.

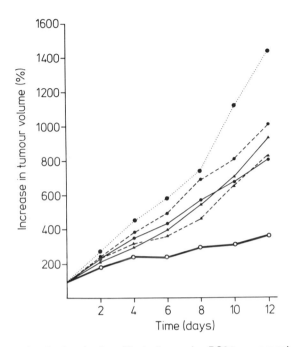

FIG. 15. Athymic nude mice bearing logarithmically growing PC3 tumors received im injections of the various treatments every 48 hours over a 12-day period. The dose of MTX, both in the free form and the conjugate preparations was 1 mg/kg body weight and the amount of free or conjugated immunoglobulin was 498 μg per injection. Tumor size was measured before each injection and the data represented as the mean percentage increase from 16 animals per group following injections of saline only (··•··), nonimmune IgG-MTX conjugates (--•--), anti-membrane immunoglobulin alone (-▲-), antimembrane immunoglobulin plus MTX (--▲--), MTX (—•—) or antimembrane immunoglobulin-MTX conjugates (—○—).

body alone, antibody and MTX combined but not conjugated, and nonimmune IgG-MTX conjugates at doses of 1 mg MTX/kg body weight. Tissue distribution studies (Fig. 16) using [³H]MTX in both free and conjugated form revealed that the MTX-antibody conjugate preferentially accumulated in the PC3 tumor. Such preliminary investigations indicate that although the polyclonal antibody used in this study was not specific for human prostatic tissue, antibodies to cell membranes that have been conjugated to cytotoxic agents such as methotrexate can have significant antitumor action.

The procedures for the management of patients with carcinoma of the prostate have advanced quite dramatically during the past decade. Current data indicate that the administration of an LH-RH analogue such as Zoladex provides a most effective medical castration with limited side effects and as such, in the absence of economic issues, probably would be the treatment of choice for primary endocrine therapy. Although there are reports in the literature of a 25% to 30% response rate for patients given second-line hormone therapy, antiandrogens, aminoglutethimide, or progestogens, these generally are subjective responses and insufficient dose of the

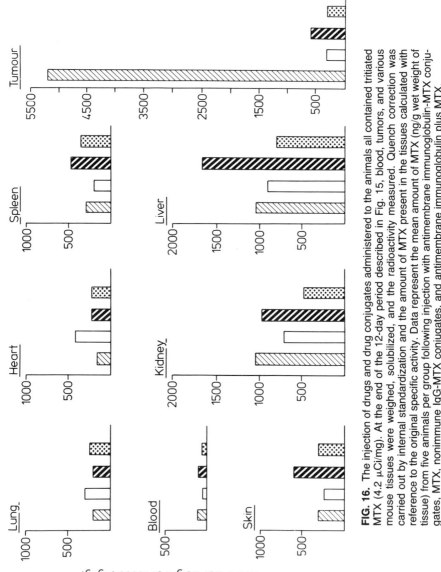

FIG. 16. The injection of drugs and drug conjugates administered to the animals all contained tritiated MTX (4.2 μCi/mg). At the end of the 12-day period described in Fig. 15, blood, tumors, and various mouse tissues were weighed, solubilized, and the radioactivity measured. Quench correction was carried out by internal standardization and the amount of MTX present in the tissues calculated with reference to the original specific activity. Data represent the mean amount of MTX (ng/g wet weight of tissue) from five animals per group following injection with antimembrane immunoglobulin–MTX conjugates, MTX, nonimmune IgG-MTX conjugates, and antimembrane immunoglobulin plus MTX.

drug used in the primary treatment (312) or lack of patient compliance could be reasons for this effect.

It seems very reasonable to consider new, more aggressive treatment for the high-risk patient with poor prognosis—and research continues in this area. With ultra-sonography gaining wider acceptance in the confirmation of "digital diagnosis" of prostatic cancer, together with its considerable value in both staging the disease and in identifying specific areas of the gland from which to obtain a tissue biopsy, then the even more sophisticated gene technology can be brought to bear on the identification of aggressive cancer. Such a form of analysis to determine specific oncogene expression for individual tumor characterization should provide greater insight into cancer diagnosis and a better appreciation of cancer biology and treatment.

Effective communication between cells by means of chemical information, the accurate deciphering of that information, and the precise response elicited to it are part of the complex processes concerned with the physiology of life. Any impairment of these molecular mediators could produce serious biological consequences, a fact highlighted by the relatively recent discovery that the true oncogenes of the acutely transforming retroviruses apparently were transduced cognates of cellular genes, which in their normal unaltered state were concerned with growth regulation or differentiation. Oncogenes, therefore, are normal growth regulatory genes in which alterations of structure or expression occur. It has become recognized that as well as the homologues of the retroviral oncogenes, all other cellular genes-encoding components of growth or differentiation-regulating systems—growth factors, growth factor receptors, or proteins concerned in the transduction of growth factor signals in either the cytoplasm or the nucleus of the cell—must be considered proto-oncogenes. Moreover, amplification, mutation, or translocation of these genes could lead to malignant transformation of cells harboring the altered genes or oncogenes. These concepts have been frequently reviewed over the past few years (313–320).

A greater understanding of the biological systems integrating these processes is imperative. Cancer therapy previously has not been particularly selective for cancer cells, whereas biochemical intervention to counteract oncogene activation to induce differentiation or to inhibit growth factor action could be considered, although somewhat optimistically as yet, more cell specific.

The search for aberrant genes in prostatic cancer can appear daunting, yet it is very reasonable to believe that a judicious screening of tumor biopsy specimens could pinpoint anomalies in the expression of genes that are fundamental to the cascade of processes mobilized by the growth factors that influence the tissue in question. In the case of the prostate gland, gene alterations that could be implicated in the initiation of cancer and in the escape from hormone dependence can be located in the pathways of androgen-imprinted growth regulation and of androgen-repressed cell death, outlined earlier in this chapter. Undoubtedly, however, other genetic lesions will contribute to cancer progression.

Such relationships between hormones and growth factors have been identified in breast cancer (321–323) and in the pattern of expression of the HER-2/neu/erbB-2 oncogene (324,325). It remains to be determined whether usurpation of its own growth regulatory processes confers upon a cell the distinct advantage of operating in an autocrine mode, not only producing, but also responding to its own growth factors (326). In doing so, the scope widens in support of the concept that the cell as such provides a target for biotechnology-based therapy.

Observations on growth factors and their receptors in relation to prostatic cancer have been outlined earlier and brief comments directed at those genes involved in the transmission of growth regulatory signals would seem relevant to complete this chapter.

Rijnders and his colleagues (327) investigated protooncogene expression in the poorly differentiated prostatic cancer cell lines PC3, PC133 and PC138 and the more differentiated androgen-dependent PC82 cell line that grows only in male immune-deficient mice. A consistently high expression of c-Ha-ras and c-myc was observed. The expression of c-fos correlated positively with androgenic status of the PC82 cells. Similarly, while screening clinical specimens of human prostatic tissue, studies in the Tenovus Institute (301) demonstrated a correlation between c-fos mRNA and AR content. This and another report (328) described an elevated level of c-myc mRNA in cancer tissues of all grades of differentiation, whereas Buttyan and coworkers (329) found increased c-myc expression only in less differentiated tissue. In a survey of lineages of the Dunning tumor (330), substantial increased levels of mRNA were found for the three nuclear oncogenes, c-myc, c-fos, and p53 on the transition from the normal dorsal prostate to the androgen-dependent HI-tumor, and significantly decreased levels during progression to the androgen-independent HI-tumor and also as metastatic cancer developed from the parent sublines. Levels of neu and c-sis mRNA also were elevated in the well-differentiated androgen-dependent tumor. Cooke and colleagues (330) concluded that in the Dunning tumor at least, increased expression of c-myc, c-fos, and p53 were indicative of neoplastic change. It is tempting to relate the possible implication of the first two to their repression by androgens in rat ventral prostate, and to attribute the correlation between androgen receptor and c-fos in diseased prostate to a dysfunctional AR. These things have yet to be ascertained, but both c-myc and c-fos are obviously prime candidates for further study. They are rapidly induced in response to a wide range of mitogens (331), the protein product of c-myc has been ascribed a role in initiation of DNA synthesis (332) and production of the c-fos protein is considered a key event in the transmission of extracellular stimuli into the diverse intracellular processes (333) by interaction with other regulatory molecules.

The Tenovus Institute study found increasing levels of c-Ha-ras mRNA with tumor dedifferentiation, but an equivocal expression of c-Ki-ras and c-sis. The suggestion that high levels of the ras p21 protein could be used as a marker for tumor progression in prostatic cancer (334) has been challenged (335,336). Although transfection of an activated ras oncogene can increase the metastatic potential of prostate cancer cells (337), activation of ras oncogene *in situ* is a rare event in prostate cancer (338) and in the Dunning tumor, the level of c-Ha-ras did not reflect aggressive tumor growth, nor was increased expression related to hormone independence (330).

Studies in cellular oncogenes undoubtedly will provide a greater understanding of the biological processes concerned with prostatic carcinogenesis and a greater insight into their potential value as prognostic indicators. Identification of prostatic growth factors, facultatively expressed under androgenic influence, or constitutively expressed when autonomy is realized, could promote the inception of new, possibly curative and precisely targeted forms of therapy. We enter a new and most exciting period as we extensively increase our understanding of the endocrine and biochemical processes that regulate prostatic growth and function.

Acknowledgments

The support and collaboration of our colleagues in the British Prostate Study Group, and the financial assistance provided by the Tenovus Organization are gratefully acknowledged.

REFERENCES

1. Alderson MR. Epidemiology in prostate cancer. In: Duncan W, ed. Recent Results in Cancer Research. No. 78, Heidelberg: Springer-Verlag, 1981;1–19.
2. Office of Population Census Statistics. Mortality Statistics 1976. Series DH2, No. 3: London: HMSO 1978.
3. Carter HB, Coffey DS. Prostate cancer: the magnitude of the problem in the United States. In: Coffey DS, Resnick MI, Dorr FA, Karr JP, eds. *A Multidisciplinary analysis of Controversies in the management of prostate cancer*. New York: Plenum Press, 1988;1–7.
4. Sondik E. Incidence, survival and mortality trends in prostate cancer in the United States. In: Coffey DS, Resnick MI, Dorr FA, Karr JP, eds. *A Multidisciplinary analysis of Controversies in the management of prostate cancer*. New York: Plenum Press, 1988;9–16.
5. Sommers SC. Endocrine changes with prostatic carcinoma. *Cancer* 1957;10:345–358.
6. Armenian HK, Lilienfeld AM, Diamond EL, Bross IDJ. Relation between benign prostatic hypertrophy and cancer of the prostate. A prospective and retrospective study. *Lancet* 1974;ii:115–117.
7. Blacklock NJ. Surgical anatomy of the prostate. In: Williams DI, Chisholm GD, eds. *Scientific Foundation of Urology, Vol II*. London: Heinemann, 1976;113–125.
8. McNeal JE. Age related changes in prostatic epithelium associated with carcinoma. In: Griffiths K, Pierrepoint CG, eds. *Some aspects of the aetiology and biochemistry of prostatic cancer, 3rd Tenovus workshop*. Cardiff: Alpha Omega Pub, 1970;23–32.
9. McNeal JE. The prostate and prostatic urethra, a morphologic synthesis. *J Urol* 1972;107:1008–1016.
10. McNeal JE. Structure and pathology of the prostate. In: Goland M, ed. *Normal and abnormal growth of the prostate*. Springfield, IL: Thomas, 1975;55–65.
11. McNeal, JE. New morphological findings relevant to the origin and evolution of carcinoma of the prostate and BPH. In: Coffey DS, Isaacs JT, eds. *UICC technical report series, vol. 48*. Geneva: UICC 1979;24–37.
12. Peeling WB, Griffiths K. Prostatic cancer. In: Lumley J, Craven J, eds. *Surgical review, vol. 1* London: Pitman Medical, 1978;303–327.
13. Skeet RG. Epidemiology of urological tumours. In: Williams DI, Chisholm GD, eds. *Scientific foundation of urology, vol. II*. London: Heinemann, 1976;199–211.
14. Miller JG. Diagnosis of stage A prostate Cancer in the People's Republic of China. In: Coffey DS, Resnick MI, Dorr FA, Karr JP, eds. *A Multidisciplinary analysis of Controversies in the management of prostate cancer*. New York: Plenum Press, 1988;17–24.

15. Huben R, Mettlin C, Natarajan N, Smart CR, Pontes E, Murphy GP. Carcinoma of prostate in men less than 50 years old. *Urology* 1982;20:585–588.
16. Rotkin ID. Epidemiological factors associated with prostatic cancer. In: Coffey DS, Isaacs JT, eds. *UICC technical report series, vol. 48*. Geneva: UICC, 1979;56–60.
17. Haenzel W, Kurihara M. Studies of Japanese migrants. I. Mortality from cancer and other diseases among Japanese in the United States. *J Natl Cancer Inst* 1968;40:43–68.
18. Wynder EL, Mabuchi K, Whitmore WF. Epidemiology of cancer of the prostate. *Cancer* 1971;28:344–360.
19. Rich AR. On frequency of occurrence of occult carcinoma of prostate. *J Urol* 1935;33:215–223.
20. Oota K, Misu Y. A study of latent carcinoma of the prostate in Japanese. *Gann* 1958;49:283–293.
21. Griffiths K, Davies P, Eaton CL, et al. Cancer of the prostate: endocrine factors. In: Clarke JR, ed. *Oxford reviews of reproductive biology, vol. 9*. Oxford: Oxford University Press, 1988;192–259.
22. Griffiths K, Davies P, Harper ME, Peeling WB, Pierrepoint CG. The etiology and endocrinology of prostatic cancer. In: Rose D, ed. *Endocrinology of cancer vol. 2*. Boca Raton: CRC Press 1979;1–55.
23. Baird DT, Uno A, Melby JC. Adrenal secretion of androgens and oestrogens. *J Endocrinol* 1969;45:135–136.
24. Lipsett MB. Steroid secretion by the human testis. In: Paulsen CA, ed. *The human testis* New York: Plenum Press, 1970;407–421.
25. Huggins C, Stevens RE Jr, Hodges CV. Studies on prostatic cancer II. The effects of castration on advanced carcinoma of the prostate gland. *Arch Surg* 1941;43:209–223.
26. Peeling WB, Griffiths K. Endocrine treatment of prostatic cancer. In: Blandy JP, Lytton B, eds. *The prostate*. London: Butterworths 1986;188–207.
27. Turkes AO, Peeling WB, Griffiths K. Treatment of patients with advanced cancer of the prostate: phase III trial, Zoladex against castration. *J Steroid Biochem* 1987;27:543–549.
28. Turkes AO, Peeling WB, Wilson DW, Griffiths K. Evaluation of different endocrine approaches in the treatment of prostatic carcinoma. In: Klosterhalfen H, ed. *New developments in biosciences 4. Endocrine management of prostatic cancer*. Berlin/New York: Walter de Gruyter & Co., 1988;75–86.
29. Mainwaring WIP. The mechanism of action of androgens. In: *Monographs in endocrinology Vol. 10*. New York: Springer-Verlag, 1977.
30. King RJB. Structure and function of steroid receptors. *J Endocrinol* 1987;114:341–349.
31. Schrader WT. New model for steroid hormone receptors? *Nature* 1984;308:17–18.
32. Heyns W, DeMoor P. Prostatic binding protein: a steroid binding protein secreted by rat prostate. *Eur J Biochem* 1977;78:221–230.
33. Lea OA, Petrusz P, French FS. Prostatein. A major secretory protein of the rat ventral prostate. *J Biol Chem* 1979;254:6196–6202.
34. Pousette A, Bjork P, Carlstrom K, Forsgren B, Gustafsson JA, Hogberg B. On the presence of prostatic secretion protein in different species. *Acta Chem Scand* 1980;334:155–156.
35. Forsgren B, Bjork P, Carlstrom K, Gustafsson JA, Pousette A, Hogberg B. Purification and distribution of a major protein in rat prostate that binds estramustine, a nitrogen mustard derivative of estradiol-17β. *Proc Natl Acad Sci U S A* 1979;76:3149–3153.
36. Heyns W, Peeters B, Mous J, Rombauts W, DeMoor P. Purification and characterisation of prostatic binding protein and its subunits. *Eur J Biochem* 1978;89:181–186.
37. Peeters B, Heyns W, Mous J, Rombauts W. Structural studies on rat prostate binding protein. The primary structure of component C1 from subunit F. *Eur J Biochem* 1982;123:55–62.
38. Peeters B, Rombauts W, Mous J, Heyns W. Structural studies on rat prostate binding protein. The primary structure of its glycosylated component C3. *Eur J Biochem* 1981;115:115–121.
39. Parker M, Needham M, White R. Prostatic steroid binding proteins: gene duplication and steroid binding. *Nature* 1982;298:92–94.
40. Carter DB, Yamada K, Harris SE. Developmental aspects of androgen-dependent mRNA from rat ventral prostate using cloned cDNA. *Mol Cell Endocrinol* 1983;31:199–214.
41. Heyns W, Peeters B, Mous J. Influence of androgens on the concentration of prostatic binding protein (PBP) and its mRNA in rat prostate. *Biochem Biophys Res Commun* 1977;77:1492–1499.
42. Parker M, Scrace, GT. Regulation of protein synthesis in rat ventral prostate: cell-free translation of mRNA. *Proc Natl Acad Sci U S A* 1979;76:1580–1584.
43. Parker MG, Scrace GT, Mainwaring WIP. Testosterone regulates the synthesis of a major protein in rat ventral prostate. *Biochem J* 1978;170:115–121.

44. Parker MG, White R, Williams JG. Cloning and characterisation of androgen-dependent mRNA from rat ventral prostate. *J Biol Chem* 1980;255:6996–7001.
45. Mous J, Peeters B, Rombauts W, Heyns W. Synthesis of rat prostatic binding protein in Xenopus oocytes and in wheat germ. *Biochem Biophys Res Commun* 1977;79:1111–1116.
46. Parker MG, Scrace GT. The androgenic regulation of abundant mRNA in rat ventral prostate. *Eur J Biochem* 1978;85:399–406.
47. Page MJ, Parker MG. Androgen-regulated expression of a cloned rat prostatic C3 gene transfected into mouse mammary tumor cells. *Cell* 1983;32:395–502.
48. Zhang YL, Parker MG. Regulation of prostatic steroid binding protein mRNAs by testosterone. *Mol Cell Endocrinol* 1985;43:151–154.
49. Davies P, Rushmere NK. Regulatory regions of androgen-responsive genes. *Biochem Soc Trans* 1988;16:695–698.
50. Evans RM. The steroid and thyroid hormone receptor superfamily. *Science* 1988;240:889–895.
51. Green S, Chambon P. Nuclear receptors enhance our understanding of transcription regulation. *Trend Genet* 1988;4:309–314.
52. Parker MG. Mechanism of steroid hormone action. *Cancer Surv* 1986;5:625–633.
53. Yamamoto T, Ikawa S, Akiyama T, et al. Similarity of protein encoded by the human c-erb-B-2 gene to epidermal growth factor receptor. *Nature* 1986;230:231–234.
54. Chang C, Kokontis J, Liao S. Molecular cloning of human and rat complementary DNA encoding androgen receptor. *Science* 1988;240:324–327.
55. Chang C, Kokontis J, Liao S. Structural analysis of complementary DNA and amino acid sequences of human and rat androgen receptors. *Proc Natl Acad Sci U S A* 1988;85:7211–7215.
56. Tan J, Joseph DR, Quarmby VE, et al. The rat androgen receptor: primary structure, autoregulation of its messenger ribonucleic acid, and immunocytochemical localization of the receptor protein. *Mol Endocrinol* 1988;2:1276–1285.
57. Lubahn DB, Joseph DR, Sar M, et al. The human androgen receptor: complementary deoxyribonucleic acid cloning, sequence analysis and gene expression in prostate. *Mol Endocrinol* 1988;2:1265–1275.
58. Lubahn DB, Joseph DR, Sullivan PM, Willard HF, French FS, Wilson EM. Cloning of human androgen receptor complementary DNA and localisation to the X chromosome. *Science* 1988;240:327–330.
59. Trapman J, Klaassen P, Kuiper GGJM, et al. Cloning, structure and expression of a cDNA encoding the human androgen receptor. *Biochem Biophys Res Commun* 1988;153:241–248.
60. Giguere V, Hollenberg SM, Rosenfeld MG, Evans RM. Functional domains of the human glucocorticoid receptor. *Cell* 1986;46:645–652.
61. Kumar V, Green S, Stack G, Berry M, Jin JR, Chambon P. Functional domains of the human estrogen receptor. *Cell* 1987;51:941–951.
62. Webster NJG, Green S, Jin JR, Chambon P. The hormone-binding domains of the estrogen and glucocorticoid receptors contain an inducible transcription activation function. *Cell* 1988;54:199–207.
63. van Laar JH, Bolt-de-Vries J, Voorhorst-Ogink MM, Brinkmann AO. The human androgen receptor is a 110 kDa protein. *Mol Cell Endocrinol* 1989;63:39–44.
64. Kuiper GGJM, Faber PW, van Rooij HCJ, et al. Structural organization of the human androgen receptor gene. *J Mol Endocrinol* 1989;3:R1–R4.
65. French FS, Lubahn DB, Brown TR, et al. The molecular basis of androgen insensitivity. *Rec Prog Hormone Res* 1990; (in press).
66. Huckaby CS, Conneely OM, Beattie WG, Dobson ADW, Tsai MJ, O'Malley BW. Structure of the chromosomal chicken progesterone receptor gene. *Proc Natl Acad Sci U S A* 1987;84:8380–8384.
67. Ponglikitmongkol M, Green S, Chambon P. Genomic organization of the human oestrogen receptor gene. *EMBO J* 1988;7:3385–3388.
68. Faber PW, Kuiper GGJM, van Rooij HCJ, van der Korput JAGM, Brinkmann AO, Trapman J. The N-terminal domain of the human androgen receptor is encoded by one, large exon. *Mol Cell Endocrinol* 1989;61:257–262.
69. Brown TR, Lubahn DB, Wilson EM, et al. Deletion of the steroid-binding domain of the human androgen receptor gene in one family with complete androgen insensitivity syndrome: evidence for further genetic heterogeneity in this syndrome. *Proc Natl Acad Sci U S A* 1988;85:8151–8155.
70. Beato M. Gene regulation by steroid hormones. *Cell* 1989;56:235–344.
71. Klein-Hitpass L, Ryffel GU, Heitlinger E, Cato ACB. A 13bp palindrome is a functional estrogen-

responsive element and interacts specifically with estrogen receptor. *Nucleic Acids Res* 1988;16: 647–663.

72. Kumar V, Chambon P. The estrogen receptor binds tightly to its responsive element as a ligand-induced homodimer. *Cell* 1988;55:145–156.

73. Denison SH, Sands A, Tindall DJ. A tyrosine aminotransferase glucocorticoid response element also mediated androgen enhancement of gene expression. *Endocrinology* 1989;124:1091–1093.

74. Cato ACB, Henderson D, Ponta H. The hormone response element of the mouse mammary tumour virus DNA mediates the progestin and androgen induction of transcription in the proviral long terminal repeat region. *EMBO J* 1987;6:363–368.

75. Ham J, Thomson A, Needham M, Webb P, Parker M. Characterization of response elements for androgens, glucocorticoids and progestins in mouse mammary tumour virus. *Nucleic Acids Res* 1988;16:5263–5277.

76. Rushmere NK, Parker MG, Davies P. Comparative binding of androgen-receptor complexes by elements of mouse mammary tumour virus and prostate genes. *Mol Cell Endocrinol* 1990; (in press).

77. Perry ST, Viskochil DH, Ho KC, et al. Androgen receptor binding to the C3(i) subunit gene of rat prostatein, In: Bruchovsky A, Chapdelaine A, Neumann F, eds. *Regulation of androgen action*. Berlin: Congressdruck R. Brückner, 1985;159–164.

78. Rushmere NK, Parker MG, Davies P. Androgen receptor-binding regions of an androgen-responsive gene. *Mol Cell Endocrinol* 1987;51:259–265.

79. Parker MG, Webb P, Needham M, White R, Ham J. Identification of androgen response elements in mouse mammary tumour virus and rat prostate C3 gene. *J Cell Biol* 1987;35:285–292.

80. Claessens F, Rushmere NK, Peeters B, Davies P, Rombouts W. Characterisation of androgen response elements in the C1 gene of prostate binding protein. *Arch Int Physiol Biochem* 1989; 97:B15.

81. Martinez E, Givel F, Wahli W. The estrogen-responsive element as an inducible enhancer: DNA sequence requirements and conversion to a glucocorticoid-responsive element. *EMBO J* 1987;6: 3719–3727.

82. Davies P, Elford C, Manning D, Phillips MEA, Rushmere N, Thomas P. Regulatory significance of receptor-chromatin associations. In: Bruchovsky A, Chapdelaine A, Neumann F, eds. *Regulation of androgen action*. Berlin: Congressdruck R. Bruckner, 1985;159–164.

83. Davies P, Thomas P, Manning DL. Correlations between prostate chromatin structure and transcriptional activity and acceptor site distribution. *Prostate* 1986;8:151–166.

84. Jantzen, HM, Strahle U, Gloss B, et al. Cooperativity of glucocorticoid response elements located far upstream of the tyrosine aminotransferase gene. *Cell* 1987;49:29–38.

85. Klein-Hitpass L, Kaling M, Ryffel GU. Synergism of closely adjacent estrogen-responsive elements increases their regulatory potential. *J Mol Biol* 1988;201:537–544.

86. Tsai SY, Tsai MJ, O'Malley BW. Cooperative binding of steroid hormone receptors contributes to transcriptional synergism at target enhancer elements. *Cell* 1989;57:443–448.

87. Miksicek R, Borgmeyer U, Nowock J. Interaction of the TGGCA-binding protein with upstream sequences is required for efficient transcription of mouse mammary tumour virus. *EMBO J* 1987;6:1355–1360.

88. Schule R, Muller M, Kaltschmidt C, Renkawitz R. Many transcription factors interact synergistically with steroid receptors. *Science* 1988;242:1418–1420.

89. Schule R, Muller M, Otsuka-Murakami H, Renkawitz R. Cooperativity of the glucocorticoid receptor and the CACCC-box binding factor. *Nature* 1988;332:87–90.

90. Strahle U, Schmid W, Schutz G. Synergistic action of the glucocorticoid receptor with transcription factors. *EMBO J* 1988;7:3389–3395.

91. Rushmere NK, Davies P. Requirements for binding of androgen-receptor complexes to androgen response elements. *Mol Endocrinol*, submitted.

92. Berry M, Nunez AM, Chambon P. Estrogen responsive element of the human pS2 gene is an imperfectly palindromic sequence. *Proc Natl Acad Sci U S A* 1989;86:1218–1222.

93. Klock G, Strahle U, Schutz G. Oestrogen and glucocorticoid response elements are closely related but distinct. *Nature* 1987;329:734–736.

94. Davies P, Griffiths K. Hormonal control of the prostate gland. In: *The management of prostatic carcinoma*, edited by D. Kirk & J. Edson. Boston: Chapman and Hall, 1989.

95. Barrack ER, Coffey DS. Biological properties of the nuclear matrix: steroid hormone binding. *Recent Prog Horm Res* 1982;38:133–189.

96. Rennie PS, Bruchovsky N, Cheng H. Isolation of 3S androgen receptors from salt-resistant frac-

tions and nuclear matrices of prostatic nuclei after mild trypsin digestion. *J Biol Chem* 1983;258: 7623–7630.

97. Chapdelaine P, Paradis G, Tremblay RR, Dube JY. High level of expression in the prostate of a human glandular kallikrein mRNA related to prostate-specific antigen. *FEBS Lett* 1988;236:205–208.

98. Dube JY, Frenette G, Paquin R, et al. Isolation from human seminal plasma of an abundant 16-kDa protein originating from the prostate, its identification with a 94-residue peptide originally described as β-inhibin. *J Androl* 1987;8:182–189.

99. Frenette G, Dubé JY, Lazure C, Paradis G, Chretien M, Tremblay RR. The major 40-kDa glycoprotein in human prostatic fluid is identical to Zn-α-glycoprotein. *Prostate* 1987;11:257–270.

100. Lilja H, Abrahamsson, PA. Three predominant proteins secreted by the human prostate gland. *Prostate* 1988;12:29–38.

101. Tremblay J, Frenette G, Tremblay RR, Dupont A, Thabet M, Dubé JY. Excretion of three major prostatic secretory proteins in the urine of normal men and patients with benign prostatic hypertrophy or prostatic cancer. *Prostate* 1987;10:235–243.

102. Digby M, Zhang XY, Richards RI. Human prostate specific antigen (PSA) gene: structure and linkage to the kallikrein-like gene, hGK-1 *Nucleic Acids Res* 1989;17:2137.

103. Henttu P, Vihko P. cDNA coding for the active human prostate specific antigen shows high homologies to the human tissue kallikrein genes. *Biochem Biophys Res Commun* 1989;160:903–910.

104. Lundwall A, Lilja H. Molecular cloning of human prostate specific antigen cDNA. *FEBS Lett* 1987;214:317–322.

105. Mbikay M, Nolet S, Fournier S, et al. Molecular cloning and sequence of the cDNA for a 94-amino-acid seminal plasma protein secreted by the human prostate. *DNA* 1987;6:23–29.

106. Riegman PHJ, Vlietstra RJ, Klaassen P, et al. The prostate-specific antigen gene and the human glandular kallikrein-1 gene are tandemly located on chromosome 19. *FEBS Lett* 1989;247:123–126.

107. Riegman PHJ, Vlietstra RJ, van der Korput JAGM, Romijn JC, Trapman J. Characterization of the prostate-specific antigen gene: a novel human kallikrein-like gene. *Biochem Biophys Res Commun* 1989;159:95–102.

108. Schulz P, Stucka R, Feldmann H, Combriato G, Klobeck HG, Fittler F. Sequence of a cDNA clone encompassing the complete mature human Prostate Specific Antigen (PSA) and an unspliced leader sequence. *Nucleic Acids Res* 1988;16:6226.

109. Sharief FS, Lee H, Leuderman MM, et al. Human prostatic acid phosphatase: cDNA cloning, gene mapping and protein sequence homology with lysosomal acid phosphatase. *Biochem Biophys Res Commun* 1989;160:79–86.

110. Vihko P, Virkkunen P, Henttu P, Roiko K, Solin T, Huhtala ML. Molecular cloning and sequence analysis of cDNA encoding prostatic acid phosphatase. *FEBS Lett* 1988;236:275–281.

111. Yeh LCC, Lee, AJ, Lee NE, Lam KW, Lee JC. Molecular cloning of cDNA for human prostatic acid phosphatase. *Gene* 1987;60:191–196.

112. Berry SJ, Isaacs JT. Comparative aspects of prostatic growth and androgen metabolism with aging in the rat versus the dog. *Endocrinology* 1984;114:511–520.

113. Isaacs JT. Antagonistic effect of androgen on prostatic cell death. *Prostate* 1984;5:545–557.

114. Cunha GR, Donjacour AA, Cooke PS, et al. The endocrinology and development biology of the prostate. *Endocr Rev* 1987;8:338–362.

115. Takeda H, Mizuno T, Lasnitzki I. Autoradiographic studies of androgen-binding sites in the rat urogenital sinus and postnatal prostate. *J Endocrinol* 1985;104:87–92.

116. Wilson JD, Lasnitzki I. Dihydrotestosterone formation in fetal tissues of the rabbit and rat. *Endocrinology* 1971;89:659–668.

117. Imperato-McGinley J. 5α-Reductase deficiency in man. *Prog Cancer Res Ther* 1984;31:491–504.

118. Ohno S. Major sex determining genes. New York: Springer-Verlag, 1979;1.

119. Bruchovsky N, Lesser B, van Doorn E, Craven S. Hormonal effects on cell proliferation in rat prostate. *Vit Horm* 1975;33:61–102.

120. Butler WWS III, Schade AL. The effects of castration and androgen replacement on the nucleic acid composition, metabolism and enzymatic capacities of the rat ventral prostate. *Endocrinology* 1958;63:271–279.

121. Coffey DS, Shimazaki J, Williams-Ashman HG. Polymerization of deoxyribonucleotides in relation to androgen-induced prostatic growth. *Arch Biochem Biophys* 1968;124:184–198.

122. Stanisic T, Sadlowsky R, Lee C, Grayhack JT. Partial inhibition of castration induced ventral prostate regression with actinomycin D and cycloheximide. *Invest Urol* 1978;16:19–22.
123. Anderson KM, Baranowski J, Economou SG, Rubenstein M. A qualitative analysis of acidic proteins associated with regressing, growing or dividing rat prostate cells. *Prostate* 1983;4:151–166.
124. Lee C, Sensibar J. Proteins of the rat prostate. II. Synthesis of new proteins in the ventral lobe during castration-induced regression. *J Urol* 1987;138:903–908.
125. Lee C, Tsai Y, Harrison H, Sensibar J. Proteins of the rat prostate. I. Preliminary characterization by two-dimensional gel electrophoresis. *Prostate* 1985;7:171–182.
126. Leger JG, Le Guellec R, Tenniswood MPR. Treatment with antiandrogens induces an androgen-repressed gene in the rat ventral prostate. *Prostate* 1988;13:131–142.
127. Leger JG, Montpetit ML, Tenniswood MP. Characterization and cloning of androgen-repressed mRNAs from rat ventral prostate. *Biochem Biophys Res Commun* 1987;147:196–203.
128. Montpetit ML, Lawless KR, Tenniswood M. Androgen-repressed messages in the rat ventral prostate. *Prostate* 1986;8:25–36.
129. Quarmby VE, Beckman WC Jr, Wilson EM, French FS. Androgen regulation of c-myc messenger ribonucleic acid levels in rat ventral prostate. *Mol Endocrinol* 1987;1:865–874.
130. Buttyan R, Zakeri Z, Lockshin R, Wolgemuth D. Cascade induction of c-fos, c-myc, and heat shock 70k transcripts during regression of the rat ventral prostate gland. *Mol Endocrinol* 1988;2:650–657.
131. Engel G, Lee C, Grayhack JT. Acid ribonuclease in rat prostate during castration-induced involution. *Biol Reprod* 1980;22:827–831.
132. Kyprianou N, Isaacs JT. Activation of programmed cell death in the rat ventral prostate after castration. *Endocrinology* 1988;122:552–562.
133. Tanabe E, Lee C, Grayhack JT. Activities of cathepsin D in rat prostate during castration-induced involution. *J Urol* 1982;127:826–828.
134. Kyprianou N, English HF, Isaacs JT. Activation of a C2 + -M2-dependent endonuclease as an early event in castration-induced prostatic cell death. *Prostate* 1988;13:103–117.
135. Rennie PS, Bouffard R, Bruchovsky N, Cheng H. Increased activity of plasminogen activators during involution of the rat ventral prostate. *Biochem J* 1984;221:171–178.
136. Rennie PS, Bowden JF, Bruchovsky N, Cheng H. The relationship between inhibition of plasminogen-activator activity and prostatic involution. *Biochem J* 1988;252:759–764.
137. Connor J, Sawczuk IS, Benson MC, et al. Calcium channel antagonists delay regression of androgen-dependent tissues and suppress gene activity associated with cell death. *Prostate* 1988;13:119–130.
138. Humphries JE, Isaacs JT. Unusual androgen sensitivity of the androgen-independent Dunning R-3327-G rat prostatic adenocarcinoma: androgen effect on tumour cell loss. *Cancer Res* 1982;42:3148–3156.
139. McKeehan WL, Adams PS, Rosser MP. Direct mitogenic effects of insulin, epidermal growth factor, glucocorticoid, cholera toxin, unknown pituitary factors and possibly prolactin, but not androgen, on normal prostate epithelial cells in serum-free, primary cell cultures. *Cancer Res* 1984;44:1998–2010.
140. Chung LWK, Coffey DS. Biochemical characterization of prostate nuclei. II Relationship between DNA synthesis and protein synthesis. *Biochem Biophys Acta* 1971;247:584–596.
141. Coffey DS. The effects of androgens on DNA and RNA synthesis in sex accessory tissue. In: Brandes D, ed. *Male accessory sex organs: structure and function.* New York: Academic Press, 1974;307–328.
142. Davies P, Thomas P. Heterogeneity of nuclear androgen receptors, in relation to growth and macromolecular synthesis. In: Navarro Moreno MA, ed. *Advances in human receptors. Methodological and clinical aspects.* Madrid: Jarpyo Editoros, 1984;66–75.
143. Van Doorn E, Craven S, Bruchovsky N. The relationship between androgen receptor and the hormonally controlled responses of the rat ventral prostate. *Biochem J* 1976;160:11–21.
144. Kyprianou N, Isaacs, JT. Quantal relationship between prostatic dihydrotestosterone and prostatic cell contents: critical threshold content. *Prostate* 1987;11:41–50.
145. De Larminat MA, Rennie PS, Bruchovsky N. Radioimmunoassay measurements of nuclear dihydrotestosterone in rat prostate. Relationship to androgen receptors and androgen-regulated responses. *Biochem J* 1981;200:465–474.
146. Griffiths K, Davies P, Eaton CL, Harper ME, Pierrepoint CG. Oestrogens and the Prostate. In: Khoury S, Chatelain C, eds. *Oestrogens and the prostate.* FIIS et RPG, 1988;308–332.

147. Stone NN, Fair WR, Fishman J. Estrogen formation in human prostatic tissue from patients with and without benign prostatic hyperplasia. *Prostate* 1986;9:311–318.
148. Brendler CB, Berry SJ, Ewing LL, et al. Spontaneous benign prostatic hyperplasia in the beagle. Age-associated changes in serum hormone levels, and the morphology and secretory function of the canine prostate. *J Clin Invest* 1983;71:1114–1123.
149. De Klerk DR, Coffey DS, Ewing LL, et al. Comparison of spontaneous and experimentally induced canine prostatic hyperplasia. *J Clin Invest* 1979;64:842–849.
150. Walsh PC. Human benign prostatic hyperplasia: Etiological considerations. In: Kimball FA, Buhl AE, Carter DB, eds. *New approaches to the study of benign prostatic hyperplasia*. New York: Alan R. Liss, 1984;1–25.
151. Wilson JD. The pathogenesis of benign prostatic hyperplasia. *Am J Med* 1980;68:745–756.
152. Nicholson RI, Walker KJ, Davies P. Hormone agonists and antagonists in the treatment of hormone sensitive breast and prostate cancer. *Cancer Surv* 1986;5:463–486.
153. Bashirelahi N, Young JD Jr, Sidh SM, Sanefuji H. Androgen, oestrogen and progestogen and their distribution in epithelial and stromal cells of human prostate. In: Schroder FH, de Voogt HJ, eds. *Steroid Receptors, Metabolism and Prostatic Cancer*. Amsterdam: Excerpta Medica, 1980;240–255.
154. Bruner-Lorand J, Mechaber D, Zwick A, et al. Characteristics of separated epithelial and stromal subfractions of prostate. I. Rat ventral prostate. *Prostate* 1984;5:231–254.
155. Mobbs BG, Johnson IE. Relationships between estrogen intake, serum testosterone, and tumour androgen, estrogen and progesterone receptor levels in diethylstilboestrol-treated rats bearing the R3327 prostatic adenocarcinoma. *Prostate* 1985;7:293–304.
156. Mobbs BG, Johnson IE. Quantitative relationships between cytosol and nuclear estrogen and progesterone receptors in the R3327 prostate adenocarcinoma of rats treated with diethylstilbestrol. *Prostate* 1986;8:256–264.
157. Eaton CL, Hamilton TC, Kenvyn K, Pierrepoint CG. Studies of androgen and estrogen binding in normal canine prostatic tissue and in epithelial and stromal cell lines derived from the canine prostate. *Prostate* 1985;7:377–388.
158. Ekman P, Barrack ER, Greene GL, Jensen EV, Walsh PC. Estrogen receptors in human prostate. Evidence for multiple binding sites. *J Clin Endocrinol Metab* 1983;57:166–176.
159. Swaneck GE, Alvarez JM, Sufrin G. Multiple species of estrogen binding sites in the nuclear fraction of the rat prostate. *Biochem Biophys Res Commun* 1982;106:1441–1447.
160. Swaneck GE, Alvarez JM. Specific binding of 3H-estradiol to rat prostate nuclear matrix. *Biochem Biophys Res Commun* 1985;128:1381–1387.
161. Barrack ER, Berry SJ. DNA synthesis in the canine prostate: effects of androgen and oestrogen treatment. *Prostate* 1987;10:45–56.
162. Chaisiri N, Pierrepoint CG, Examination of the distribution of oestrogen receptor between stromal and epithelial compartments of the canine prostate. *Prostate* 1980;1:357–366.
163. Krieg M, Bartsch W, Thomsen M, Voigt KD. Androgens and oestrogens: their interaction with stroma and epithelium of human benign prostatic hyperplasia and normal prostate. *J Steriod Biochem* 1983;19:155–161.
164. Krieg M, Klotzl G, Kaufmann J, Voigt KD. Stroma of human benign prostatic hyperplasia: preferential tissue for androgen metabolism and oestrogen binding. *Acta Endocrinol* 1981; (Copenh) 96:422–432.
165. Purvis K, Morkas L, Rui H, Attramadal A. Estrogen receptors in stromal and epithelial fractions of the rat ventral prostate of rats. *Arch Androl* 1985;15:143–151.
166. Geller J, Albert JD, Kirshner M, Liu J. Tamoxifen decrease human prostate CPK concentration. *Prostate* 1985;7:283–285.
167. Geller J, Liu J, Albert JD, Fay W, Berry CC. Effect of antiandrogen and/or antiestrogen blockage on human prostate epithelial and stromal cell protein synthesis. *J Steroid Biochem* 1986;25:759–763.
168. Liu J, Albert JD, Geller J, Faber LE. Effect of tamoxifen on stromal protein synthesis in the human prostate. *J Clin Endocrinol Metab* 1984;55:710–713.
169. Schulze H, Barrack ER. Immunocytochemical localization of oestrogen receptors in spontaneous and experimentally induced canine benign prostatic hyperplasia. *Prostate* 1987;11:145–162.
170. McNeal JE. Origin and evolution of benign prostatic enlargement. *Invest Urol* 1978;15:340–345.
171. Eaton CL, Pierrepoint CG. Epithelial and fibroblastoid cell lines derived from the normal canine prostate: II. Cell proliferation in response to steroid hormones. *Prostate* 1982;3:493–506.
172. Huggins C, Clark PJ. Quantitative studies of prostatic secretion. II. The effects of castration and of

estrogen injection on the normal and on the hyperplastic prostatic glands of dogs. *J Exp Med* 1940;72:747–762.

173. Mawhinney MG, Neubauer BL. Actions of estrogens in the male. *Invest Urol* 1979;16:409–420.
174. Walsh PC, Wilson JD. The induction of prostatic hypertrophy in the dog with androstanediol. *J Clin Invest* 1976;57:1093–1097.
175. Chang C, Kokontis J, Chang CT, Liao S. Cloning and sequence analysis of the rat ventral prostate glucocorticoid receptor cDNA. *Nucleic Acids Res* 1987;15:9603.
176. Rennie PS, Bowden JF, Freeman SN, et al. Cortisol alters gene expression during involution of the rat ventral prostate. *Mol Endocrinol* 1989;3:703–708.
177. Martikainen P, Harkonen P, Vanhala T, Makela S, Viljanen M, Suominen J. Multihormonal control of synthesis and secretion of prostatein in cultured rat ventral prostate. *Endocrinology*, 1987; 121:604–611.
178. Omukai Y, Nakamura N, Hiraoka D, et al. Growth-stimulating effect of pharmacological doses of glucocorticoid on androgen-responsive Shionogi carcinoma 115 in vivo in mice and in cell culture. *Cancer Res* 1987;47:4329–4334.
179. Rennie PS, Bruchovsky N, Buttyan R, Benson M, Cheng H. Gene expression during the early phases of regression of the androgen-dependent Shionogi mouse mammary carcinoma. *Cancer Res* 1988;48:6309–6312.
180. Davies P, Rushmere NK. Association of glucocorticoid nucleic receptors with prostate nucleic sites for androgen receptors and with androgen response elements. *J Mol Endocrinol* 1990; 5: (in press).
181. Claessens F, Celis L, Peeters B, Heyns W, Verhoeven G, Rombauts W. Functional characterization of an androgen response element in the first intron of the C3(1) gene of prostatic binding protein. *Biochem Biophys Res Commun* 1989;164:833–840.
182. Meyer ME, Gronemeyer H, Turcotte B, Bocquel MT, Tasset D, Chambon P. Steroid hormone receptors compete for factors that mediate their enhancer function. *Cell* 1989;57:433–442.
183. De Klerk DP, Coffey DS. Quantitative determination of prostatic epithelial and stromal hyperplasia by a new technique: biomorphometrics. *Invest Urol* 1978;16:240–245.
184. Bartsch G, Daxenbichler G, Rohr HP. Correlative morphological and biochemical investigation on the stromal tissue of the human prostate. *J Steroid Biochem* 1983;19:147–154.
185. Harper ME, Pike A, Peeling WB, Griffiths K. Steroids of adrenal origin metabolised by human prostatic tissue in vivo and in vitro. *J Endocrinol* 1974;60:117–125.
186. Schweikert HU, Totzauer P, Rohr HP, Bartsch G. Correlated biochemical and stereological studies on testosterone metabolism in the stromal and epithelial compartment of human benign prostatic hyperplasia. *J Urol* 1985;134:403–407.
187. Orlowski J, Bird CE, Clark AF. Androgen 5α-reductase and 3α-hydroxysteroid dehydrogenase activities in ventral prostate epithelial and stromal cells from immature and mature rats. *J Endocrinol* 1983;99:131–139.
188. Bruchovsky N, Dunstan-Adams E. Regulation of 5α-reductase activity in stroma and epithelium of human prostate. In: Bruchovsky A, Chapdelaine A, Neumann F, eds. *Regulation of androgen action*. Berlin: Congressdruck R. Brückner, 1985;31–35.
189. Krieg M. Biochemical endocrinology of human prostatic tumours. In: King RJB, Lippman ME, eds. *Progress in cancer research therapy: hormones and cancer 2.vol. 31*. New York: Raven Press, 1984;425–440.
190. Kyprianou N, Davies P. Association states of androgen receptors in nuclei of human benign hypertrophic prostate. *Prostate* 1986;8:363–380.
191. Chung LWK, Cunha GR. Stromal-epithelial interactions. II. Regulation of prostatic growth by embryonic urogenital sinus mesenchyme. *Prostate* 1983;4:503–511.
192. Chung LWK, Matsuura J, Runner MN. Tissue interactions and prostatic growth. I. Induction of adult mouse prostatic hyperplasia by fetal urogenital sinus implants. *Biol Reprod* 1984;31:155–165.
193. Thompson TC, Chung LWK. Regulation of overgrowth and expression of prostate binding protein in rat chimeric prostate gland. *Endocrinology* 1986;118:2437–2444.
194. Buchanan LJ, Riches AC. Proliferative responses of rat ventral prostate: effects of variations in organ culture media and methodology. *Prostate* 1986;8:63–74.
195. Sandberg AA, Kadohama N. Regulation of prostate growth in organ culture. *Prog Clin Biol Res* 1980; 37:9–29.
196. Santti RS, Johansson R. Some biochemical effects of insulin and steroid hormones on the rat prostate in organ culture. *Exp Cell Res* 1973;77:111–120.

197. Peehl DM, Stamey TA. Growth response of normal, benign hyperplastic, and malignant human prostatic epithelial cells in vitro to cholera toxin, pituitary extract, and hydrocortisone. *Prostate* 1986;8:51–61.
198. Davies P, Thomas P, Giles MG. Responses to androgens of rat ventral prostate nuclear androgen-binding sites sensitive and resistant to micrococcal nuclease. *Prostate* 1982;3:439–457.
199. Jacobs SC, Pinka D, Lawson RK. Prostatic osteoblastic factor. *Ivest Urol* 1979;17:195–199.
200. Hierowski MT, McDonald MW, Dunn L, Sullivan JW. The partial dependency of human prostatic growth factor on steroid hormones in stimulating thymidine incorporation into DNA. *J Urol* 1987;138:909–912.
201. Jacobs SC, Lawson RK. Mitogenic factor in human prostate extracts. *Urology* 1980;16:488–493.
202. Jinno H, Udea K, Otaguro K, Kato T, Ito J, Tanaka R. Prostate growth factor in the extracts of benign prostatic hypertrophy *Eur Urol* 1986;12:41–48.
203. Lawson RK, Story MT, Jacobs SC. A growth factor in extracts of human prostate tissue. In: Kimball FA, Buhl AE, Carter DB, eds. *New approaches to the study of benign prostatic hyperplasia.* New York: Alan R. Liss, 1984;325–336.
204. Maehama S, Li D, Nanri H, Leykam JF, Deuel TF. Purification and partial characterization of prostate-derived growth factor. *Proc Natl Acad Sci U S A* 1986;83:8162–8166.
205. Matuo Y, Nishi N, Wada F. Growth factors in the prostate. *Arch Androl* 1987;19:193–210.
206. Matuo Y, Nishi N, Matsui S, Sandberg AA, Isaacs JT, Wada F. Heparin binding affinity of rat prostatic growth factor in normal and cancerous prostates: partial purification and characterization of rat prostatic growth factor in the Dunning tumor. *Cancer Res* 1987;47:188–190.
207. Mydlo JH, Bulbul MA, Richon VM, Heston WDW, Fair WR. Heparin-binding growth factor isolated from human prostatic extracts. *Prostate* 1988;12:343–355.
208. Nishi N, Matuo Y, Wada F. Partial purification of a major type of rat prostatic growth factor: characterization as an epidermal growth factor-related mitogen. *Prostate* 1988;13:209–220.
209. Nishi N, Matuo Y, Kumtomi K, et al. Comparative analyses of growth factors in normal and pathologic human prostates. *Prostate* 1988;13:39–48.
210. Parrish RF, Heston WDW, Pletscher LS, Tackett R, Fair WR. Prostate derived growth factors. In: Kimball FA, Buhl AE, Carter DB, eds. *New approaches to the study of benign prostatic hyperplasia.* New York: Alan R. Liss, 1984;181–195.
211. Story MT, Jacobs SC, Lawson RK. Partial purification of a prostatic growth factor. *J Urol* 1984;132:1212–1215.
212. Tackett RE, Heston WDW, Parrish RF, Pletscher LS, Fair WF. Mitogenic factors in prostatic tissue and expressed prostatic secretions. *J Urol* 1985;133:45–48.
213. Story MT, Jacobs SC, Lawson RK. Epidermal growth factor is not the major growth-promoting agent in extracts of prostatic tissue. *J Urol* 1983;130:175–179.
214. Story MT, Esch F, Shimasaki S, Sasse J, Jacobs SC, Lawson RK. Amino-terminal sequence of a large form of basic fibroblast growth factor isolated from human benign prostatic hyperplastic tissue. *Biochem Biophys Res Commun* 1987;142:702–709.
215. Story MT, Sasse J, Jacobs SC, Lawson RK. Prostatic growth factor: purification and structural relationship to basic fibroblast growth factor. *Biochemistry* 1987;26:3843–3849.
216. Koutsilieris M, Rabbani SA, Goltzman D. Selective osteoblast mitogens can be extracted from prostatic tissue. *Prostate* 1987;9:109–115.
217. Koutsilieris M, Rabbani SA, Goltzman D. Effects of human prostatic mitogens on rat bone cells and fibroblasts. *J Endocrinol* 1987;115:447–454.
218. Koutsilieris M, Rabbani SA, Bennett HPJ, Goltzman D. Characteristics of prostate-deprived growth factors for cells of the osteoblast phenotype. *J Clin Invest* 1987;80:941–946.
219. Simpson E, Harrod J, Eilon G, Jacobs JW, Mundy GR. Identification of a messenger ribonucleic acid fraction in human prostatic cancer cells coding for a novel osteoblast-stimulating factor. *Endocrinology* 1985;117:1615–1620.
220. Mydlo JH, Michaeli J, Heston WDW, Fair WR. Expression of basic fibroblast growth factor mRNA in benign prostatic hyperplasia and prostatic carcinoma. *Prostate* 1988;13:241–247.
221. Sitaras NM, Sariban E, Bravo M, Pantazis P, Antoniades HN. Quantitative production of platelet-derived growth factor-like proteins by human prostate carcinoma cell lines. *Cancer Res* 1988;48:1930–1935.
222. Ikeda T, Lioubin MN, Marquadt M. Human transforming growth factor β type 2: production by a prostatic adenocarcinoma cell line, purification and initial characterization. *Biochemistry* 1987;26:2406–2410.

223. Tsong SD, Phillips D, Halmi N, Liotta AS, Margioris A, Bardin CW. ACTH and beta-endorphin related peptides are present in multiple-sites in the reproductive tract of the male rat. *Endocrinology* 1982;110:2204–2206.

224. Cameron DF, Corton GL, Larkin LH. Relaxin-like antigenicity in the armadillo prostate gland. *Ann NY Acad Sci* 1982;380:231–240.

225. Adashi E, Hseuh AJW. Direct inhibition of testicular androgen biosynthesis revealing antigonadal activity of neurohypophysial hormones. *Nature* 1981;293:650–656.

226. Sathe VS, Sheth NA, Phadke MA, Sheth AR, Zaveri, JP. Biosynthesis and localization of inhibin in human prostate. *Prostate* 1987;10:33–43.

227. Di Sant Agnese PA, de Messey Jensen JL. Somatostatin-like immunoreactive endocrine-paracrine cells in human prostate gland. *Arch Pathol Lab Med* 1986;108:693–696.

228. Harper GP, Barde YA, Burnstock G, et al. Guinea pig prostate is rich source of nerve growth factor. *Nature* 1979;279:160–162.

229. Pekary AE, Sharp B, Briggs J, Carlson HG, Hershman JM. High concentrations of D-Glu-His-Pro-NH2-(thyrotropin-releasing hormone) occur in rat prostate. *Peptides* 1983;4:915–919.

230. El Etreby MP, Mahrous AT. Immunocytochemical technique for detection of prolactin (PRL) and growth hormone (GH) in hyperplastic and neoplastic lesions of dog prostate and mammary gland. *Histochemistry* 1979;64:279–286.

231. Harper ME, Sibley PEC, Peeling WB, Griffiths K. The immunocytochemical detection of growth hormone and prolactin in human prostatic tissue. In: Murphy GP, Sandberg AA, Karr JP, eds. *The prostate cell: structure and function-part B*. New York: Alan R. Liss, 1981;115–128.

232. Sibley PEC, Harper ME, Peeling WR, Griffiths K. Growth hormone and prostatic tumours: localization using a monoclonal human growth hormone antibody. *J Endocrinol* 1986;102:311–315.

233. Stahler MS, Panskey B, Budd GC. Immunocytochemical demonstration of insulin or insulin-like immunoreactivity in the rat prostate gland. *Prostate* 1988;13:189–198.

234. Jacobs SC, Story MT, Sasse J, Lawson RK. Characterization of growth factors derived from the rat ventral prostate. *J Urol* 1988;139:1106–1110.

235. Shikata H, Utsumi N, Hiramatsu N, Minami M, Nemoto N, Shikata T. Immunohistochemical localization of nerve growth factor and epidermal growth factor in guinea pig prostate gland. *Histochemistry* 1984;80:411–413.

236. Elson SD, Browne CA, Thornburn GD. Identification of epidermal growth factor-like activity in human male reproductive tissue and fluids. *J Clin Endocrinol Metab* 1984;58:589–594.

237. Gregory H, Willshire IR, Kavanagh JP, Blacklock NJ, Chowdury S, Richards RC. Urogastrone-treated normal individuals and patients with benign prostatic hypertrophy. *Clin Sci* 1986;70:359–363.

238. Hiramatsu M, Kashimata M, Minami N, Sato A, Murayama M, Minami N. Androgenic regulation of epidermal growth factor in the mouse ventral prostate. *Biochem Int.* 1988;17:311–317.

239. Jacobs SC, Story MT, Lawson RK. Effect of orchiectomy on rat prostatic growth factor levels. In: Benign Prostatic Hyperplasia Vol. II, NIH Publication No: 87–2881, 1987;228–290.

240. Jacobs SC, Story MT. Exocrine secretion of epidermal growth factor by the rat prostate: effect of adrenergic agents, cholinergic agents, and vasoactive intestinal peptide. *Prostate* 1988;13:79–87.

241. Eaton CL, Davies P, Phillips MEA. Growth factor involvement and oncogene expression in prostatic tumours. *J Steroid Biochem* 1988;30:341–345.

242. McKeehan WL, Adams PS, Fast D. Different hormonal requirements for androgen-independent growth of normal and tumor epithelial cells from rat prostate. *in Vitro Cell Dev Biol* 1987;23:147–152.

243. Wilding G, Zugmeier G, Knabbe C, Flanders K, Gelmann, E. Differentiated effects of transforming growth factor β on human prostate cancer cells in vitro. *Mol Cell Endocrinol* 1989;62:79–87.

244. Syms AJ, Harper ME, Griffiths K. The effect of prolactin on human BPH epithelial cell proliferation. *Prostate* 1985;6:145–153.

245. Chaproniere DM, McKeenan WL. Serial culture of single adult human prostatic epithelial cells in serum-free medium containing low calcium and a new growth factor from bovine brain. *Cancer Res* 1986;46:819–820.

246. Crabb JW, Armes LG, Carr SA, et al. Complete primary structure of prostatropin, a prostate epithelial cell growth factor. *Biochemistry* 1986;25:4988–4993.

247. Davies P, Eaton CL. Binding of epidermal growth factor by human normal hypertrophic and carcinomatous prostate. *Prostate* 1989;14:123–132.

248. Schuurmans ALG, Bolt J, Mulder E. Androgens stimulate both growth rate and epidermal growth factor receptor activity of the human prostate tumor cell line LNCaP. *Prostate* 1988;12:55–63.
249. Traish AM, Wotiz HH. Prostatic epidermal growth factor receptors and their regulation by androgens. *Endocrinology* 1987;121:1461–1467.
250. Carmena MJ, Fernandez MD, Prieto JC. Characterization of insulin receptors in isolated epithelial cells from rat ventral prostate: Effect of fasting. *Cell Biochem Funct* 1986;4:19–24.
251. France TD, Phillips MEA, Eaton CL, Davies P. Regulation of prostatic growth. *Biochem Soc Trans* 1988;16:389–390.
252. Aragona C, Freisen H. Specific prolactin binding sites in the prostate and testis of rats. *Endocrinology* 1975;97:677–684.
253. Kyprianou N, Isaacs JT. Identification of a cellular receptor for transforming growth factor-β in rat ventral prostate and the negative regulation by androgens. *Endocrinology* 1988;123:2124–2131.
254. St. Arnaud R, Poyet P, Walker P, Labrie F. Androgens modulate epidermal growth factor receptor levels in the rat ventral prostate. *Mol Cell Endocrinol* 1988;56:21–27.
255. Schuurmans ALG, Bolt J, Mulder E. Androgens and transforming growth factor β modulate the growth response to epidermal growth factor in human prostatic tumor cells (LNCaP). *Mol Cell Endocrinol* 1988;60:101–104.
256. Boni-Schnetzler M, Pilch PF. Mechanism of epidermal growth factor receptor autophosophorylation and high affinity binding. *Proc Natl Acad Sci U S A* 1987;84:7832–7836.
257. Yarden Y, Schlessinger J. Epidermal growth factor induces rapid, reversible aggregation of the purified epidermal growth factor receptor. *Biochemistry* 1987;26:1443–1451.
258. Yarden Y, Schlessinger J. Self-phosphorylation of epidermal growth factor receptor: Evidence for a model of intermolecular allosteric activation. *Biochemistry* 1987;26:1434–1442.
259. Basu A, Raghunath M, Bishayee S, Das M. Inhibition of tyrosine kinase activity of the epidermal growth factor (EGF) receptor by a truncated receptor form that binds to EGF: Role for interreceptor interaction in kinase regulation. *Mol Cell Biol* 1989;9:671–677.
260. Sorkin A, Kornilova E, Teslenko L, Sorokin A, Nikolsky N. Recycling of epidermal growth factor—receptor complexes in A431 cells. *Biochem Biophys Acta* 1989;1011:88–89.
261. Huggins C, Hodges CV. Studies on prostatic cancer. The effect of castration, of estrogen and of androgen injection on serum phosphatases in metastatic carcinoma of the prostate. *Cancer Res* 1941;1:293–297.
262. Cabot AT. The question of castration for enlarged postate. *Ann Surg* 1896;24:265–309.
263. White JW. The results of double castration in hypertrophy of the prostate. *Ann Surg* 1895;22:1–80.
264. Peeling WB, Griffiths K. The Prostate. In: Mundy AR, ed. *Scientific Basis of Urology*. Avon: Churchill Livingston, 1987;263–295.
265. Resnick MI, Grayhack JT. Treatment of Stage IV carcinoma of the prostate. *Urol Clin N Am* 1975;2:141–161.
266. Jordan WB Jr, Blackard CE, Byar DP. Reconsideration of orchiectomy in the treatment of advanced prostatic carcinoma. *Southern Med J* 1977;70:1411–1413.
267. Whitmore WF. The natural history of prostatic cancer. *Cancer* 1973;321:104–1112.
268. McNeal JE. Anatomy of the prostate and morphogenesis of benign prostatic hyperplasia. In: Kimball FA, Buhl AE, Carter DB, eds. *New approaches to the study of benign prostatic hyperplasia*. New York: Alan R. Liss, 1984;27–64.
269. Koppel M, Heranze DR, Shimkin MB. Characteristics of patients with prostatic carcinoma: a control case study on 83 autopsy pairs. *J Urol* 1967;98:229–233.
270. Baba S. Epidemiology of cancer of the prostate: analysis of countries of high and low incidence. In: Jacobi GH, Hohenfellner R, eds. *Prostate Cancer, International Perspectives in Urology 3*, Baltimore: Williams & Wilkins, 1982;11–28.
271. Hirst AE Jr, Bergman RT. Carcinoma of the prostate in men 80 or more years old. *Cancer* 1954;7:136–141.
272. Peeling WB, Griffiths GJ. Imaging of the prostate by ultrasound. *J Urol* 1984;132:217–224.
273. Arduino LJ. Veterans Administration Cooperative Urological Research Group. Carcinoma of the prostate. Treatment and comparisons. *J Urol* 1967;98:516–522.
274. Mellinger GT. Veterans Administration Cooperative Urological Research Group. Carcinoma of the prostate: A continuing co-operative study. *J Urol* 1964;91:590–594.
275. Burge PD, Harper ME, Hartog M, Gingell JC. Subcapsular orchidectomy—an effective operation? *Proc R Soc Med* 1976;69:663–664.

276. Vermeulen A, Schelfhout W, De Sy W. The treatment for prostatic cancer: Plasma androgen levels after subcapsular orchidectomy or estrogen. *Prostate* 1982;3:115–121.

277. Jonsson G, Olsson AM, Luttrop W, Cekan Z, Purvis K, Diczfalusy E. Treatment of prostatic carcinoma with various types of oestrogen derivatives. *Vitamins and Hormones V* 1975;33:351–376.

278. Corbin A. From contraception to cancer: A review of the therapeutic applications of LH-RH analogues as antitumour agents. *Yale J Biol Med* 1982;55:27–47.

279. Schally AV, Arimura A, Coy DH. Recent approaches to fertility control based on derivatives of LH-RH. *Vitamins and Hormones* 1980;38:257–323.

280. Schally AV, Comaru-Schally AM, Redding TW. Antitumour effects of analogues of hypothalamic hormones in endocrine-dependent cancers. *Proc Soc Exp Biol Med* 1984;175:259–281.

281. Auclair C, Kelly PA, Labrie F, Coy DH, Schally AV. Inhibition of testicular LH/HCG receptor levels by treatment with a potent LH-RH agonist or HCG. *Biochem Biophys Res Commun* 1977;76:855–862.

282. Maynard PV, Nicholson RI. Effect of high doses of a series of new luteinizing hormone releasing hormone analogues in intact female rats. *Br J Cancer* 1979;39:274–279.

283. Nicholson RI, Walker KJ, Maynard PV. Antitumour potential of a new luteinizing hormone releasing hormone analogue ICI 118630. In: Mourisden HT, Palshof T, eds. *Breast cancer: experimental and clinical aspects*. New York: Pergamon Press, 1980;296–299.

284. Pierrepoint CG, Turkes AO, Walker KJ, Harper ME, Wilson DW, Peeling WB, Griffiths K. Endocrine factors in the treatment of prostatic cancer. In: Schroder FH, Richards B, eds. *Therapeutic principles in metastatic prostatic cancer. EORTC genitourinary group monograph 2 part A.* New York: Alan R. Liss, 1985;51–72.

285. Walker KJ, Nicholson RI, Turkes AO, et al. Therapeutic potential of the LHRH agonist, ICI 118630 in the treatment of advanced prostatic carcinoma. *Lancet* 1983;II:413–416.

286. Walker KJ, Turkes AO, Turkes A, et al. Treatment of patients with advanced cancer of the prostate using a slow-release (depot) formulation of the LHRH agonist ICI 118630 (Zoladex). *J Endocrinol* 1984;103:R1–R4.

287. Peeling WB. A phase III trial comparing ICI. 118630 (Zoladex) with orchidectomy in the management of advanced prostatic cancer. In: Chisholm GD, ed. *Zoladex, a new treatment for prostatic cancer*. London: Royal Society of Medicine Service, 1987;27–44.

288. Kaisary A, Tyrrell CJ, Peeling WB, Griffiths K, (on behalf of the study group). A randomised trial comparing the LHRH analogue 'Zoladex' with orchidectomy in patients with metastatic prostatic carcinoma. *Br J Urol* 1990; (in press).

289. Labrie F, Dupont A, Belanger A, et al. New approach in the treatment of prostate cancer: complete instead of partial withdrawal of androgens. *Prostate* 1983;4:579–594.

290. Harper ME, Peeling WB, Griffiths K. Adrenal androgens and the prostate. In: Motta M, Serio M, eds. *Hormonal therapy of prostatic diseases: basic and clinical aspects*. Netherlands: Medicom Europe, 1988:81–104.

291. Huggins C, Bergenstal D. Effect of bilateral adrenalectomy on certain human tumors. *Proc Natl Acad Sci U S A* 1952;38:73–76.

292. Brendler H. Andrenalectomy and hypophysectomy for prostatic cancer. *Urology* 1973;2:99–102.

293. Schulze H, Oesterling JE, Isaacs JT, Coffey DS. Hormonal Therapy of Prostate Cancer: Limitations in the Total Androgen Ablation Concept. In: Coffey DS, Resnick MI, Dorr FA, Karr JP, eds. *A Multidisciplinary analysis of Controversies in the management of prostate cancer*. New York: Plenum Press, 1988;9–16.

294. Schroeder FH. Total androgen suppression in the management of prostatic cancer. A critical review. In: Richards B, Schroeder FH, eds. *EORTC Genitourinary Group Monograph 2, Part A: Therapeutic Principles in Metastatic Prostate Cancer*, New York: Alan R. Liss, 1985;307–319.

295. Geller J, Albert JD. Comparison of various hormone therapies for prostatic carcinoma. *Semin Oncol* 1983;10:34–42.

296. Labrie F, Dupont A, Belanger A. Spectacular response to combined antihormonal treatment in advanced prostate cancer. In: Labrie F, Proulx L, eds. *Endocrinology, international congress series 655*. Amsterdam: Excerpta Medica, 1984:450–453.

297. Labrie F, Dupont A, Belanger A. Complete androgen blockade for the treatment of prostate cancer. In: DeVita VT, Hellman S, Rosenberg SA, eds. *Important advances in oncology*. Philadelphia: JB Lippincott, 1985;193–217.

298. Labrie F, Dupont A, Belanger A, et al. Combination therapy with flutamide and castration (LHRH

agonist or orchidectomy) in advanced prostate cancer: a marked improvement in response and survival. *J Steroid Biochem* 1985;23:833–841.

299. Wilson DW, Harper ME, et al. A Prognostic index for the clinical management of patients with advanced prostatic cancer. *Prostate* 1985;7:131–141.

300. Rannikko S, Kairento AL, Karonen SL, Adlercreutz H. Hormonal patterns in prostatic cancer 1. Correlation with local extent of tumour, presence of metastases and grade of differentiation. *Acta Endocrinol (Copenh)* 1981;98:625–633.

301. Phillips MEA, Ferro MA, Smith PJB, Davies P. Intranuclear androgen receptor deployment and protooncogene expression in human diseased prostate. *Urol Int* 1987;42:115–119.

302. Murphy GP. Is chemotherapy effective in the treatment of prostatic cancer? In: *Bailliere clinical oncology*, Vol 2: 1988; pp. 641–645.

303. Griffiths K, Davies P, Harper ME, Nicholson RI. Biochemical effects of cytotoxic estrogens and cytotoxic antioestrogens. In: Raus J, Martens H, Leclercq G, eds. *Cytotoxic Estrogens in Hormone Receptive Tumors*. New York: Academic Press, 1980;205.

304. Jonsson G, Hogberg B. Treatment of advanced prostatic carcinoma with Estracyt: a preliminary report. *Scand J Urol Nephrol* 1971;5:103–107.

305. Jonsson G, Hogberg B, Nilsson T. Treatment of advanced prostatic carcinoma with estramustine phosphate (Estracyt). *Scand J Urol Nephrol* 1977;11:231–238.

306. Leistenschneider W, Nagel R. Estracyt therapy of advanced prostatic cancer with special reference to control of therapy with cytology and DNA-cytophotometry. *Eur Urol* 1980:6:111–117.

307. Veronesi A, Zattoni F, Frustaci S, et al. Estramustine phosphate (Estracyt) treatment of T3–T4 prostatic carcinoma. *Prostate* 1982;3:159–164.

308. Edsmyr F, Anderson L, Konyves I. Estramustine phosphate (Estracyt): experimental studies and clinical experience In: Jacobi GH, Hohenfeller R, eds. *Prostate cancer: international perspectives in urology, vol 3*. Baltimore: Williams & Wilkens, 1982;253–266.

309. Ghose T, Blair AH. Antibody-linked cytotoxic agents in the treatments of cancer: current status and future prospects. *J Natl Cancer Inst* 1978;61:657–676.

310. Rowland AJ, Harper ME, Wilson DW, Griffiths K. The effect of a methotrexate-antimembrane antibody conjugate and antibody targeted liposomes on the human prostatic tumour line. *PC3. Abst. 263, Proceedings of the Sixth NCI-EORTC Symposium on New Drugs in Cancer Therapy*. Amsterdam, 1989.

311. Rowland AJ, Harper ME, Wilson DW, Griffiths K. The effect of an anti-membrane antibody-methotrexate conjugate on the human prostatic tumour line PC3. *Br J Cancer* 1990;61:702–708.

312. Kemp HA, Read GF, Fahmy DR, et al. Measurement of diethylstilboestrol in plasma from patients with cancer of the prostate. *Cancer Res* 1981;41:4693–4697.

313. Bishop JM. Cellular oncogenes and retroviruses. *Ann Rev Biochem* 1983;52:301–354.

314. Bishop JM. The molecular genetics of cancer. *Science* 1987;235:305–311.

315. Deuel TF. Polypeptide growth factors: roles in normal and abnormal cell growth. *Ann Rev Cell Biol* 1987;3:443–492.

316. Duesberg PH. Cancer genes: rare recombinants instead of activated oncogenes. *Proc Natl Acad Sci U S A* 1987;84:2117–2124.

317. Goustin S, Leof EB, Shipley GD, Moses HL. Growth factors and cancer. *Cancer Res* 1986;46:1015–1029.

318. Roberts AB, Sporn MB, eds. Growth factors and malignancy. *Cancer Surv* 1985;4:627–815.

319. Varmus H, Bishop JM, eds. Biochemical mechanisms of oncogene activity: proteins encoded by oncogenes. *Cancer Surv* 1986;5:153–430.

320. Weinberg RA. The action of oncogenes in the cytoplasm and nucleus. *Science* 1985;230:770–776.

321. Bates SE, Davidson NE, Valverius E, et al. Expression of transforming growth factor α and its messenger ribonucleic acid in human breast cancer: its regulation by estrogen and its possible functional significance. *Mol Endocrinol* 1988;2:543–555.

322. Dickson RB, Lippman ME. Estrogenic regulation of growth and polypeptide growth factor β secretion in human breast carcinoma. *Endocrinol Rev* 1987;8:29–43.

323. Knabbe C, Lippman ME, Wakefield LM, et al. Evidence that transforming growth factor- is a hormonally regulated negative growth factor in human breast cancer cell. *Cell* 1987;48:417–428.

324. Slamon DJ, Clark GM, Wong SG, Levin WJ, Ullrich A, McGuire WL. Human breast cancer: correlation of relapse and survival with amplification of the HER-2/neu oncogene. *Science* 1987;325:177–182.

325. Varley JM, Swallow JE, Brammar WJ, Whittaker JL, Walker RA. Alterations to either c-erbB-2

(neu) or c-myc proto-oncogenes in breast carcinomas correlate with poor short-term prognosis. *Oncogene* 1987;1:423–430.

326. Sporn MB, Roberts AB. Autocrine growth factors and cancer. *Nature* 1985;313:745–747.
327. Rijnders AWM, van der Korput JAGM, van Steenbrugge GJ, Romijn JC, Trapman J. Expression of cellular oncogenes in human prostatic carcinoma cell lines. *Biochem Biophys Res Commun* 1985;132:548–554.
328. Fleming WH, Hamel A, MacDonald R, et al. Expression of the c-myc protooncogene in human prostatic carcinoma and benign prostatic hyperplasia. *Cancer Res* 1986;46:1535–1538.
329. Buttyan R, Sawczuk IS, Benson MC, Siegal JD, Olsson CA. Enhanced expression of the c-myc protooncogene high-grade human prostate cancers. *Prostate* 1987;11:327–337.
330. Cooke DB, Quarmby VE, Mickey DD, Isaacs JT, French FS. Oncogene expression in prostate cancer: Dunning R3327 rat dorsal prostate adenocarcinoma system. *Prostate* 1988;13:263–272.
331. Curran T, Bravo R, Muller R. Transient induction of c-fos and c-myc is an immediate consequence of growth factor stimulation. *Cancer Surv* 1985;4:655–681.
332. Alt FW, Harlowe E, Ziff EB. Introduction. In: *Nuclear Oncogenes. CSH Current Communications in Molecular Biology.* New York: Cold Spring Harbor, 1987;1–26.
333. Marx JL. The fos gene as "master switch". *Science* 1987;237:854–856.
334. Viola MV, Fromowitz F, Oravez, et al. Expression of ras oncogene p21 in prostate cancer. *N Engl J Med* 1986;314:133–137.
335. Chesa PG, Rettig W, Melamed MR, Old JJ, Nirrian HL. Expression of p21 ras in normal and malignant tissues—lack of association with proliferation and malignancy. *Proc Natl Acad Sci U S A* 1987;84:3234–3238.
336. Varma VA, Austin GE, O'Connell AC. Antibodies to ras oncogenes p21 proteins lack immunohistochemical specificity for neoplastic epithelium in human prostate tissue. *Arch Pathol Lab Med* 1989;113:16–19.
337. Treiger B, Isaacs J. Expression of a transfected v-Harvey-ras oncogene in a Dunning rat prostate adenocarcinoma and the development of high metastatic ability. *J Urol* 1988;140:1580–1586.
338. Peehl DM, Wehner N, Stamey TA. Activated Ki-ras oncogene in human prostatic adenocarcinoma. *Prostate* 1987;10:281–289.

Endocrine Dependent Tumors, edited by
Klaus-Dieter Voigt and Cornelius Knabbe.
Raven Press, Ltd., New York © 1991.

5

Biochemical Endocrinology of Prostate Cancer

*Hartmut Klein, †Max Bressel, ‡Hartwig Kastendieck, and
*Klaus-Dieter Voigt

*Department of Clinical Chemistry, Medical Clinic, University of Hamburg, D-2000
Hamburg 20, Federal Republic of Germany, and †Departments of Urology and
‡Pathology, Harburg General Hospital, D-2100 Hamburg 90,
Federal Republic of Germany

HORMONE DEPENDENCY OF PROSTATE CANCER: HISTORY AND PRESENT STATE

Prostatic functional and proliferative activities essentially depend on stimulation by androgens and consequently on the regular function of the gonads. This endocrine mechanism has been principally known at least since the eighteenth century (1), though its biochemical basis remained unclear until the hormone testosterone (for review see (2)) and its utilization by the prostate (3–8) could be identified. Even without any knowledge about its molecular mechanisms, first proposals to use the hormonal regulation of prostatic proliferation as an objective of therapeutical intervention against tumor diseases of the prostate, for example, by orchiectomy, were made during the last decade of the nineteenth century (9–11). At that time, however, the idea aimed at the palliation of severe cases of benign prostatic hyperplasia, though some of the clinically enlarged prostates seen in these early studies might have contained carcinomas.

Some decades later, several pioneering studies reviewed by Sharifi and Kiefer (12) which culminated in the famous papers of Charles Huggins and coworkers (13, 14), definitively established the benefits of androgen withdrawal in patients with cancer of the prostate. Since that time, the diminuation of androgenic stimuli by endocrine manipulations such as orchiectomy, treatment with estrogens, progestins, or antiandrogens, chemical castration by LHRH superagonists, as well as combinations of these techniques became the generally accepted therapeutical strategy for carcinomas of the prostate that can no more be cured by surgery (15–18).

Frequent failures of these therapeutical attempts to sufficiently control proliferative activities of prostatic carcinomas are still one of the most pressing problems in the field of urology. Most of the respective studies reported objective initial response rates in the order of 80% to 90% of the patients without detectable systematic differences between the various treatment modalities. In contrast, the intervals of response differed substantially, the shortest of them being less than half a year (19–31). From the point of view of clinical medicine, the remaining 10% to 20% initial nonresponders as well as the later relapses from endocrine treatment mark the so-called androgen-independent progress of prostate cancer. Though cursory and unsatisfying from a biochemical point of view, this clinical classification still represents the best-founded empirical definition of the states of androgen dependency or homone sensitivity in human prostate cancer.

As a consequence of the frequent relapses from hormonal treatment, survival rates of prostate cancer patients progressively decline beyond one year after the beginning of endocrine manipulations. These observations underline the limits of endocrine treatment despite all improvements achieved during the last fifty years. Insofar, the state of the art in prostate cancer therapy has only gradually but not fundamentally changed since Maximilian Bruch one and a half centuries ago characterized this disease as "serious, of bad prognosis, commonly lethal, and rarely cured, even with excision." Concerning the chances of treatment he already wrote "the cure employed is palliative" (32).

It is quite clear and generally accepted that progress in the field of endocrine management of prostate cancer essentially depend on and consequently demand for an improved insight in the behavior of these malignant cells *in vivo*. Their mechanisms of growth control and androgen utilization, as well as the linkages between these two fields of cellular biology are of particular interest. These aspects, however, are still objectives of controversial considerations.

A variety of mechanisms is discussed to explain failures of the endocrine control of prostate cancer. The two hypotheses that are focused on emphasize either the presence of androgen-independent cells in heterogenous carcinomas (33–37) or a continuated androgenic stimulation in spite of hormonal treatment (38–42). Insufficient antiandrogenic potencies or intrinsic androgeneities of antiandrogens (43), adaptation processes of androgen target cells to the conditions of androgen deficiency, principal limitations in the capacity of hormone depletion to kill prostatic target cells (44), and androgen-hypersensitive tumor cells (45) are other hypothetical mechanisms that are discussed to contribute to survival and progression of prostatic carcinomas under endocrine therapy.

Particularly the two first hypotheses mentioned deserve a more detailed reflection. From a theoretical point of view, two alternative definitions of androgen-independent cells are possible. Independence of hormonal stimulation could be defined by the capacity of cells to survive the absence of androgen or by their capacity to proliferate without androgenic stimuli. Because systemic treatment of cancer principally aim at an inhibition of cancer cell proliferation and at the death of these cells, both of these possible elements of hormone independence would counteract therapeutical successes. Animal studies with rat prostate and its tumors indicate the existence of both phenomenons, the androgen-independent proliferation being observed with malignant (46,47), an androgen-independent survival even with benign epithelial cells of the prostates (44,48).

Assuming the presence of androgen-independent clones in original tumor cell populations of human prostates, these cells can become predominant as a consequence of the selection pressure during therapeutical androgen withdrawal or even during the prediagnostic and pretreatment phase of tumor development, thus explaining relapses from endocrine treatment as well as the phenomenon of initial nonresponding. There is still no direct proof, however, for the factual existence of these kinds of androgen-independent clones in human prostate cancer tissues *in vivo*, it is still unclear how such clones arise (preformation in the benign mother tissue, spontaneous mutation, other forms of dedifferentiation, adaptation processes?), and also the cellular and molecular mechanisms of an androgen-independent growth are still unknown. Regarding the latter, first steps to clarification might have been done. Recent studies with cultured human prostate cancer cells *in vitro* indicate that auto- and paracrine effects of growth factors are involved in the proliferation of androgen-dependent as well as of androgen-independent cell lines (49,50) and that in androgen-dependent cells at least some growth factors and growth factor receptors are controlled by androgens (51,52), thus linking the cellular mechanisms of androgen utilization and growth control. Presuming an androgenic control of growth factor mechanisms in normal cells of the prostate, it can be hypothesized that cancer cells could reach an autonomous state of proliferation by switching to an androgen-independent production of and/or response to these growth factors. Further studies on the endocrine control of peptide growth factors in human prostatic carcinomas might clarify cellular mechanisms of treatment-resistant proliferation. At this point, however, possible contributions of autonomous growth factor-related processes to this phenomenon remain to be established.

The alternative idea that orchiectomy or comparable endocrine manipulations might achieve an only incomplete control of androgenic stimuli and that remaining hormonal influences on the carcinomas might contribute to further tumor growth was first considered by Huggins when he introduced the additional adrenalectomy in the treatment of advanced prostate cancer (53). Since these first trials, the elimination of adrenal endocrine activities by surgical or functional adrenalectomy, the latter achieved by hypophysectomy or by pharmacological means, has been repeatedly used as a second-line intervention in patients with progressive tumor growth in spite of previous orchiectomy (54–71). Individually impressive but generally limited successes of these measures supported the idea that hormonal effects might be involved at least in some of the cases of the so-called androgen-independent progression of relapsing tumors, though the more frequent failures to achieve at least transient palliative effects by adrenalectomy indicate that the majority of these advanced stages of prostate cancer proliferate due to other mechanisms. The idea was later boostered by very optimistic reports about successes of the so-called "total androgen withdrawal" that combines surgical or functional castration with additional antiandrogen treatment (40–42). Moreover, the detection of steroid metabolizing enzymes in benign prostatic tissues (72,73) and prostatic carcinomas (74) that could metabolize steroids of adrenal origin along the pathway to DHT further supported the concept of residual androgens that continuate hormonal stimulation subsequent to orchiectomy. Possessing these kinds of enzymes, tumor cells of patients treated by androgen ablation are possibly not restricted to the utilization of the small amounts of testosterone that circulate in the blood of castrated men, but might gain access to the substantial amounts of testosterone precursors that might be converted to DHT directly in the malignant androgen target cells. Principal capacities of these steroids to replace deficient testosterone could be established by animal studies with rats (75–77). Their real involvement in the androgenic stimulation of prostatic carcinomas under conditions of endocrine treatment and consequently in the failures of this therapeutical strategy, however, are not established.

All of the hypotheses concerning failures of the endocrine management of prostate cancer are nearly exclusively based on model studies and *in vitro* experiments. Comparable data from original human cancer tissues that could support or disprove one or another aspect of these hypotheses are naturally rare (38,74–88). Many studies dealing with hormone utilization of prostate cancer were hampered by the well-known difficulties of obtaining sufficient amounts of pure cancer tissues from a substantial number of patients. The recent establishment of the tumor line PC-82 for the first time allowed an extension of only descriptive studies on original human tumor tissues to functional experiments (85–87). Though particularly promising as a model system without the principal disadvantages of *in vitro* cultured and clonally selected cell lines, one should also bear in mind that this tumor line as descendant of an individual carcinoma cannot represent prostate cancer as a whole. This purpose needs precise descriptive characterizations of larger groups of carcinomas belonging to various types of differentiation.

Recently, we established experimental techniques that allow a broad characterization of functions of steroid utilization in prostate cancer primary tumors (73). These procedures involved: (1) The acquisition of tumor tissues by total prostatectomies that were routinely done to cure the respective cancer patients by surgical means. (2) The isolation of sufficient amounts of tumor tissues from these totally excised organs by step sections. This technique obtained pure or nearly pure cancer samples in the order of 1.5 g per patient as well as sufficient amounts of tissue from benign parts of the prostates. On this basis, an individual comparison between the respective tumor and its individual benign surrounding tissue became possible. (3) Analytical procedures that quantified enzymes involved in the synthesis of DHT from testosterone or alternative precursor steroids as well as enzymes of DHT desactivation, procedures that quantified the steroids involved in these pathways as substrates or products of the enzymes, and procedures that quantified the subcellular distribution of DHT as a measure of androgen receptor (AR) function. Working on the basis of 1.5 g of tissue, these techniques give an opportunity to analyze most of the functions of androgen utilization that are of interest for the discussion of endocrine aspects of prostate cancer. This chapter summarizes endocrine characteristics of 23 carcinomas that were evaluated by these techniques and discusses their biological implications. Moreover, fundamental aspects of the analytical work with prostate cancer tissues and of the interpretation of resulting data will be discussed.

TUMOR CHARACTERISTICS AND BASIC ASPECTS OF EVALUATION

Before dealing with functions of steroid utilization and their biological implications in prostate cancer, some aspects of fundamental importance in these kinds of studies will be outlined. These aspects are selecting samples for evaluation and selecting reference points for the data's subsequent interpretation.

One major problem regarding selecting samples results from the dissiminated spread of carcinomas in the prostate. Because of this frequent type of growth, many carcinomas of the prostate are forming tissue areas of mixed benign and malignant cells. Though representing a substantial percentage of all prostatic carcinomas, these tissue mixtures are principally unsuitable to characterize the respective tumor and consequently have to be excluded from appropriate studies to prevent misinterpretations. Only prostatic carcinomas that show the compact type of tumor growth and that are consequently devoid of substantial contamination by benign epithelial cells are suitable for biochemical characterization. Unfortunately, these tumors represent only a minority of the prostatic carcinomas, and this fact seriously limits the access to tumor samples. Aiming at reliable data, however, this limitation must be accepted.

Our study was consequently restricted to prostates with compact growing tumors that allowed the isolation of entirely—or at least nearly—pure tumor tissues, the latter being samples with benign contaminations of less than 10% of the tissue volume. The 23 primary tumors that fulfilled this postulate and that were selected for the present study from much larger series of prostatectomies comprised all common types of histological differentiation and grades of malignancy (Table 1), including some cases of extraordinary characteristics (Fig. 1). Their unequal distribution between the various morphological types of prostate cancer reflects corresponding frequencies of these types of differentiation being found in patients, most of them naturally belonging to the typical pluriform (mixed glandular-cribriform) type and being of medium malignancy. Insofar, this group of tumors might be representative of prostate cancer. Their unequal distribution on the morphological subclasses, however, hampers the search for correlations between biochemical and morphological characteristics of the evaluated tumors. From this point of view, interest in a substantial extension of the evaluated tumor series that would allow the acquisition of more samples of the rare types of prostate cancer competes with the previously mentioned problems of sample acquisition, and even the unique tumor series presented here represents a compromise between the desirable and the possible. Again, pragmatism demands for the acceptance of the possible and of its inherent limitations. Despite these limitations, however, our group of 23 compact grown prostatic carcinomas allows a survey of the mechanisms of androgen utilization within the complex field of this tumor disease, at least with respect to the developmental stage of cancer cell populations that are represented by these primary tumors.

A variety of aspects have to be discussed concerning points of reference for the interpretation of data obtained from cancerous samples. First, and regarding the

TABLE 1. *Morphological and basic biochemical characteristics of the evaluated primary tumors*

Case no.	Grading *			Histological** type	DNA		Hydroxiproline	
	(A)	(B)	(C)		Cancer	Benign	Cancer	Benign
1	2–3	II b	I b	1	2.29	2.50	5.56	5.06
2	2–2	II a	I b	1	1.66	1.31	n.d.	3.27
3	1–2	I b	I b	1	2.39	1.59	2.83	4.42
4	3–2	III a	II a	2	3.84	1.55	5.11	5.24
5	3–3	III b	II a	2	3.52	2.07	3.84	2.68
6	2–3	II b	II a	2	3.32	2.45	1.93	4.02
7	2–2	II b	II a	2	3.35	1.35	3.32	5.73
8	2–3	III a	II a	2	1.83	1.50	4.00	3.84
9	3–3	III a	II b	2	3.87	2.12	4.41	3.22
10	5–3	III a	II b	4	3.74	2.14	3.10	5.10
11	3–5	III b	II b	2	3.17	1.75	3.74	3.35
12	3–4	III a	II b	2	2.58	1.96	2.27	3.62
13	3–3	III a	II b	2	4.60	3.37	3.16	3.66
14	3–3	III a	II b	2	3.17	2.37	4.16	2.79
15	3–3	III a	II b	2	2.67	1.57	4.46	5.46
16	3–3	III a	II b	2	3.22	1.43	5.05	4.79
17	4–3	II b	II b	3	3.60	2.64	2.42	3.78
18	4–4	III b	III a	3	3.12	1.87	3.54	5.02
19	5–3	III b	III a	2	3.63	1.20	3.59	4.50
20	4–5	III b	III a	2	1.63	0.91	3.69	5.26
21	5–5	III a	ill a	3	1.76	1.31	3.22	3.27
22	4–5	III b	III b	2	2.60	1.94	3.38	4.06
23	4–3	III b	III b	4	2.02	0.77	n.d.	n.d.

Primary tumors compared to data from the benign prostatic tissues of the same patients.
*Grading according to Gleason (88) (A), according to Helpap (98) (B), and modified for quantitative aspects (C) as outlined on page 155.
**Types of histological differentiation: (1) uniform glandular, (2) typical pluriform (mixed glandular/cribriform), (3) uniform cribriform, (4) pluriform (mixed cribriform/solid). The concentrations of DNA and hydroxiproline are given as mg/g of tissue wet weight; n.d., not determined.

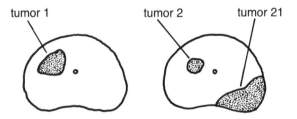

FIG. 1. Atypical central and ventral positions of the tumors no. 1 and 2 as compared to the typical peripheral and dorsolateral localization of prostatic carcinomas shown by tumor no. 21. Regarding this atypical localization as well as their high differentiation, these tumors are transition zone carcinomas (89) that resembled the incidental type of prostate cancer. Views on central sections through the prostate perpendicular to the urethra. Notice the simultaneous presence of two carcinomas (nos. 2 and 21) of completely different morphological characteristics within the same prostate.

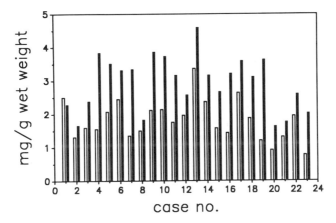

FIG. 2. DNA contents of prostatic carcinomas (filled columns) as compared to their individual benign surrounding tissues (open columns). Notice regularly inceased DNA contents of the carcinomas and the exceptional character of tumor no. 1.

internal point of reference, enzyme activities and steroid concentrations can be expressed in relation to the tissue weight or to its DNA content. In principle, data related to DNA are thought to parallel the cellular contents. From a biological point of view, this way of expression seems to be particularly useful for benign tissues that are formed by identical cells with uniform degree of ploidy. Contents expressed per DNA of these tissues consequently approximate the identical cellular contents of all of their individual cells. Tissues of this type can be compared by data expressed per DNA. Malignant tissues, however, frequently are composed of cells that differ from benign cells as well as from each other with respect to their degree of ploidy. Regularly increased DNA contents of carcinomas (Fig. 2) consequently reflect the sum of two effects, that is, an increased density of cells within the tumor tissues and an increased average DNA content per cell. Because of the shift in the cellular amount of DNA, effects of an increased density of cells on data obtained from carcinomas cannot be balanced by an expression in relation to the tissue's DNA content. Moreover, and because of the cancer's heterogeneous ploidy, contents expressed per DNA of malignant tissues would only represent average but not individual cellular contents, and even this value would still be a function of the distribution curves of cellular DNA in particular tumors. Accordingly, tumor tissue data expressed per DNA are neither comparable with each other nor with data from nonmalignant samples, and any attempt to ignore this problem would lead to an increased confusion. Only intranuclear concentrations of biological materials, for example, nuclear DHT, can be expressed in relation to the nuclear DNA content and compared to each other without falsification by incomparable points of reference.

The alternative type of expression in relation to the wet weight of the tissue avoids these problems of DNA references. Comparisons of benign and malignant tissues of the human prostate on this basis, however, are hampered by different densities of cells in these two types of tissue. Expressing data per tissue weight, an increased density of epithelial cells per tissue volume could easily simulate an increased activity of cellular functions, for example, of enzyme activities or steroid accumulation capacities. Obviously, neither DNA nor tissue weight represent an ideal point of reference for cancer data. Without this ideal internal point of reference and balancing advantages and disadvantages of both nonideal alternatives against each other, we preferred the expression per tissue weight as the less problematical kind of data presentation. Though superior in causing easier identifiable and thus easier controlable artifacts, the limitations of this type of expression have to be considered when dealing with the tumor data presented in the following chapters.

An appropriate external point of reference for the steroid utilization in prostatic carcinomas should ensure the identification of cancer-typical alterations and clearly differentiate these kinds of changes from methods-related phenomenons and artifacts. Materials to be considered for this task are the blood of cancer patients, benign areas of their cancerous prostates, and noncancerous prostates from other men, for example, BPH patients or organ donors. Aspects to be evaluated during these considerations are influences of plasma steroids on the intratissular steroid concentrations, effects of the surgical procedure and of the sampling technique on tissue steroid levels and enzyme activities, and possible differences between benign areas of cancerous and noncancerous prostates, that is, whether or not cancerous organs might be characterized by cancer-associated changes even outside the tumor.

The external endocrine milieu as reflected by plasma steroid patterns influences assessable intratissular, and this includes the intracarcinomatous, steroid concentrations by its regular steroid supply function, as well as by unavoidable plasma contaminations of the excised tissues. Any use of steroid tissue levels as markers of the tissue-specific steroid metabolism and binding *in vivo*, however, essentially depend on the predominance of these intratissular factors that should be exclusively or at least predominantly reflected by the tissue steroid concentrations. To exclude substantial effects of external factors on intraprostatic steroid patterns or, alternatively, to balance them by using steroid plasma concentrations as reference points, we have compared intraprostatic steroid concentrations with those of appropriate blood samples that were taken immediately before the prostatectomies. These experiments did not reveal any correlation between plasma and tissue levels of the particular steroids, neither for malignant nor for benign areas of the prostates (data not shown). This finding confirms the predominant role of the intraprostatic enzyme apparates and AR system in regulating intraprostatic steroid levels in the carcinomas as well as in the regular prostate. On the other hand, the obvious absence of decisive effects of the external steroidal milieu on intraprostatic steroid patterns excludes the use of plasma steroid levels as reference points, even to balance some substantial interindividual variations that could be observed, for example, for prostatic DHT contents.

In contrast to the plasma-tissue relationship, excellent correlations were found

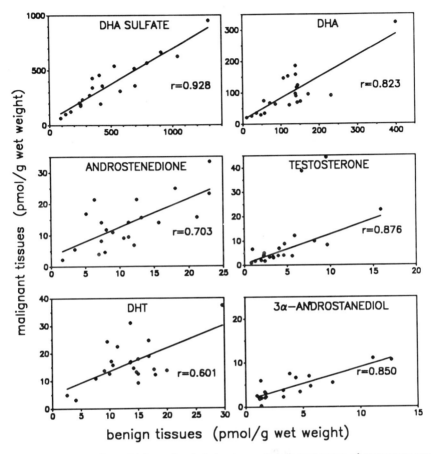

FIG. 3. Correlation of steroid tissue levels in benign and malignant areas of cancerous prostates. Excluding two or one exceptional testosterone and androstanediol values, respectively, from the calculation, most of the correlation coefficients exceeded 0.8, thus underlining the parallelism of factors that influence or control steroid levels in both compartments. Slightly lower coefficients of correlation for DHT and androstenedione indicate more substantial differences in metabolism and binding of these steroids by the corresponding benign and malignant parts of the prostates.

between steroid concentrations in the carcinomas and those in their individual benign surrounding tissues (Fig.3). This indicates that all factors that determine steroid levels in the carcinomas exert equal influences on steroids in the benign compartments of the prostates, including all artificial shifts in steroid content caused by the surgical procedure and the sampling technique (e.g., consequences of continuated steroid metabolism during the interval between surgical interruption of blood circulation and consequently of its steroid supply function and the subsequent freezing of tissues in liquid nitrogen that finally blocks all further metabolic processes). The obviously exceptional value of individual reference tissues in these kinds of

TABLE 2. *Steroid levels and enzyme activities in benign parts of cancerous prostates (n = 22) as compared to data from noncancerous prostates of BPH patients and organ donors (n = 12)*

Steroid or enzyme	Cancerous prostates	Noncancerous prostates
DHA sulfate	294 ± 53	199 ± 126
DHA	70.5 ± 10.9	55.4 ± 30.9
4-androstenedione	6.62 ± 0.90	5.25 ± 2.31
Testosterone	2.86 ± 0.57	3.45 ± 1.99
DHT	7.81 ± 0.94	6.18 ± 0.84
3α-androstanediol	2.23 ± 0.43	2.37 ± 0.37
Sulfatase	24.6 ± 2.1	31.4 ± 10.1
17β-HSDH	7.41 ± 0.60	11.2 ± 1.8
5α-reductase	2.25 ± 0.27	2.52 ± 0.42

(The data are expressed as pmol/mg DNA and nmol/h·mg DNA for steroids and enzymes, respectively. Means ± SEM.)

studies that balance all artificial influences on the carcinomas, however, essentially depends on the absence of cancer-associated changes in these benign mother tissues. To ensure this absence of cancer-associated changes in benign areas of cancerous prostates, we compared their steroid levels and enzyme activities with those measured by identical techniques in other prostates that were free of cancerous alterations. As from comparisons with previously published steroid concentrations in noncancerous prostates (90–92), no evidence for systematic cancer associated changes in the benign neighborhood of prostatic carcinomas derived from these experiments (Table 2), thus revealing the individual benign surrounding tissues in fact being ideal external points of reference for the steroid utilization in prostatic carcinomas. The following description of functions of steroid utilization in prostate cancer primary tumors consequently will be based on the permanent and direct comparison between benign and malignant prostatic compartments of individual patients.

FORMATION, ACCUMULATION, AND DESACTIVATION OF DHT

It is generally accepted that the androgenic stimulation of prostatic target cells is mediated through the binding of DHT to the androgen receptor and the intranuclear activities that are subsequently exerted by these steroid-receptor complexes. All factors participating in the control of intracellular DHT levels therefore should be of particular interest also in carcinomas of the prostate. Under the conditions of physiological hormonal environment, that is, regular function of the gonads and corresponding high plasma concentrations of testosterone, the intraprostatic level of DHT results from the equilibrium of three biochemical functions. These are the formation of DHT from testosterone by the enzyme 5α-reductase (EC 1.3.99.5), its subsequent desactivation by the enzymes 3α- and 3β- hydroxysteroid dehydrogenase (3α/β-HSDH, EC 1.1.1.50 and 1.1.1.51) and the transient sequestration of

TABLE 3. *Activities of steroid metabolizing enzymes in human prostate carcinomas and their individual benign surrounding tissues*

Case no.	Sulfatase		17β-HSDH		5α-reductase		3αβ-HSDH	
	Cancer	Benign	Cancer	Benign	Cancer	Benign	Cancer	Benign
1	32,1	46,1	11,8	9,54	2,68	2,93	11,1	11,8
2	n.d.	n.d.	9,00	7,00	2,40	2,64	n.d.	8,69
3	50,0	36,9	14,0	11,3	2,80	3,28	9,77	6,35
4	70,4	39,8	12,0	14,9	1,99	3,42	12,7	10,6
5	38,3	33,0	9,96	12,2	3,12	3,88	9,94	8,39
6	18,9	25,9	7,20	5,61	2,06	1,68	7,00	5,95
7	35,4	46,4	6,15	n.d.	1,86	4,46	3,67	5,45
8	26,8	31,5	13,9	11,4	2,08	2,34	3,84	6,28
9	65,4	77,4	10,3	14,0	1,04	3,00	11,4	7,73
10	124,6	61,9	11,0	12,7	2,17	4,48	9,78	11,2
11	64,8	45,0	11,2	13,6	1,43	5,47	9,62	10,2
12	45,9	51,6	7,20	19,0	0,94	6,16	8,42	13,6
13	32,4	59,2	9,56	24,8	1,48	6,92	6,81	11,0
14	34,8	31,8	6,00	12,6	1,80	4,73	5,76	8,63
15	32,1	53,7	6,56	12,9	1,07	3,56	6,89	7,24
16	27,6	25,2	10,8	15,4	0,64	3,29	8,17	4,28
17	41,5	35,8	10,5	13,2	2,50	3,14	8,00	7,86
18	24,0	31,8	8,46	10,0	1,82	3,29	6,63	7,76
19	32,7	54,0	16,1	11,6	0,51	3,17	8,72	8,36
20	30,4	21,0	4,81	9,70	1,12	1,72	2,26	6,20
21	27,6	36,4	13,4	7,00	1,30	2,64	4,39	8,69
22	41,6	36,3	19,0	17,0	1,65	3,03	10,3	12,6
23	38,8	35,6	9,16	11,5	0,84	5,78	5,10	6,35

(The data are expressed as nmol/h·g of tissue; n.d., not determined.)

DHT by high affinity binding to androgen receptors that temporarily protects this active androgen from an immediate enzymatic desactivation (92,93).

Regarding the formation of DHT from testosterone, 5α-reductase activities (Table 3) were found to be systematically (22/23 patients) and substantially (1.71 ± 0.15 vs. 3.70 ± 0.28 nmol/h·g, means ± sem) lower in the carcinomas as compared to surrounding benign areas of the prostates (Fig. 4). This highly significant loss of enzyme activity in the tumors (p<0.0001, paired two-tailed t-test) appeared to be even more impressive when the data were related to tissue DNA contents (0.63 ± 0.07 vs. 2.25 ± 0.27 nmol/h·mg DNA). Comparable effects of the use of DNA as point of reference also could be observed for other enzymes of the prostatic steroid metabolism. Though these data do not only reflect ratios of cellular activities, they might still indicate diminished efficiacies of the enhanced DNA contents of malignant cells to express specific cellular functions.

Because substantial amounts of the prostatic 5α-reductase are located in the stromal and particularly muscular elements of the organ, the question raises whether these losses of enzyme activity observed in malignant tissues are the result of decreased activities in the epithelial compartment, that is, in the real malignant cells, or additionally involve the intracarcinomatous but itself nonmalignant stroma. Re-

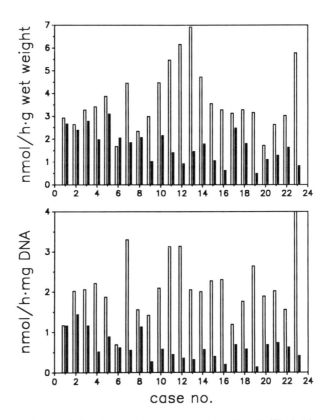

FIG. 4. 5α-Reductase activities in prostate cancer primary tumors (filled columns) as compared to their individual benign surrounding tissues (open columns). Enzyme activities are related to the tissue wet weight (upper panel) or to its DNA content (lower panel). Notice regular though quantitatively different losses of 5α-reductase in the carcinomas, their more impressive appearance when the data are related to DNA, and the obvious exception of the transition zone cancer no. 1. 5α-Reductase activities were found identical in this tumor and its benign surroundings even when the data are related to tissue DNA contents.

garding the latter, overall losses of 5α-reductase in prostate cancer could reflect factually decreased cellular enzyme activities in the stromal compartment. Alternatively, a shift in the intracarcinomatous ratio of malignant epithelium and benign stroma, the latter possibly being partially displaced by the proliferating tumor cells, has to be considered.

For an approximative quantification of stromal contributions to overall tumor volumes, intratissular hydroxiproline concentrations were used as biochemical marker of the collagen content. Comparing hydroxiproline contents in malignant and benign parts of the prostates (see Table 1), we found a small but statistically significant decrease in the group of carcinomas (3.66 ± 0.20 vs. 4.23 ± 0.20 mg/g, $p < 0.05$) that could be seen in 14/22 evaluated tumors (Fig. 5). These comparatively

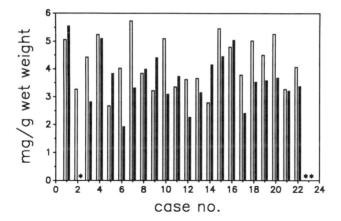

FIG. 5. Hydroxiproline contents of prostate cancer primary tumors (filled columns) as compared to their individual benign surrounding tissues (open columns). Notice generally similar hydroxiproline contents in both types of samples and less systematical deviations of the tumor data as compared to the tissue DNA concentrations. The hydroxiproline concentrations in the group of tumors (3.66 ± 0.20) were nevertheless found to be significantly lower (p<0.05) than those in benign parts of the prostates (4.23 ± 0.20), thus indicating a tendency to slightly lower amounts of stroma in cancerous areas of the prostates. (*no data available.)

small differences in overall stromal contributions to tissue volumes, however, cannot account for the substantial differences between the 5α-reductase activities in benign and malignant tissues. Accordingly, no correlation could be found between individual decreases in 5α-reductase activities and hydroxiproline contents (data not shown). Moreover, semiquantitative histological examinations of tissue slices revealed comparable amounts of muscular stroma being present in nearly all of the carcinomas and their benign surrounding tissues, with the only exception of tumor no. 12. This tumor showed one of the most prominent losses of 5α-reductase activity as compared to its benign neighborhood (see Fig. 4) and was nearly devoid of muscular stroma. Obviously, the losses of 5α-reductase activity observed in carcinomas cannot be explained by decreased overall amounts of stroma in these tissues or (with one exception) particular losses of muscular stroma from the primary tumors. Therefore, other and predominantly cellular factors have to be considered. Quantifications of the 5α-reductase distribution between malignant epithelium and nonmalignant stroma in prostate cancer primary tumors revealed parallel contributions of both compartments to the overall losses of enzyme activity (Fig. 6). Obviously, the characteristic losses of 5α-reductase in malignant tissues of the prostate are not restricted to the malignant cells but comparatively involve also the stromal compartment. Though speculative at this point, this phenomenon might reflect changes in the interactions of epithelial and stromal cells in prostate carcinomas. The exact mechanism of the parallel losses of 5α-reductase from cancer cells and intracarcinomatous stroma, however, remains to be elucidated.

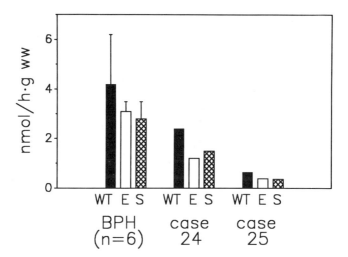

FIG. 6. 5α-reductase activities in whole tissue homogenates (filled columns) and separated epithelial (open columns) and stromal fractions (hatched columns). Mechanical separations of epithelium and stroma were performed by the standard techniques of Cowan and associates (93) as modified by Krieg and colleagues (95). The tumors no. 24 and 25 were obtained from prostates that were nearly completely filled with malignant tissue. Therefore, no benign prostatic tissues could be obtained from these patients for individual comparisons and in place of that kind of reference tissues, a group of samples from benign hyperplastic organs served for comparison. Tumor no. 24 was characterized by moderate, tumor no. 25 by substantial losses of 5α-reductase. Notice the involvement of both tissue fractions in the overall losses of enzyme activity and the parallelism of these losses in both tissue compartments. (ww = tissue wet weight.)

In contrast to the DHT-forming 5α-reductase pathway, capacities of DHT desactivation appeared to be essentially unchanged in the investigated group of carcinomas (see Table 3). No systematic or significant difference could be found between the 3αβ-HSDH activities measured in the cancer tissues and those detected in the surrounding benign parts of the respective prostates (7.74 ± 0.59 vs. 8.48 ± 0.53 nmol/h·g). Some variation, however, occurred and there were individual carcinomas with 3αβ-HSDH activities equal to those in their benign surroundings (5/22) as well as other tumors with higher (6/22) or lower (11/22) enzyme activities.

In the context of an unchanged DHT desactivation, one should expect that the partial but nevertheless substantial losses of the enzyme 5α-reductase would result in decreased tissue concentrations of its product DHT with a parallel increase in the tissue levels of the substrate testosterone. In fact, the latter phenomenon could be found, but no decrease in the tissue concentrations of DHT could be detected (Table 4). As expected, testosterone tissue concentrations (Fig. 7) were found to be significantly higher in the malignant samples (9.11 ± 2.46 vs. 4.66 ± 0.77 pmol/g, 16/23 cases, $p < 0.05$). But in contrast to the expectation, DHT concentrations measured

TABLE 4. *Concentrations of androgens and of their desactivation product 3α-androstanediol in human prostate carcinomas and benign tissues from the same prostates*

Case no.	Testosterone		5α-DHT		3α-androstanediol	
	Cancer	Benign	Cancer	Benign	Cancer	Benign
1	8,35	9,65	14,6	14,2	2,24	3,29
2	n.d.	15,9	17,9	15,0	23,5	5,65
3	5,10	2,29	15,7	10,6	6,61	4,38
4	8,85	4,69	22,4	11,4	2,00	1,37
5	3,71	2,23	24,6	16,9	n.d.	n.d.
6	9,98	8,19	24,3	9,62	2,55	0,96
7	1,77	2,39	17,1	10,3	3,42	1,65
8	3,55	3,33	3,11	4,09	2,10	1,15
9	3,06	3,39	13,7	20,0	5,53	7,57
10	7,03	4,05	12,6	10,0	3,22	1,71
11	6,68	0,92	31,1	13,7	6,99	5,53
12	1,72	1,25	9,22	15,0	5,98	1,30
13	4,27	2,25	18,9	16,9	n.d.	n.d.
14	44,3	9,62	37,3	29,7	3,46	4,74
15	4,11	4,58	16,6	13,6	10,6	12,7
16	3,38	2,92	16,9	13,7	7,53	3,84
17	2,05	1,94	13,7	9,10	2,09	1,68
18	38,7	6,76	13,2	14,7	3,80	3,27
19	1,09	0,78	9,60	3,90	2,30	1,75
20	3,98	3,95	10,9	7,60	0,27	1,34
21	22,7	15,9	12,5	15,0	4,73	5,65
22	3,84	5,58	14,1	17,8	11,0	11,1
23	12,2	5,87	12,2	18,0	1,82	1,20

(The data are expressed as pmol/g of tissue; n.d., not determined.)

in cancerous tissues (Fig. 8) were not decreased but found even higher as compared to the benign parts of the prostates (16.4 ± 1.6 vs. 13.5 ± 1.2 pmol/g, 15/23 cases, $p<0.05$). Only 3/23 evaluated tumors (nos. 9, 12, 23) showed substantial reductions in their total capacities for DHT accumulation (Fig. 8), tumor no. 12 being the most prominent among them with a 40% loss of DHT accumulation as compared to its benign neighborhood (Table 4). A tendency to higher levels of the DHT-desactivation product 3α-androstandiol (Table 4) in the tumors (5.32 ± 1.10 vs. 3.90 ± 0.72 pmol/g, 14/21 cases) additionally reflects the increased tissue concentrations of DHT found in most of the carcinomas.

Unchanged or even increased levels of DHT in the cancer tissues elucidate the hierarchy of mechanisms that participate in the regulation of intracellular DHT concentrations. Under normal *in vivo* conditions, amount or activity of the 5α-reductase obviously do not limit the accumulation of DHT, at least not as long as minimal 5α-reductase capacities are preserved. Though some alternative factors that also might contribute to the maintenance of DHT accumulation in prostate cancer principally have to be considered (e.g., an excess of cellular 5α-reductase capacity in normal prostatic tissues or contributions of circulating DHT that might be accumulated from the blood and bound to ARs without involving the intraprostatic 5α-reduc-

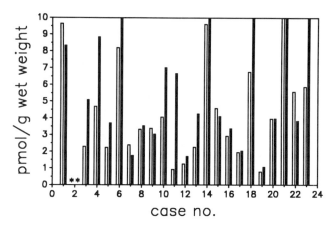

FIG. 7. Testosterone tissue concentrations in prostate cancer primary tumors (filled columns) and their benign surroundings (open columns). Notice frequently increased levels of testosterone in the carcinomas.

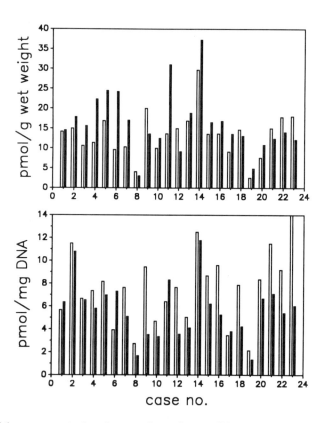

FIG. 8. DHT tissue concentrations in prostatic carcinomas (filled columns) and in surrounding benign areas of the prostates (open columns). Amounts of steroids are related to the tissue wet weight (upper panel) or to the DNA contents (lower panel). Notice the generally preserved or even increased DHT accumulation in the tumors and the only few exceptions (tumors no. 9 and 12).

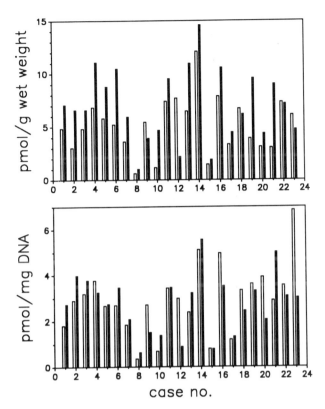

FIG. 9. Nuclear DHT concentrations in prostatic carcinomas (filled columns) and in surrounding benign areas of the prostates (open columns) related to the tissue wet weight (upper panel) or to the DNA contents of the nuclear fractions (lower panel). Notice that the nuclear accumulation of DHT is preserved or even increased in most of the tumors and the particular loss of nuclear DHT accumulation in carcinoma no. 12.

tion), this finding impressively underlines the pivotal role of the androgen receptor system and of its DHT sequestration capacity in the regulation of intracellular DHT levels. The regularly normal capacity of DHT accumulation in the carcinomas strongly indicate the presence of quantitatively unchanged and functionally intact ARs in these tumors. Moreover, essentially unchanged or even increased capacities of nuclear DHT accumulation (Fig. 9) that can be concluded from the DHT concentrations measured in nuclear fractions of the tumor tissues and from ratios of intranuclear and total tissue DHT in these tumors (Table 5) support the hypothesis of an intact AR system in the majority of these carcinomas. Obviously, an intact AR system maintains the normal accumulation of DHT in tumor tissues in spite of substantial losses of 5α-reductase, at least under the conditions of physiological hormonal environment from which these primary tumors have been obtained. Comparing nuclear DHT concentrations (Fig. 9) and ratios of nuclear and total DHT in the tumors and benign surrounding tissues (Table 5), only 1/23 evaluated tumors revealed a substantial loss of nuclear DHT accumulation capacity. It suggests itself

TABLE 5. *Comparison of DHT concentrations in nuclear fractions prepared from human prostate primary tumors and benign prostatic tissue areas from the same patients*

Case no.	(A) Cancer	(A) Benign	(B) Cancer	(B) Benign	(C) Cancer	(C) Benign
	Nuclear DHT					
1	7,10	4,84	2,74	1,81	48.6	34.1
2	6,62	3,02	3,99	2,90	37.0	20.1
3	6,62	4,81	3,78	3,19	42.2	45.4
4	11,1	6,84	3,26	3,76	49.6	60.0
5	8,81	5,81	2,75	2,67	35.8	34.4
6	10,5	5,22	3,47	2,69	43.2	54.3
7	5,97	3,60	2,09	1,84	34.9	35.0
8	1,03	0,61	0,64	0,35	33.1	14.9
9	3,95	5,45	1,52	2,71	28.8	27.3
10	4,69	1,16	1,38	0,68	37.2	11.6
11	9,57	7,41	3,47	3,43	30.8	54.1
12	2,20	7,70	0,89	2,98	23.9	51.3
13	11,0	6,48	3,23	2,38	58.2	38.3
14	14,6	12,1	5,57	5,11	39.1	40.7
15	1,92	1,45	0,79	0,79	11.6	10.7
16	10,6	7,88	3,53	4,96	62.7	57.5
17	4,49	3,33	1,32	1,19	32.8	36.6
18	6,21	6,72	2,46	3,33	47.1	45.7
19	4,95	2,55	1,71	2,36	51.6	65.4
20	4,37	3,09	2,07	3,91	40.1	40.7
21	9,03	3,02	5,02	2,90	72.2	20.1
22	7,18	7,31	3,09	3,55	50.9	41.1
23	4,76	6,10	3,03	6,85	39.0	33.9

(The data are expressed as pmol/g of tissue (A), pmol/mg DNA (B), and % of the respective total tissue DHT content (C).)

that this tumor (no. 12) lost its ARs at least partially. Though the mechanism of this receptor loss remains unclear at this point, the remarkable parallels between apparent loss of ARs, loss of DHT accumulation capacity, and exceptional high loss of 5α-reductase activity in this carcinoma gains further attention and will be discussed later.

Summarizing these findings, the great majority of prostate cancer primary tumors that had not undergone previous endocrine manipulations possesses principally identical mechanisms of DHT formation, accumulation, and desactivation. Quantitatively, the carcinomas are characterized by gradual losses of 5α-reductase without systematic deviations in the desactivation of DHT. In spite of this shift in the balance between DHT forming and desactivating enzyme activities, overall capacities of DHT accumulation are still normal, obviously because of intact ARs in these tumors. This regularly normal system of androgen metabolism and accumulation in prostatic carcinomas corresponds to the clinical experience that most of the carcinomas initially respond to androgen ablation treatment. It consequently might be concluded that an essentially unchanged system of androgen metabolism and accumulation indicate androgen-dependence of the respective tumor.

ADRENAL ANDROGENS

In the presence of testes with normal endocrine function, testosterone dominates the androgenic stimulation of peripheral tissues. Steroids of adrenal origin are not thought to contribute to androgenic effects on androgen target cells under these conditions. Following an elimination of the testicular testosterone secretion by therapeutic means, however, the situation might be different. Under these conditions of testosterone deficiency, adrenal androgens have been suggested to stimulate the proliferation of prostatic carcinomas via peripheral conversion to testosterone and DHT, for example, directly in the tumor cells.

Considering principal pathways of steroid metabolism (Fig. 10), four of the steroids secreted by the adrenals are of particular interest in this context, that is, 5-androstenediol, 4-androstenedione, DHA, and DHA sulfate. These compounds are precursors of each other and of testosterone in the biochemical cascade that subse-

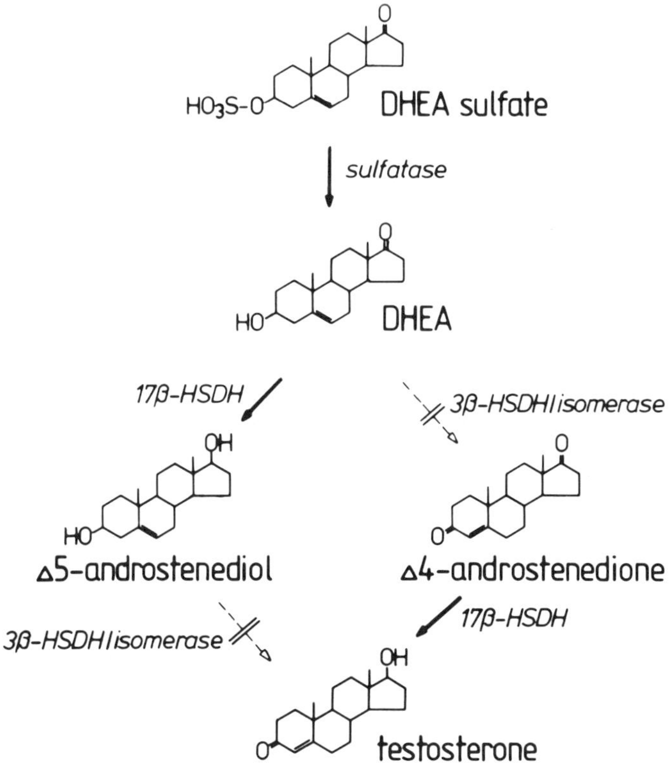

FIG. 10. Biochemical pathways from adrenal precursor steroids to testosterone in benign tissues of the human prostate.

quently involves three enzymes, that is, the steroid sulfate sulfatase (EC 3.1.6.2, production of free DHA by cleavage of DHA sulfate), the 3β-HSDH- Δ^{4-5}-isomerase complex (EC 1.1.1.145, formation of androstenedione from DHA and of testosterone from androstenediol), and the 17β-hydroxisteroid dehydrogenases (17β-HSDH, EC 1.1.1.63 and 1.1.1.64, conversion of DHA to androstenediol and of androstenedione to testosterone) (93). Benign tissues of the human prostate are well characterized for this enzymatic apparatus. They possess substantial activities of 17β-HSDH (72) and steroid sulfate sulfatase (73) which allow the conversion of DHA sulfate to DHA and 5-androstenediol as well as the formation of testosterone from androstenedione (Fig. 10). In contrast, only very low activities of the 3β-HSDH-Δ^{4-5}-isomerase complex could be detected (9). Biologically, these low isomerase activities in the order of the detection limit of a highly sensitive procedure obviously are irrelevant and do not link the enormous amounts of circulating DHA sulfate to the intraprostatic formation of testosterone via the 17β-HSDH pathway and the intermediate metabolites androstenedione or 5-androstenediol. The well-known involution of the prostate following castration confirms the practical absence of isomerase in human prostates, because otherwise this organ would be independent of testicular androgens. As a consequence of the missing enzymatic link between sulfatase and 17β-HSDH, the metabolic capacities of benign tissues of the prostate do only allow the use of androstenedione as substrate of an intraprostatic testosterone formation under conditions of testosterone deficiency.

In malignant tissues of the human prostate, this enzyme apparatus might maintain the androgenic stimulation on a reduced level and compensate at least partially the lack of testosterone that follows orchiectomy or chemical castration. Any contribution of these kinds of processes to the progression of prostatic carcinomas essentially depends on the availability of substantial amounts of precursor steroids in the circulating blood even under the conditions of androgen-ablative treatment, the presence of sufficient activities of the respective enzymes in the cancer tissues, and androgen-dependent growth control mechanisms in the cancer cells that allow proliferation only in response to available androgens. Concerning the last of these postulates, our extremely limited knowledge about the mechanisms of androgenic growth control in prostatic cells has to be kept in mind. Moreover, not only the principal linkages of steroids and growth control in the prostate would have to be known for an estimation of the role of adrenal androgens in stimulation of prostate cancer, but also the fate of these mechanisms during tumor initiation, tumor progression, and endocrine treatment. At this point, no answers are available to these questions and therefore all aspects related to the other two postulates only can be discussed on the understanding that the principal linkages between androgens and cellular growth control are preserved during the malignant transformation of prostatic epithelium as well as during the subsequent progression of the resulting tumor.

Concerning plasma levels of androgen precursors under conditions of therapeutical androgen ablation, that is, following an elimination of the testicular endocrine activities, substantial concentrations of androstenedione, DHA, and DHA sulfate are maintained in the circulating blood (96). Figure 11 illustrates this situation and

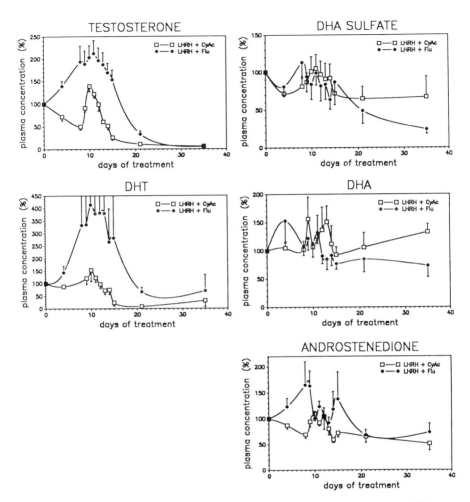

FIG. 11. Response of steroid plasma concentrations to chemical castration by LHRH treatment in combination with antiandrogens (so-called total androgen ablation). During these trials, the antiandrogen treatment (either cyproterone acetate 200 mg/d or flutamide 750 mg/d p.o.) was begun 7 days before the first s.c. depot injection of the LHRH agonist Zoladex (3.6 mg/month) in order to prevent or to attenuate possible flare phenomenons. Notice the different effects of the two antiandrogens on the initially increasing testosterone concentrations during the first phase of LHRH treatment and the obvious superiority of the progestional drug cyproterone acetate in this context as compared to the pure antiandrogen flutamide. In contrast to the excessively decreasing concentrations of testosterone and DHT, both modalities of endocrine treatment had only minor effects on the plasma levels of the possible testosterone precursors androstenedione, DHA, and DHA sulfate. Means ± SEM of 5 patients per group.

the different effects of castration (in this case chemical castration) on plasma levels of active androgens and of their biochemical precursors. This treatment reduces the plasma concentrations of testosterone and of its metabolite DHT to 5% and 10%, respectively, of their initial levels (corresponding to about 1 nmol/1 testosterone and 0.1 nmol/1 DHT). In contrast, plasma concentrations of androstenedione, DHA, and DHA sulfate are less influenced by LHRH treatment or remain essentially unchanged. Under castration conditions, plasma levels in the order of 1 nmol/1 androstenedione, 3 nmol/1 DHA, and 1μmol/1 DHA sulfate are still available for the peripheral formation of testosterone, provided that appropriate enzymes are active in the respective tissue.

Primary tumors of prostate cancer did not substantially differ from benign prostatic tissues in their enzymatic apparatus for conversion of these precursor steroids to testosterone. Steroid sulfate sulfatase activities in the carcinomas (see Table 3) equaled those in the benign surrounding tissues (42.6 ± 4.9 vs. 41.7 ± 2.9 nmol/h·g), and similar 17β-HSDH activities (see Table 3) were found in the malignant and benign parts of cancerous prostates (10.5 ± 0.7 vs. 12.6 ± 0.9 nmol/h·g). A tendency to lower activities of 17β-HSDH in the carcinomas (14/22 cases), however, could be observed (Fig. 12). With regard to the activity of the 3β-HSDH-Δ^{4-5}-isomerase complex in the human prostate, controversial results have been published (72,97). Using improved and highly sensitive techniques, we recently measured very low activities of this enzyme in samples of cancerous prostates without significant differences between the benign areas of the organs and the carcinomas (92). The

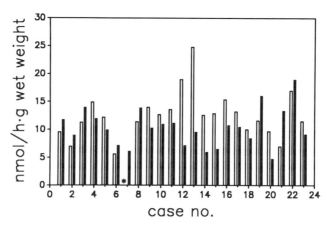

FIG. 12. 17β-HSDH activities in prostate cancer primary tumors (filled columns) as compared to benign tissue areas of the same prostates (open columns). The tendency to lower enzyme activities in the malignant tissues (14/22 cases) was near the level of significance. (*not determined.)

TABLE 6. *Tissue concentrations of adrenal steroids in benign and malignant parts of cancerous prostates*

Case no.	DHA-sulfatase		DHA		Androstenedione		5-androstenediol	
	Cancer	Benign	Cancer	Benign	Cancer	Benign	Cancer	Benign
1	313	577	72,6	151,4	6,82	12,1	2,90	1,97
2	n.d.	130	n.d.	35,4	9,48	11,3	n.d.	n.d.
3	566	798	153,1	119,1	4,62	7,83	n.d.	n.d.
4	235	270	67,7	70,8	14,1	7,34	0,33	0,14
5	360	431	95,1	171,9	4,02	6,96	1,17	1,30
6	179	255	30,0	46,9	n.d.	n.d.	2,78	2,40
7	125	172	35,1	56,9	n.d.	n.d.	1,70	2,75
8	655	911	117,4	141,7	11,8	8,04	n.d.	n.d.
9	950	1295	322,9	400,7	16,9	5,14	7,57	9,83
10	191	254	69,4	142,7	33,4	23,1	2,24	2,62
11	204	244	90,3	139,6	24,9	18,1	2,07	1,93
12	200	248	96,9	138,5	21,4	6,36	2,48	2,86
13	274	329	146,9	107,6	21,4	12,5	1,54	1,51
14	196	417	158,3	139,2	15,7	21,2	2,50	1,82
15	458	408	185,8	138,9	15,6	13,2	3,81	7,12
16	343	351	26,6	22,6	9,13	10,6	3,43	1,47
17	540	530	75,3	54,9	2,20	1,64	2,80	3,84
18	429	352	64,2	85,4	14,0	15,7	1,65	2,82
19	626	1044	91,0	231,2	23,2	23,0	1,10	1,00
20	67	90	21,5	9,7	8,22	7,31	n.d.	n.d.
21	102	130	35,8	35,4	14,1	11,3	n.d.	n.d.
22	516	695	124,3	144,1	11,0	8,99	6,17	7,10
23	360	699	61,1	122,6	5,59	3,46	n.d.	n.d.

(The data are expressed as pmol/g of tissue wet weight. Means ± sem; n.d., not determined.)

metabolic capacities of these primary tumors to form testosterone from steroids of adrenal origin therefore should correspond to those of benign tissues of the human prostate (see Fig. 10). Consequently, androstenedione, but not 5-androstenediol, DHA, or DHA sulfate might be utilized for an intraprostatic formation of testosterone under conditions of androgen deficiency though substantial amounts of all of these steroids are available in the tumor tissues (Table 6).

Factual contributions of an intraprostatic conversion of adrenal steroids to the prostatic accumulation of DHT under conditions of androgen deficiency are not easy to establish. It is particularly difficult to differentiate this kind of DHT formation from the extraprostatic steroid metabolism that also forms testosterone from adrenal precursors. Overall effects, however, of the adrenal steroid secretion on prostatic DHT contents under these conditions could be quantified in patients with an LHRH/antiandrogen treatment before prostatectomy (Table 7). In these patients, chemical castration decreased total tissue levels of DHT in the prostates to the order of 15% and the nuclear DHT concentrations to the order of 30% of concentrations

TABLE 7. *DHT tissue concentrations in cancerous prostates of patients treated by an LHRH agonist (Zoladex 3.6 mg/month s.c.) and an antiandrogen (cyproterone acetate 150 mg/d p.o.) during 8 weeks before the total prostatectomy*

Case	Total DHT		Nuclear DHT		Nuclear DHT (%)	
no.	Cancer	Benign	Cancer	Benign	Cancer	Benign
26	2.71	2.48	1.88	2.48	69	100
27	2.44	n.d.	2.38	n.d.	98	n.d.
28	1.67	0.67	1.21	0.48	72	71

(The data are expressed as pmol/g of tissue and % of the total DHT content, respectively. n.d., not determined.)

measured in prostates of untreated cancer patients. Compared to 5% remaining testosterone in the blood, this observation indicates an increased efficacy of the prostatic DHT accumulation under castration conditions. The high percentage of residual DHT found in the nuclear fractions of evaluated tissue samples illustrates again the role of androgen receptors in the prostatic DHT accumulation. Moreover, these data reflect the limited potency of the antiandrogen to block the ARs completely and to compete successfully with the residual amounts of DHT. Obviously, the antiandrogen did not prevent remaining DHT from the binding to androgen receptors and from subsequent translocation to the nuclei. It has to be concluded that even combinations of castration and antiandrogen treatment do not achieve a state of total androgen withdrawal from prostatic tumor cells. The biological consequences of these residual amounts of androgen on the proliferative activities of prostate tumor tissues remain to be elucidated. Principally, failures of combination therapies to sufficiently control the proliferation of prostatic carcinomas might be explained by these residual amounts of androgen and therefore do not establish an androgen-independent character of treatment-resistant tumor progression.

LINKAGES OF MORPHOLOGY AND BIOCHEMISTRY

Parallels between biochemical and morphological characteristics of prostate cancer could be derived from the systematic variation of parameters within the group of evaluated tumors as well as from particular properties of some exceptional carcinomas. Before dealing with these parallels, some aspects of the morphological classification of cancer and of their consequences for biochemical evaluations have to be discussed.

In principle, developmental capacities of prostatic carcinomas and the prognostic consequences of these capacities are read from morphological characteristics of the tumor tissues. Because the aspect of prognosis naturally dominates the interest in tumor classification from the clinical point of view, morphological grading systems are focussed on the description of characteristics that allow an assessment of the patient's presumable fate. Aiming at optimal prognostic statements, the grading system of Helpap and coworkers (97) handles the heterogeneous morphology of prostatic carcinomas by fixing overall grades of malignancy at the most malignant areas of the tumor that are thought to determine the patient's fate. Quantitative contributions of different tissue areas to the overall tumor volume do not play any role in this grading system that is exclusively based on qualitative classifications. For biochemical evaluations of tissue homogenates, however, quantitative aspects are of obvious importance. Under the perspective of prognosis, for example, a morphologically heterogenous carcinoma that is composed of tissue areas belonging to grades IIb and IIIb and contributing 95% and 5% of the total tissue volume, respectively, had to be graded as IIIb tumor. However, the contributions of these small IIIb areas to homogenates produced from larger amounts of tumor tissue are negligible, and the homogenates and all data derived from these materials will nearly exclusively represent grade IIb tissues. To avoid misinterpretations during the comparison of morphological and biochemical data, we introduced a variant of the Helpap grading based on the original qualitative rules for classification of morphological characteristics but fixes overall grades of malignancy at the quantitatively predominant parts of the tumors and not at their most malignant areas. In cases without obvious predominance of one grade of malignancy, an average grade was used for the correlation of biochemical and morphological data. This variant of the Helpap grading (see Table 1) proved to be particularly useful for the identification of parallels between morphological and biochemical characteristics of prostate cancer. For this purpose and *only* for this intention, it was clearly superior to the original grading system.

The alternative grading system introduced by Gleason (88) handles the morphological heterogeneity of prostatic carcinomas in a different way. This system separately classifies the two quantitatively predominant types of differentiation being found in an individual tumor. The tumor's overall grade of malignancy subsequently derives from the combination of these two subclassifications and consequently represents some quantitative information, though the factual contributions of the respective tumor areas and particularly of the second type of differentiation to the total tissue volume remain open to question. Comparing correlations of biochemical and morphological data based on these Gleason scores with those based on the particular Gleason classification of the quantitatively predominant tumor areas, even the Gleason grading confirms the superiority of quantification-based morphological classifications in these kinds of studies. Figure 13 clearly demonstrates that the tendency of individual 5α-reductase losses to parallel the respective tumor's morphological grade of malignancy is equally shown by the two grading systems of Helpap and colleagues and of Gleason, provided that the grading is exclusively based on morphological characteristics of the quantitatively predominant tumor area. Any inclusion of other parts of the tumors in morphological classifications of these tissues results in lower coefficients of correlation between enzyme activity and morphological grading (Fig. 13). Aiming at an elucidation of parallels between histo/cytological and biochemical changes in prostate cancer, our considerations consequently were based on the morphological classification of the respective predominant type of differentiation.

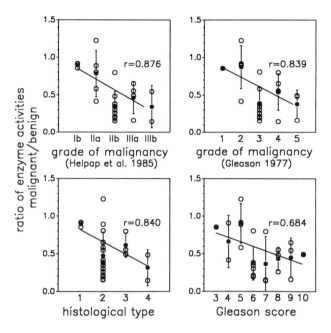

FIG. 13. Comparison of 5α-reductase activities with morphological characteristics of prostatic carcinomas. Aiming at an evaluation of individual changes, 5α-reductase activities in tumor samples were expressed in relation to the enzyme activities in their individual benign surrounding tissues. The resulting ratios of enzyme activity were compared to predominant grades of malignancy in the respective tumors and to predominant types of histological differentiation (1 uniform glandular, 2 typical pluriform, 3 uniform cribriform, 4 mixed cribriform/solid). Coefficients of correlation were calculated from the means of the respective groups. Notice comparable correlations of enzyme activities with the tumor classifications of different grading systems and a lower correlation with Gleason scores as compared to Gleason classifications of quantitatively predominant tumor areas.

Using this strategy, the losses of 5α-reductase activity in the carcinomas revealed to be quantitatively correlated with increasing grade of malignancy and decreasing histological differentiation (Fig. 13). Although not systematically decreased in the tumors, a corresponding tendency also could be observed for DHT concentrations in the tumor tissues (Fig. 14). This might reflect the losses of 5α-reductase at the level of the steroid, but also could indicate a general decline in the capacities of DHT accumulation with progression of dedifferentiation. Regarding the nuclear DHT concentrations as a more specific measure of receptor function, less systematic variations with morphological changes were found (Fig. 15). Obviously, the factors that influence AR functions and the resulting nuclear accumulation of DHT are more complex than those acting on the 5α-reductase, and particularly some tumors with high grades of malignancy and prominent dedifferentiation do not follow the rule of parallelism between morphological dedifferentiation and loss of specific functions

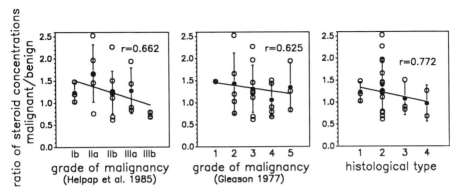

FIG. 14. Comparison of prostate cancer tissue DHT concentrations with morphological characteristics of prostatic carcinomas. For further explanations, see caption of Fig. 13.

in the cellular system of androgen utilization. In principle and considering some exceptional tumors, however, also the nuclear DHT accumulation declined gradually as a function of progressive morphological dedifferentiation.

Corresponding to the losses of 5α-reductase, the tendency to lower 17β-HSDH activities in tumors followed morphological characteristics of dedifferentiation, at least in the subgroups of carcinomas with moderate histological or cytological deviations from benign prostatic tissues. However, some tumors with high grades of malignancy did not follow this rule (Fig. 16).

The carcinomas no. 1 and 12 represent the full spectrum of this variation. Tumor no. 1 was a highly differentiated glandular carcinoma with low grade of malignancy and other characteristics of a transition zone carcinoma (89). This tumor did not

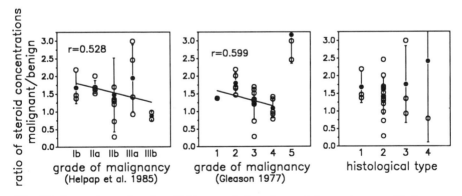

FIG. 15. Comparison of nuclear DHT concentrations in prostatic carcinomas with the morphological characteristics of these tumors. Presentation of data as outlined for Fig. 13. Notice exceptional high accumulation of DHT in the nuclei of some tumors with high grade of malignancy.

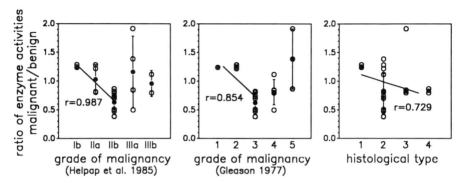

FIG. 16. Comparison of 17β-HSDH activities in prostatic carcinomas with the morphological characteristics of these tumors. Presentation of data as outlined in the legend of Fig. 13. In contrast to the 5α-reductase, parallel decreases of this enzyme activity and of the morphological differentiation could be observed only for tumors of lower grades of malignancy.

show any change found in the other carcinomas of the prostate, that is, no increase in DNA content and no losses of 5α-reductase, 17β-HSDH, and DHT accumulation. In contrast, the pluriform and low differentiated carcinoma no. 12 with morphological characteristics of a high malignant cancer was one of the tumors with the most prominent losses of 5α-reductase (See Fig. 4) and 17β-HSDH (see Fig. 12) and the tumor with the most substantial decrease in nuclear DHT accumulation (see Fig. 9). Moreover, this tumor demonstrated signs of periglandular stroma sclerosis with a nearly complete loss of smooth muscular tissue elements and alterations that resembled morphological reactions to androgen withdrawal, that is, vacuolization of the tumor cells, apparent ruptures of cellular membranes and nuclear pyknoses. This loss of muscular stroma and the cytological alterations are morphological correlates of the decreases in 5α-reductase activity and capacity for nuclear DHT accumulation.

Taken together, the data on 17β-HSDH, 5α-reductase, and DHT accumulation indicate that both enzymes and the androgen receptors that all revealed to be androgen-dependent proteins in animal experiments (44, 99–103) are gradually lost from prostate cancer tissues with increasing morphological dedifferentiation. These observations are in accordance with two hypotheses: a biochemical dedifferentiation of the cancer cells that might be all and equally involved in these changes; or a mixture of two types of cells that correspond either to normal prostatic cells or represent a completely different state that do no more possess these specific cellular functions. The last-mentioned hypothetical type of cells might then represent an androgen-independent subpopulation and higher grades of malignancy defined by morphological characteristics consequently would be associated with increasing contents of these androgen-independent tumor cells. Under this hypothesis, tumor no. 12 should be predominantly composed of the androgen-independent type of cells and tumor no. 1 should be devoid of them and consequently represent the prototype of androgen-dependent carcinomas. The proliferation of tumor no. 12

despite its only residual functions of androgen utilization and its resulting DHT deficiency supports the idea of an androgen-independent character of this carcinoma. Further information about possible biochemical heterogeneities of prostatic carcinomas will be derived from analyses of metastatic tumors that are in progress.

CONCLUSIONS

Carcinomas of the prostate generally possess the complete system of androgen metabolism and accumulation. Consequently, androstenedione represents the only relevant adrenal source for synthesis of testosterone directly in the tumor tissues. Biological consequences of this pathway are still open to question.

Although the functions of steroid utilization in prostate cancer principally correspond to those in benign prostatic tissue, dedifferentiation is associated with gradual loss of pivotal functions of androgen utilization, that is, 5α-reductase, DHT accumulation and nuclear translocation, eventually leading to the expression of an androgen-independent phenotype. The discrepancy between substantial loss of 5α-reductase and essentially unchanged DHT accumulation suggests a defect in the cellular utilization of available androgen, that is, an insufficient formation of the androgen-dependent enzyme protein despite regular amounts of hormone. The loss of 5α-reductase in prostatic carcinomas is qualitatively correlated with losses of two other hormone-dependent prostatic enzyme proteins—the 17β-HSDH and the BB isoenzyme of creatine kinase (73). Moreover, the AR as another androgen-dependent protein also is gradually lost in particular tumors. Taken together, these findings indicate a reduced formation of androgen regulated proteins in tumor cells despite normal nuclear DHT contents. This can be interpreted as sign of biochemical dedifferentiation.

Acknowledgments

This study was supported by the Deutsche Forschungsgemeinschaft (grant K1 582/1). The excellent technical assistance of Mrs. Jutta Bahn and Miss Caren Warnecke is gratefully acknowledged.

REFERENCES

1. Hunter R. *Observations on certain parts of the animal oeconomy.* London: Bibliotheka Osteriana, 1786.
2. Voigt KD, Schmidt H. *Sexual Hormones* Reinbek: Rowohlt, 1968.
3. Bruchovsky N, Wilson JD. The conversion of testosterone to 5α-androstan-17β-ol-3-one by rat prostate in vivo and in vitro. *J Biol Chem* 1968,243:2012–2021.
4. Bruchovsky N, Wilson JD. The intranuclear binding of testosterone and 5α-androstan-17β-ol-3-one by rat prostate. *J Biol Chem* 1968;243:5953–5960.
5. Fang S, Liao S. Androgen receptors. Steroid- and tissue-specific retention of a 17β-hydroxy-5α-androstan-3-one-protein complex by the cell nuclei of ventral prostate. *J Biol Chem* 1971;246:16–24.
6. Fang S, Anderson KM, Liao S. Receptor proteins for androgens: on the role of specific proteins in

selective retention of 17β-hydroxy-5α-androstan-3-one by ventral prostate in vivo and in vitro. *J Biol Chem* 1969;244:6584–6595.

7. Mainwaring WIP. The binding of 1,2 ^{3}H-testosterone within nuclei of the rat prostate. *J Endocr* 1969;44:323–333.

8. Mainwaring WIP. A soluble androgen receptor in the cytoplasm of rat prostate. *J Endocr* 1969; 45:531–541.

9. Cabot AT. The question of castration for enlarged prostate. *Ann Surg* 1896;24:265–309.

10. Ramm F. *Kastrationens betydning: prostata-hypertrofiens behandling.* Kristiana: H. Aschehoug, 1894.

11. White JW. The results of double castration in hypertrophy of the prostate. *Ann Surg* 1895;22:1–80.

12. Sharifi R, Kiefer J. History of endocrine manipulation in the treatment of carcinoma of the prostate—who was first? *J Endocrinol Invest* 1987;(Suppl) 10:2,91.

13. Huggins C, Hodges CV. Studies on prostatic cancer. I. The effect of castration, of estrogen and of androgen injection on serum phosphatases in metastatic carcinoma of the prostate. *Cancer Res* 1941;1:293–297.

14. Huggins C, Stevens RE, Hodges CV. Studies on prostatic cancer. II. The effects of castration on advanced carcinoma of the prostate gland. *Archive of Surgery* 1941;43:209–223.

15. Di Silverio F, Sciarra F. Therapeutic approaches in prostatic cancer. *J Steroid Biochem* 1986;25: 773–779.

16. Morse MJ, Whitmore WF. Clinical management of advanced prostatic cancer. In: Hollander VP, ed. *Hormonally Responsive Tumors.* New York: Academic Press, 1985;431–468.

17. Murphy GP. A current review of the clinical experience with Estracyt. In: Murphy GP, et al. eds. *Prostate cancer, Part B: Imaging techniques, radiotherapy, chemotherapy and management.* New York: Alan R. Liss, 1987;521–525.

18. Scott WW. Historical overview of the treatment of prostatic cancer. *Prostate* 1983;4:435–440.

19. Blackard CE. The Veterans Administration Cooperative Urological Research Groups' studies of carcinoma of the prostate: a review. *Cancer Chemother Rep* 1975;59:225–246.

20. Byar DP. The Veterans Administration Cooperative Urological Research Groups' studies of cancer of the prostate. *Cancer* 1973;32:1126–1140.

21. Jacobi GH, Altwein JE, Kurth KH, Basting R, Hohenfellner R. Treatment of advanced prostatic cancer with parenteral Cyproterone acetate: a phase III randomised trial. *Br J Urol* 1980;52:208–215.

22. Jacobi GH, Wenderoth UK, Ehrenthal W, et al. Endocrine and clinical evaluation of 107 patients with advanced prostatic carcinoma under long term pernasal buserelin or intramuscular decapeptyl depot treatment. In: Klijn JGM, ed. *Hormonal manipulation of cancer.* New York: Raven Press, 1987;235–248.

23. Kraljic A, Tarle M. Evaluation of endocrine therapy of prostate cancer by assessing tumor markers and hormone parameters. Hormonal "cross-over" treatment of false endocrine independent tumors. In: Murphy GP, et al., eds. *Prostate cancer, Part B: Imaging techniques, radiotherapy, chemotherapy and management.* New York: Alan R. Liss, 1987;521–525.

24. Lepor H, Ross A, Walsh PC. The influence of hormonal therapy on survival of men with advanced prostatic cancer. *J Urol* 1982;128:335–340.

25. Leuprolide Study Group. Leuprolide versus diethylstilbestrol for metastatic prostatic cancer. *N Engl J Med* 1984;311:1281–1286.

26. Murphy GP, Beckley S, Brady MF. Treatment of newly diagnosed metastatic prostate cancer patients with chemotherapy agents in combination with hormones versus hormones alone. *Cancer* 1983;51:1264–1272.

27. Narayama AS, Loening SA, Culp DA. Flutamide in the treatment of metastatic carcinoma of the prostate. *Br J Urol* 1981;53:152–153.

28. Prout GR, Irwin RJ, Kliman B, Daly JJ, Maclaughin RA, Griffin PP. Prostatic cancer and SCH-13251: II. Histological alterations and the pituitary gonadal axis. *J Urol* 1975;113:834–840.

29. Robinson MRG, Shearer RJ, Fergusson JD. Adrenal suppression in the treatment of carcinoma of the prostate. *Br J Urol* 1974;46:555–559.

30. Sogani PC, Vagaiwala MR, Whitmore WF. Experience with Flutamide in patients with advanced prostatic cancer without prior endocrine therapy. *Cancer* 1984;54:744–750.

31. Trachtenberg J. Ketoconazole therapy in advanced prostatic carcinoma. *J Urol* 1984;132:61–63.

32. Manci EM, Gardner WA. Bruch's De Morbis Glandulae Prostatae: An early account of prostatic diseases (1835). *Prostate* 1986;8:103–121.
33. Bruchovsky N, Brown EM, Coppin CM, et al. The endocrinology and treatment of prostate tumor progression. In: Coffey DS, et al., eds. *Current concepts and approaches to the study of prostate cancer*. New York: Alan R. Liss, 1987;347–387.
34. Coffey DS, Pienta KJ. New concepts in studying the control of normal growth of the prostate. In: Coffey DS, et al., eds. *Current concepts and approaches to the study of prostate cancer*. New York: Alan R. Liss, 1987;1–73.
35. Hechter O. Susceptibility of the prostate cancer cell to different physical, hormonal, and chemical agents: present status and theoretical prospects for improved prostate cancer therapy. *Prostate* 1984;5:159–180.
36. Isaacs JT. Mechanisms for resistance of prostatic cancers to androgen ablation therapy. In: Bruchovsky N, et al., eds. *Regulation of androgen action*. Berlin: Congressdruck R. Brückner 1985;71–75.
37. Isaacs JT, Schulze H, Coffey DS. Development of androgen resistance in prostate cancer. In: *Prostate cancer. Part A: Research, endocrine treatment and histopathology*. New York: Alan R. Liss, 1987;21–31.
38. Geller J, Albert J, de la Vega D, Loza D, Stoeltzing W. Dihydrotestosterone concentration in prostate cancer tissue as a predictor of tumor differentiation and hormonal dependency. *Cancer Res* 1978;38:4349–4352.
39. Geller J, Albert JD. BPH and prostate cancer—results of hormonal manipulation. In: Bruchovsky N, Chapdelaine A, Neumann F, eds. *Regulation of Androgen Action*. Berlin: Congressdruck R. Brückner, 1985;51–57.
40. Labrie F, Dupont A, Belanger A, et al. New approach in the treatment of prostate cancer: complete instead of partial withdrawal of androgens. *Prostate* 1983;4:579–594.
41. Labrie F, Dupont A, Belanger A, et al. Combined antihormonal treatment in prostate cancer: a new approach using an LHRH agonist or castration and an antiandrogen. In: Bresciani F, et al., eds. *Hormones and cancer 2, progress in cancer research and therapy, vol 31*. New York: Raven Press, 1984;533–547.
42. Labrie F, Dupont A, Belanger A, et al. Combination therapy with Flutamide and castration (LHRH agonist or orchiectomy) in advanced prostate cancer: a marked improvement in response and survival. *J Steroid Biochem* 1985;23:833–841.
43. Poyet P, Labrie F. Comparison of the antiandrogenic/androgenic activities of flutamide, cyproterone acetate and megestrol acetate. *Mol Cell Endocrinol* 1985;42:283–288.
44. Klein H, Steinhoff KR, Reinpold WM, Berndt C, Voigt KD. Prostatic target cell reactions to androgen withdrawal and replenishment: the rat model. *Exp Clin Endocrinol (Life Sci Adv)* 1989;8:185–220.
45. Labrie F, Veilleux R. A wide range of sensitivities to androgens develops in cloned Shionoge mouse mammary cells. *Prostate* 1986;8:293–300.
46. Isaacs JT, Coffey DS. Adaptation versus selection on the mechanisms responsible for the relapse of prostatic cancer to androgen ablation therapy as studied in the Dunning R-3327-H adenocarcinoma. *Cancer Res* 1981;41:5070–5075.
47. Isaacs JT, Heston WDW, Weissman RM, Coffey DS. Animal models of the hormone-sensitive and -insensitive prostatic adenocarcinomas, Dunning R-3327-H, R-3327-HI, and R-3327-AT. *Cancer Res* 1978;38:4353–4359.
48. Sanford NL, Searle JW, Kerr JFR. Successive waves of apoptosis in the rat prostate after repeated withdrawal of testosterone stimulation. *Pathology* 1984;16:406–410.
49. Wilding G, Zugmaier G, Knabbe C, Flanders K, Gelmann EP. Differential effects of transforming growth factor β on human prostate cancer cells in vitro. *Molec Cell Endocrinol* 1984;62:79–87.
50. Wilding G, Valverius E, Knabbe C, Gelmann EP. Role of transforming growth factor α in human prostate cancer cell growth. *Prostate* 1989;15:1–12.
51. Knabbe, C. Personal communication, 1990.
52. Schuurmans ALG, Bolt J, Mulder E. Androgens stimulate both growth-rate and epidermal growth factor receptor activity of the human prostate tumor cell LNCaP. *Prostate* 1989;12:55–63.
53. Huggins C, Scott WW. Bilateral adrenalectomy in prostatic cancer: clinical features and urinary excretion of 17-ketosteroids and estrogen. *Ann Surg* 1945;122:1031–1041.
54. Baker WJ. Bilateral adrenalectomy for carcinoma of the prostate gland: preliminary report. *J Urol* 1953;70:275–281.

55. Bhanalaph T, Varkarakis MJ, Murphy GP. Current status of bilateral adrenalectomy of advanced prostatic carcinoma. *Ann Surg* 1974;179:17–23.
56. Harrison JH, Thorn GW, Jenkins D. Total adrenalectomy for reactivated carcinoma of the prostate. *N Engl J Med* 1953;248:86–92.
57. Huggins C, Bergenstal D. Effect of bilateral adrenalectomy on certain human tumors. *Proc Nat Acad Sci* 1952;38:73–76.
58. Klosterhalfen H, Becker H, Lotzin C, Kautzky R. Die Hypophysektomie als Behandlungsmöglichkeit beim Endstadium des Prostatakarzinomas. *Urologe A* 1980;19:85–88.
59. Levin AB, Benson RC, Katz J, Nielsson T. Chemical hypophysectomy for relief of bone pain in carcinoma of the prostate. *J Urol* 1978;119:517–521.
60. Macfarlane DA, Thomas LP, Harrison JH. A survey of total adrenalectomy in cancer of the prostate. *Am J Surg* 1960;99:562–572.
61. Maddy JA, Winternitz WW, Norrell H. Cryohypophysectomy in the management of advanced prostatic cancer. *Cancer* 1971;28:322–328.
62. Morales P, Brendler H, Hotchkiss RS. The role of the adrenal cortex in prostatic cancer. *J Urol* 1955;73:399–409.
63. Murphy GP, Reynoso G, Schoonees R, et al. Hypophysectomy and adrenalectomy for disseminated prostatic carcinoma. *J Urol* 1971;105:817–825.
64. Murray R, Pitt P. Treatment of advanced prostatic cancer resistant to conventional therapy, with aminogluthetimide. *Eur J Cancer Clin Oncol* 1985;21:453–458.
65. Ponder BAJ, Shearer RJ, Pocock RD, et al. Response to aminogluthetimide and cortisone acetate in advanced prostatic cancer. *Br J Cancer* 1984;50:757–763.
66. Scott WW, Schirmer HK. Hypophysectomy for disseminated prostatic cancer. In: *On Cancer and Hormones: Essays in Experimental Biology.* Chicago: University of Chicago Press, 1962;175–204.
67. Smith JA, Eyre HJ, Roberts TS, Middleton RG. Transphenoidal hypophysectomy in the management of carcinoma of the prostate. *Cancer* 1984;53:2385–2387.
68. Thiebault JB, Thurel C, Cunin G, Serie A. The role of neurosurgery in the non-specific treatment of prostate pain. In: Murphy GP, et al., eds. *Prostate cancer, Part B: Imaging techniques, radiotherapy, chemotherapy and management.* New York: Alan R. Liss, 1987;493–496.
69. Whitmore WF, Randall HT, Pearson OH, West CD. Adrenalectomy in the treatment of prostatic cancer. *Geriatrics* 1954;9:62–69.
70. Worgul TJ, Santen RJ, Samojlik E, et al. Clinical and biochemical effect of aminoglutethimide in the treatment of advanced prostatic carcinoma. *J Urol* 1983;129:51–55.
71. Van Oyen P, Vercruysse P, Denys H, Vergison R. Pain-treatment in metastatic prostatic carcinoma by radiofrequency thermolesion on the pituitary gland, preliminary report. In: Murphy GP, Khoury S, Küss R, Chatelain C, Denis L, eds. *Prostate Cancer, Part B: Imaging Techniques, Radiotherapy, Chemotherapy, and Management Issues.* New York: Alan R. Liss, 1987;497–500.
72. Bartsch W, Greeve J, Voigt KD. 17β-Hydroxysteroid dehydrogenase in the human prostate: properties and distribution between epithelium and stroma in benign hyperplastic tissue. *J Steroid Biochem* 1987;28:35–42.
73. Klein H, Molwitz T, Bartsch W. Steroid sulfate sulfatase in human benign prostatic hyperplasia: characterization and quantification of the enzyme in epithelium and stroma. *J Steroid Biochem* 1969;33:195–200.
74. Klein H, Bressel M, Kastendieck H, Voigt KD. Quantitative assessment of endogenous testicular and adrenal sex steroids and of steroid metabolizing enzymes in untreated human prostatic cancerous tissue. *J Steroid Biochem* 1988;30:119–130.
75. Klein H, Kohlsaat E, Voigt KD. The role of androstenedione in hormonal control of prostatic tissue: a model study in the rat. (In preparation).
76. Labrie C, Belanger A, Labrie F. Androgenic activity of dehydroepiandrosterone and androstenedione in the rat ventral prostate. *Endocrinology* 1988;123:1412–1417.
77. Moguilewsky M, Cotard M, Proulx L, Tournemine C, Raynaud JP. What is an antiandrogen and what is the physiological and pharmacological rationale for combined "castration" + "antiandrogen" therapy. In: Murphy GP, et al., eds. *Prostate cancer, Part A: Research, endocrine treatment, and histopathology.* New York: Alan R. Liss, 1987;315–340.
78. Barrack ER, Brendler CB, Walsh PC. Steroid receptor and biochemical profiles in prostatic cancer: correlation with response to hormonal treatment. In: Murphy GP, et al., eds. *Prostate cancer, Part A:research, endocrine treatment, and histopathology.* New York: Alan R. Liss, 1987;79–97.

79. Concolino G, Marocchi A, Margiotta G, et al. Steroid receptors and hormone responsiveness of human prostatic carcinoma. *Prostate* 1982;3:475–482.
80. Fentie DD, Lakey WH, McBlain WA. Applicability of nuclear androgen receptor quantification to human prostatic adenocarcinoma. *J Urol* 1986;135:167–173.
81. Geller J. Rationale for blockade of adrenal as well as testicular androgens in the treatment of advanced prostate cancer. *Sem Oncol* 1985;12:28–35.
82. Geller J, Candari CD. Comparison of dihydrotestosterone levels in prostatic cancer metastases and primary prostate cancer. *Prostate* 1989;15:171–175.
83. Krieg M, Bartsch W, Janssen W, Voigt KD. A comparative study of binding, metabolism and endogenous levels of androgens in normal, hyperplastic and carcinomatous human prostate. *J Steroid Biochem* 1979;11:615–624.
84. Trachtenberg J, Walsh PC. Correlation of prostatic nuclear androgen receptor content with duration of response and survival following hormonal therapy in advanced prostatic cancer. *J Urol* 1982;127:466–471.
85. Hoehn W, Schroeder FH, Riemann JF, Joebsis AC, Hermanek P. Human prostatic adenocarcinoma: some characteristics of a serially transplantable line in nude mice (PC-82). *Prostate* 1980;1:95–104.
86. Van Steenbrugge GJ, Groen M, Romijn JC, Schröder FH. Biological effects of hormonal treatment regimens on a transplantable human prostatic tumor line (PC-82). *J Urol* 1984;131:812–817.
87. Van Steenbrugge GJ, Ultee-van Gessel AM, Groen M, de Jong FH, Schröder FH. Administration of an LHRH-antagonist to male mice: effects on in vivo secretion of hormones and on the growth of a transplantable human prostatic carcinoma. *Life Sci* 1987;40:1335–1343.
88. Gleason DF. Histologic grading and clinical staging of prostatic carcinoma. In: Tannenbaum M, ed. *Urologic pathology: the prostate*. Philadelphia: Lea & Febiger, 1977;171–198.
89. McNeal JE, Redwine EA, Freiha FS, Stamey TA. Zonal distribution of prostatic adenocarcinoma. *Am J Surg Pathol* 1988;12:897–906.
90. Bartsch W, Krieg M, Becker H, Mohrmann J, Voigt KD. Endogenous androgen levels in epithelium and stroma of human benign prostatic hyperplasia and normal prostate. *Acta Endocrinol* 1982;100:634–640.
91. Bartsch W, Kozak I, Gorenflos P, Becker H, Voigt KD. Concentrations of 3β-hydroxy androgens in epithelium and stroma of benign hyperplastic and normal human prostate. *Prostate* 1986;8:3–10.
92. Bartsch W, Klein H, Schiemann U, Bauer HW, Voigt KD. Enzymes of androgen formation and degradation in the human prostate. *Ann NY Acad Sci* 1990;595:53–66.
93. Voigt KD, Bartsch W. Intratissular androgens in benign prostatic hyperplasia and prostatic cancer. *J Steroid Biochem* 1986;25:749–757.
94. Cowan RA, Cowan SK, Grant JK, Elder HY. Biochemical investigations of separated epithelium and stroma from benign hyperplastic prostatic tissue. *J Endocrinol* 1977;74:111–120.
95. Krieg M, Klötzl G, Kaufmann J, Voigt KD. Stroma of human benign prostatic hyperplasia: preferential tissue for androgen metabolism and oestrogen binding. *Acta Endocrinol* 1981;96:422–432.
96. Fiet J, Vilette JM, Bertagna C, et al. Plasma hormone levels before and after orchiectomy in prostate cancer patients. In: Murphy GP, et al., eds. *Prostate cancer, Part A: research, endocrine treatment, and histopathology*. New York: Alan R. Liss, 1987;33–44.
97. Harper ME, Pike A, Peeling WB, Griffiths K. Steroids of adrenal origin metabolized by human prostatic tissue both in vivo and in vitro. *J Endocrinol* 1974;60:117–125.
98. Helpap B, Böcking A, Dhom G, et al. Klassifikation, histologisches und zytologisches Grading sowie Regressiongrading des Prostatakarzinomas. *Pathologe* 1985;6:3–7.
99. Bartsch W, Klein H, Nehse G, Voigt KD. In vivo model for uptake, metabolism and binding of androgens in prostatic tissue. In: Bresciani F, et al., eds., *Hormones and cancer 2, progress in cancer research and therapy, vol 31*. New York: Raven Press, 1984;441–452.
100. Fjoesne HE, Sunde A. Androgen metabolism in the prostate of castrated and pituitary grafted wistar rats. *J Steroid Biochem* 1987;28:86S.
101. Moore RJ, Wilson JD. The effect of androgenic hormones on the reduced nicotinamide adenine dinucleotide phosphate Δ^4-3-ketosteroid 5α-oxidoreductase of rat ventral prostate. *Endocrinology* 1975;93:581–582.
102. Shimazaki J, Matsushita I, Furuya N, Yamanaka H, Shida K. Reduction of 5α-position of testosterone in the rat ventral prostate. *Endocrinol Jpn* 1969;16:453–458.
103. Shimazaki J, Ohki Y, Matsuoka M, Tanaka M, Shida K. Further studies on testosterone 5α-reduction in the rat ventral prostate. *Endocrinol Jpn* 1972;19:69–75.

Endocrine Dependent Tumors, edited by
Klaus-Dieter Voigt and Cornelius Knabbe.
Raven Press, Ltd., New York © 1991.

6

Regulation of Growth Inhibitory Polypeptides in Human Breast Cancer

Cornelius Knabbe

*Department of Clinical Chemistry, Medical Clinic, University of Hamburg,
D-2000 Hamburg 20, Federal Republic of Germany*

The mechanism by which transformed cells escape normal growth control is only poorly understood. New insights have been provided by the proposal of an autocrine mechanism of growth control that was postulated by Sporn and Todaro in 1980 (1): Tumor cells stimulate their own growth by their ability to produce, secrete, and respond to growth stimulatory polypeptides via receptor mediated pathways. Particular emphasis was put on this field of research in last decade when it was demonstrated that a number of growth factors, their receptors or parts of the intracellular signal transduction pathway show high similarity to proteins encoded by different cellular oncogenes (for review see 2).

Dramatic progress has been made in the area of solid tumors in breast cancer research because this malignancy provides because of its known hormonal dependence an additional advantage for studying the mechanism of growth control: Breast cancer is strongly regulated in at least one-third of clinical cases by estrogenic hormones or estrogen antagonists; breast cancer is found in women who had never functional ovaries with only 1% of the frequency of that in women with intact ovaries (for review see 3). *In vitro* as well as *in vivo* model systems can be manipulated efficiently in terms of proliferation and tumorigenicity by the use of estrogen or estrogen antagonizing agents. On the basis of these studies it has been suggested that estrogens exert their action on estrogen-dependent breast cancer through coordinated control of secreted growth factors that might act in an autocrine and paracrine fashion; members of the transforming growth factor α- and insulin-like growth factor family have been identified as major estrogen-regulated growth promoting polypeptides with autostimulatory potential and eventually represent "second messengers" of estrogen action (for review see 4). The detailed analysis of the regulatory system "transforming growth factor α - EGF-receptor - HER-2/neu protooncogene" has led to several clinical studies to improve diagnosis and treatment of breast cancer (5–9). Overexpression of the EGF-receptor and amplification of the HER-2/neu oncogene seem to correlate with increased proliferation rate and negative prognosis of the disease. Recent studies demonstrated that the interruption of this autocrine loop by the use of antibodies against the EGF-receptor could represent a new therapeutic opportunity for treatment of human breast cancer (10). The clinical significance of the insulin-like growth factor family and their corresponding receptors needs further elucidation. It has been reported that the antiestrogen tamoxifen leads to diminished secretion of IGF-like factors *in vitro* as well as *in vivo* (11,12). IGF-II seems to have a primarily paracrine role, mediating the communication between tumor cells and the surrounding stroma (13,14).

A marked shift in emphasis has occured during the past few years in growth control research. Analysis of the autoinhibitory mechanisms that prevent the normal cell from uncontrolled proliferation is now the primary focus of many research activities. The identification of several tumor suppressor genes has led to a deeper understanding of the process how malignant cells might escape normal growth control (for review see 15–17). In parallel, the hypothesis of an autocrine mechanism of growth control has been extended to include the concept that transformation also might be correlated with the failure of cells to synthesize, express, or respond to specific negative growth factors they normally release to control their own growth (18). This chapter will focus on the regulation of secreted polypeptide growth inhibitors that might be involved in growth control of human breast cancer cells.

The existence of endogenous growth inhibitors of cell division was first suggested by studies on epidermal wound healing and carcinogenesis; the term *chalone* was given to this putative class of molecules that act as inhibitory growth regulators in a tissue specific way (for review see 19). Several polypeptide growth inhibitors with different degrees of cell- and tissue specificity have been identified in mammary systems that will be discussed in the following: Transforming growth factor(s) type β (TGFβ), mammary-derived growth inhibitor (MDGI)/ mammary cell growth inhibitor (MCGI), mammastatin and other partially characterized polypeptides. Special attention will be given to the regulation of TGFβ that is the best described growth modulator with growth inhibitory potential for human breast cancer cells.

TRANSFORMING GROWTH FACTOR(S) TYPE β

The 25 kDa TGFβ peptides belong to a family of growth and differentiation factors that also include inhibins, activins, Müllerian inhibitory substance and the decapentaplegic gene complex transcript in Drosophila (for review see 20): Three known forms of human TGFβ exist. The polypeptide originally described as TGFβ (21–23) consists of two disulfide linked β-1 subunits and is now named TGFβ-1. TGFβ-1 is stored in high concentrations in human platelets and has been identified as the product of many transformed cell lines. TGFβ-2 is composed of two β-2 subunits that are highly homologous to β-1 but represent different gene products: TGFβ-1 is encoded as a 390 amino acid precursor (24), TGFβ-2 as a 412 amino acid precursor (25,26), each having an N-terminal signal peptide of 20–23 amino acids. The processed 112 amino acid chains of the two peptides are 72% identical, all 9 cysteine residues are conserved. Recently the existence of a third human TGFβ species was revealed (27).

Biological effects of TGFβ

TGFβ is the prototypical multifunctional growth factor (28). TGFβ-1 and TGFβ-2 seem to have similar biological potency (29,30) with only a few exceptions (31–33). TGFβ stimulates anchorage independent growth of murine, rat, and human fibroblasts; conversely, TGFβ inhibits growth of human megakaryocytic and erythroid precursors, keratinocytes, endothelial cells, hepatocytes and human carcinoma cell lines. TGFβ-1 is a reversible inhibitor of mammary gland growth *in vivo* (34). TGFβ-1 and TGFβ-2 are equipotent growth inhibitors of human breast cancer cell lines *in vitro*: The anchorage independent growth of the estrogen receptor negative human breast cancer cell lines MDA-MB 231, MDA-MB 468, SKBR-3 and Hs578-T is inhibited by both TGFβ-1 and TGFβ-2 (35,36). Reports about the growth inhibitory potential of TGFβ on estrogen receptor positive human breast cancer cells somewhat diverge. Whereas several investigators find a significant growth inhibition of the estrogen receptor positive human breast cancer cell lines MCF-7, ZR-75-1, T-47D by TGFβ-1 and TGFβ-2 (35–39), there has been the hypothesis that TGFβ-responsiveness might be restricted to estrogen receptor negative cells (40). However, progression of the estrogen receptor positive T47-D cells from a steroid sensitive to a steroid insensitive state has been shown to be accompanied by a change in the response to TGFβ-1: TGFβ-1 becomes even growth stimulatory in steroid insensitive cells (41). Moreover, it has been demonstrated that MCF-7 cells can be selected for resistance to growth inhibition by TGFβ under certain tissue culture conditions (36). These changes might account for different results obtained by different research groups. In other experimental systems, that is retinoblastoma and skin squamous carcinoma cells, it has been previously shown that loss of TGFβ-responsiveness might be associated with increased malignancy (42,43). Similar observations have been made in an experimental setting where different oncogene transformed human mammary epithelial cells were compared with their benzo(a)pyrene immortalized parental cells (44–46). Besides its function as growth regulator, TGFβ is an important modulator of differentiation. In the human mammary epithelial cell system, TGFβ induces the expression of the epithelial membrane antigen as an important marker of differentiation, parallel to a change in the morphology from the cobblestone epithelial appearance of normal cells to an elongated spindle shape (47). Comparable results were gained in bronchial epithelial cells (48). It can be concluded that loss of responsiveness to TGFβ-polypeptides as endogenous growth inhibitors and inducers of differentiation might contribute to the expression of the malignant phenotype in certain human breast cancer cells.

Mechanism of TGFβ Action

The mechanism how TGFβ regulates growth and differentiation is not completely understood. A complex pattern of cross-reactive ligands and receptors has been described (49). Scatchard analysis shows the existence of one high affinity site on normal and malignant mammary cells (35,36,46). TGFβ-1 and TGFβ-2 are mutually competitive for binding to this receptor species (36).

Cross-linking studies of iodinated TGFβ-1 to cell surface proteins of human breast cancer cells show the existence of at least three binding components with high (250 kDa) and low (65 and 85–110 kDa) molecular weight; correlation of the binding pattern on different cell lines with their responsiveness to TGFβ has led to the proposal that the lower molecular weight components are the active receptors (50). The TGFβ receptor is not down-regulated after having been occupied by the ligand (51). The structure of the receptor(s) is not known, the intracellular signaling pathway appears to be dissociated from the tyrosine kinase pathway taken by most other growth factors like epidermal growth factor and platelet derived growth factor. Both G protein-dependent and independent pathways seem to be involved in the mechanism of signal transduction (52,53). Several pieces of evidence have been presented that TGFβ might partially exert its action through regulation of the expression of other growth factors and growth factor receptors: It modulates the expression of the EGF-receptor and erbB-2 oncogene in the estrogen receptor-negative human breast carcinoma cell line MDA-468 (54,55). Furthermore, it induces expression of the c-sis mRNA in human breast cancer cells (Knabbe, unpublished observations) and glioblastoma cells (56). Regulation of the extracellular matrix might represent an important target of TGFβ action. Although numerous studies have been performed in other experimental systems (for review see 57) only limited data are available in human mammary systems. A recent study suggests that the paracrine communication of tumor cells and surrounding fibroblasts might be mediated through the regulation of extracellular matrix proteins by TGFβ (58). The loss of sensitivity to TGFβ induced growth inhibition can be apparently caused by several mechanisms: An MCF-7 subclone that is not inhibited by TGFβ-1 or TGFβ-2 does not show a detectable expression of TGFβ cell surface receptors suggesting that loss of receptors might cause loss of TGFβ-sensitivity (36,59). Another mechanism was found in oncogene transformed human mammary epithelial cells: The reduction of TGFβ-sensitivity in cells of full malignancy does not coincide with a change in the receptor characteristics (46); similar findings have been obtained in a human colon carcinoma cell line (60) suggesting regulatory events in the mechanism of signal transduction distal to the TGFβ receptor(s).

Regulation of TGFβ

TGFβ-peptides differ from the majority of growth factors in that they are usually synthesized and secreted by most cells in a biologically latent form that must be activated before they can exert their biological effects on target cells (61). The mechanism of activation *in vivo* is unclear, but can require a strong acidic environment or specific proteases, and eventually be dependent on cell-cell interactions (62–64). The major latent form of TGFβ-1 is represented by a high molecular weight complex, in which the active TGFβ-1 homodimer is noncovalently associated with a dimer of the remainder of its precursor "pro" region; this is linked by a disulfidebridge to a third protein of 135 kDa (65,66). After the initial description of the presence of two classes of transforming growth factors in human breast cancer cells (67,68), it became evident that, in contrast to most other cells, human breast cancer cell lines secrete a significant part of TGFβ in a biologically active form requiring no further activation, as measured by specific growth and receptor competition assays (35,40,58): TGFβ derived from MCF-7 cells competes with ^{125}I-labeled TGFβ-1 for binding to its receptor and comigrates with TGFβ-1 upon acid gel exclusion chromatography. Immunoprecipitation of ^{35}S-cysteine labeled media from MCF-7 cells with an antibody generated against platelet derived TGFβ reveals a polypeptide that comigrates with ^{125}I-labeled human platelet TGFβ upon SDS-PAGE. The expression-pattern of the three different TGFβ-peptides vary between different breast cancer cell lines as judged by analysis of the corresponding mRNAs: T-47D express all three species, ZR-75-1 TGFβ-1 and TGFβ-3, MCF-7 and MD-MB 231 TGFβ-1 and TGFβ-2 (39,69). The analysis of the corresponding proteins themselves has only been performed to a limited extent. Immunodetection and quantitation of *total* (= biologically active and latent) TGFβ-1 and TGFβ-2 has shown secretion of predominantly TGFβ-2 by MCF-7 cells (70) whereas TGFβ-1 represents the majority of *biologically active* TGFβ-peptides secreted by MCF-7 cells (69). No data are available on the TGFβ-3 protein.

The influence of growth modulatory steroids on secretion of TGFβ has been extensively studied in the estrogen-responsive MCF-7 human breast cancer cell line (35). Secretion of biologically active autoinhibitory TGFβ-peptides can be strongly induced under treatment with growth inhibitory antiestrogen. Growth stimulatory estrogen and insulin decrease secretion of TGFβ. Antiestrogen induction of TGFβ can be reversed completely by the addition of excess estrogens showing that the estrogen/antiestrogen regulation of TGFβ secretion is mediated through the estrogen receptor. The induction of TGFβ by antiestrogens is not found in the antiestrogen resistant MCF-7 variant LY 2, which, however, can be inhibited by the administration of TGFβ. Lack of induction of TGFβ by antiestrogen might contribute significantly to the antiestrogen resistant phenotype of the LY 2 variant.

The exact mechanism of this regulation remains to be elucidated. Further insights were provided by the detailed analysis of the different TGFβ-forms (35,69): Treatment of MCF-7 cells with growth inhibitory antiestrogens leads to an increased secretion of both biologically active TGFβ-1 and TGFβ-2. The steady state level of TGFβ-1 mRNA does not change, suggesting a nontranscriptional control mechanism; similar observations have been in T-47D cells under treatment with antiestrogens (71). The process of activation of latent TGFβ-1 might be a target for control of TGFβ-1 secretion, that is, regulation of specific proteases that convert TGFβ-1 into a receptor binding biologically active form: the proportion of active *vs.* latent TGFβ-1 found in conditioned medium increases under antiestrogen treatment. In the contrary, expression of TGFβ-2 mRNA is significantly induced by long term antiestrogen treatment. Time course analysis of TGFβ-2 mRNA under treatment with antiestrogen reveals a rapid down-regulation within 1 hour followed by an induction up to 10-fold above control after 48 to 72 hours. Complementary results were obtained in T-47D cells where long term treatment with growth stimulatory estrogen leads to a down-regulation of the TGFβ-2 mRNA (39). These data suggest that regulation of TGFβ-2 secretion takes place primarily at the transcriptional level. However, the biphasic regulation with an initial decrease and consecutive induction of TGFβ-2 makes a direct transcriptional control by estrogen/antiestrogen less likely and points to an involvement of other transcriptionally active factors in this mechanism. This hypothesis is supported by our finding that frequent changes of the culture medium prevent induction of TGFβ-2m RNA under antiestrogen treatment suggesting that secreted factors are necessary for induction of TGFβ-2. No induction of TGFβ-2 is seen in the antiestrogen resistant MCF-7 variant LY 2 under antiestrogen treatment. On the basis of these findings we propose the following hypothesis on the mechanism of regulation of TGFβ: Antiestrogens induce the secretion of TGFβ-1 via a nontranscriptional pathway, most likely by regulation of a specific protease that converts TGFβ-1 in a biologically active form; TGFβ-1 itself induces TGFβ-2 by a direct transcriptional mechanism; by this means TGFβ-2 can be seen as an endpoint marker of antiestrogen action.

Secretion of TGFβ-peptides by breast cancer cells is coupled to the hormonally controlled growth state. This association apparently is specific for certain classes of growth modulators, that is, to steroids, like 17β-estradiol and dexamethasone and antiestrogens, like the triphenylethylene tamoxifen and its derivatives 4-OH-tamoxifen (35) and droloxifene (72), the benzothiophene LY 117018 (73) and the steroidal antiestrogen ICI 164,384 (74). As shown in a recently published study, treatment of T-47D cells with growth inhibitory progestins leads to a dose- and time-dependent downregulation of TGFβ-1 mRNA suggesting a different mechanism of growth inhibition (71,75); however, the regulation of biologically active TGFβ-proteins was not examined, which seems to be the biologically important point of regulation. Another possible mechanism of regulation of TGFβ-1 has been recently identified: Treatment of ZR-75 cells with growth inhibitory α-interferon leads to an up-regulation of the steady state level of TGFβ-1 mRNA (76). Modulation of proliferation rate and tumorigenicity by other ways than hormonal treatment seems not to be associated with a changed pattern of TGFβ-secretion. Transfection of MCF-7 cells with the v-Ha-ras-oncogene leads to increased proliferation rate and estrogen-independent tumorigenicity but is not accompanied by a decreased secretion of biologically active TGFβ (77,78). Similar observations have been made in the human mammary epithelial system mentioned previously (46). Therefore, hormonal regulation of TGFβ-secretion exhibits relative specificity for estrogens/antiestrogens and might participate in the mediation of action of these growth modulators. A putative action of TGFβ as negative autocrine growth factors also has been postulated in a recently published study where neutralization of secreted TGFβ by a specific antibody resulted in increased proliferation of normal mammary epithelial cells (79). The biological significance of this pathway is underlined by our finding that TGFβ is the principle secreted growth inhibitor for human breast cancer cells (35): Breast cancer cells resistant to treatment with antiestrogens are still growth inhibited by TGFβ *in vitro*. Antiestrogens exert their growth inhibitory activity even on antiestrogen-insensitive MDA-MB 231 cells in coculture with antiestrogen-sensitive MCF-7 cells through an enhancement of TGFβ-secretion by MCF-7 cells, suggesting a paracrine and autocrine action of TGFβ in breast cancer. This could explain how antiestrogens inhibit initially proliferation of many breast cancers at an early stage of disease. Tumors are often heterogenous in their cellular estrogen receptor content; cells with and without detectable estrogen receptor commonly coexist in the same tumor, with the latter predominating (80). Antiestrogens can exert two tumor-inhibiting effects *in vivo*: they antagonize the estrogen stimulation of estrogen receptor-containing cells and additionally can inhibit estrogen receptor-positive and estrogen receptor-negative cells by the induction of TGFβ. The role of TGFβ as an important marker of antiestrogen action deserves particular attention. A clinical use of these findings is hampered by the fact that assays to detect biologically active TGFβ in tissue specimen are not available because extraction of TGFβ from tissue requires a transient acidification that makes the discrimination between biologically active and latent TGFβ impossible (21). This discrimination also is not possible by immunostaining. The analysis of TGFβ-1 mRNA cannot provide insights into activation processes for regulation of biologically active TGFβ within the tumor because the apparently important nontranscriptional control mechanism cannot be detected (14,81). However, our present hypothesis that TGFβ-2 might represent an endpoint marker of antiestrogen action that is regulated at the transcriptional level can allow broad clinical applications because no measurement of the biologically active fraction is necessary anymore. Responsiveness of breast cancer to antiestrogen therapy eventually could be predicted on the basis of the inducibility of TGFβ-2 in the tumor, determined in tumor tissue or even by analysis of the secreted protein in peripheral blood. This approach may be superior to the determination of the estrogen receptor content of tumor tissue by exchange assays or immunostaining.

In summary, TGFβ-peptides represent a new class of growth inhibiting and differentiation inducing factors in human mammary epithelial cells with both autocrine and paracrine potential. Defects of the regulatory system "transforming growth factor β" can be located at different sites and can contribute to the increased proliferation and dedifferentiation of cells expressing the malignant phenotype.

MAMMARY-DERIVED GROWTH INHIBITOR/MAMMARY CELL GROWTH INHIBITOR

A polypeptide growth inhibitor for Ehrlich ascites mammary carcinoma cells has been isolated from bovine mammary gland, which is antagonized by EGF and insulin (82). The highest expression of this MDGI of 13 kDa molecular weight was observed in epithelial cells of lactating mammary glands (83,84). Analysis of the amino acid sequence revealed no homology to TGFβ or interferon, but to a family of low molecular weight hydrophobic ligand-binding proteins, among them a fatty acid-binding protein from rat heart, myelin P2, a differentiation associated protein in adipocytes (p422) and the cellular retinoic acid-binding protein (85). The biological function of this protein is not known. The similarity to retinoic-acid binding proteins suggests an involvement of MDGI in the process of differentiation of mammary epithelial cells. Analysis of its growth inhibitory potential on different mammary epithelial cell lines reveals a complex pattern of response: Normal human mammary epithelial cells were inhibited as well as the breast cancer cell lines MaTu and T-47D; however, MCF-7 cells showed a slight stimulation (86). Although one could speculate that loss of responsiveness to this factor might be associated with decreased differentiation and increased malignancy, more detailed studies have to be undertaken to answer this question. Another polypeptide of similar size and identical isoelectric point isolated from human milk was initially thought to be the human counterpart of MDGI (87). This factor was termed MCGI. However, MCGI is now unequivocally identified as α-lactalbumin, which is a very potent growth inhibitor in the range of 10ng/ml for normal and some malignant mammary epithelial cell lines. It has been speculated that this product of differentiated mammary epithelium is an important negative growth regulator during lactation; its role in the process of transformation has not been elucidated.

MAMMASTATIN AND OTHER PARTIALLY CHARACTERIZED POLYPEPTIDES

Another group of polypeptides distinct from TGFβ was recently identified as the secretory product of normal human mammary epithelial cells (88). These proteins of 65 kDa and 47 kDa have been termed mammastatin and inhibit growth of human breast cancer cell lines in vitro (MCF-7, BT-20, MDA-MB 231, ZR-75-1) in a dose-dependent manner reaching their highest growth inhibitory potential at a concentration of 10–20 ng/ml. No difference between estrogen receptor postitive and negative cells in responsiveness to mammastatin was observed. Mammastatin appears to be a heat-labile protein; it shows high tissue specificity because tumor cell lines derived from other organs were not inhibited; antibodies against TGFβ did not recognize mammastatin. These findings show that mammastatin does not belong to the TGFβ family and might represent a new class of tissue specific growth inhibitors. By this means mammastatin would fulfill the requirements of a chalone-like substance. Expression of mammastatin is restricted to normal mammary epithelial cells; no mammastatin could be detected in human breast cancer cell lines. According to the hypothesis of autocrine growth regulation, a decreased production of mammastatin by transformed mammary cells might contribute to the loss of normal growth control of these cells.

The relationship of mammastatin to a previously described growth inhibitor that has been purified from human plasma-derived serum (PDS fraction) remains to be determined (89,90). The PDS fraction migrates with an apparent molecular weight of 53 kDa on SDS-PAGE whereas a similar analysis of mammastatin reveals two prominent bands at 65 kDa and 47kDa and a minor band at 63 kDa. Both proteins show a specificity for mammary cells: maximal growth inhibition is seen in MCF-7 cells, only minimal growth inhibition is found in HBL-100 cells. Consequently, it is not unlikely that both activities belong to the same family of growth modulatory peptides. The same is true for an activity we have recently identified in conditioned media from antiestrogen treated MCF-7 cells (59). This novel activity migrates on neutral S-200 gel exclusion chromatography with an apparent molecular weight of 60 kDa. Its growth inhibitory activity on human breast cancer cells is not blocked by an antibody that neutralizes the action of TGFβ-1 and TGFβ-2. It also inhibits a TGFβ-resistant MCF-7 subclone. Although mammastatin has not been detected in MCF-7 cells, it cannot be ruled out that this novel activity induced by antiestrogens might belong to the mammastatin/PDS fraction group of growth modulatory polypeptides. Mammastatin is not related to a glycoprotein that has been purified to apparent homogeneity from phorbol 12-myristate 13-acetate-treated MCF-7 cells (91). Amino-terminal sequence analysis shows that this single chain protein, which has been termed "amphiregulin," is different from any known growth factor including TGFβ. Amphiregulin is a bifunctional growth regulator like TGFβ: It stimulates growth of human fibroblasts and is a potent growth inhibitor for several human tumor cell lines. The human breast cancer cell lines HTB 132 and HTB 26 exhibit exquisite sensitivity to amphiregulin, whereas MCF-7 and ZR cells do not show significant growth inhibition under treatment with amphiregulin. The mechanism of action and biological function of amphiregulin is not known.

CONCLUSION

Several polypeptide growth inhibitors with autocrine and paracrine potential have been identified in normal and malignant human mammary cells. Interpretation of the results of these investigations is hampered by the fact that the action of these factors *in vivo* takes place in a network of communicating regulatory mechanisms that only incompletely can be imitated *in vitro*. However, research within the last decade has demonstrated clearly that defects of growth inhibitory control mechanisms contribute significantly to the expression of the malignant phenotype of human mammary epithelial cells. Several sites of defects in inhibitory mechanisms have been identified. Transformation to full malignancy by oncogenes leads to escape from growth inhibition by TGFβ. Deficient production of the growth inhibitor mammastatin has been correlated with the process of malignant transformation. Hormonal regulation of TGFβ is tightly coupled to the hormonally controlled growth state of estrogen responsive human breast cancer cells; TGFβ represents the only known endocrine-regulated growth modulator with *inhibitory* potential. A thorough knowledge of the biological function and interaction of these factors with other growth regulating pathways will certainly provide better insights into the process of malignant transformation and allow the development of improved strategies for prevention, diagnosis and treatment of human breast cancer.

Acknowledgments

The work performed in the author's laboratory and cited in this chapter was supported by a grant from the Deutsche Forschungsgemeinschaft (Ho 388/6-1/6).

REFERENCES

1. Sporn MB, Todaro GJ. Autocrine secretion and malignant transformation of cells. *N Eng J Med* 1980;303:878–880.
2. Goustin AS, Leof EB, Shipley GD, Moses HL. Growth factors and cancer. *Cancer Res* 1986;46:1015–1029.
3. Lippman ME. Endocrine responsive cancers of man. In: Williams RH, ed. *Textbook of Endocrinology*. Philadelpia: Saunders, 1985;1309–1326.
4. Dickson RB, Lippman ME. Estrogenic regulation of growth and polypeptide growth factor secretion in human breast carcinoma. *Endocrine Reviews* 1987;8:29–43.
5. Sainsbury JRC, Farndon JR, Sherbet GV, Harris AL. Epidermal growth factor receptors and oestrogen receptors in human breast cancer. *Lancet* 1985;i:364–366.
6. Sainsbury JRC, Farndon JR, Needham GK, Malcolm AJ, Harris AL. Epidermal growth factor receptor status as predictor of recurrence of and early death from breast cancer. *Lancet* 1987;i:1398–1402.
7. Slamon DJ, Godolphin W, Jones LA, et al. Studies of the HER-2/neu proto-oncogene in human breast and ovarian cancer. *Science* 1989;244:707–712.
8. Slamon DJ, Clark GM, Wong SG, Levin WJ, Ullrich A, McGuire WL. Human breast cancer: correlation of relapse and survival with amplification of the HER-2/neu oncogene. *Science* 1987;235:177–182.
9. Scott JA, McGuire WL. New molecular markers of prognosis in breast cancer. In: Voigt KD, Knabbe C eds. *Endocrine dependent tumors*. New York: Raven Press, 1990.
10. Ennis BW, Valverius EM, Bates SE, et al. Anti-epidermal growth factor receptor antibodies inhibit the autocrine-stimulated growth of MDA-468 human breast cancer cells. *Mol Endocrinol* 1989;3:1830–1838.
11. Huff KK, Knabbe C, Lindsey R, et al. Multihormonal regulation of insulin-like growth factor-I-related protein in MCF-7 human breast cancer cells. *Mol Endocrinology* 1988;2:200–208.
12. Colletti RB, Roberts JD, Devlin JT, Copland, KC. Effect of tamoxifen on plasma insulin-like growth factor I in patients with breast cancer. *Cancer Res* 1989;49:1882–1884.
13. Yee D, Cullen KJ, Paik S, et al. Insulin-like growth factor II mRNA expression in human breast cancer. *Cancer Res* 1988;48:6691–6696.
14. Travers MT, Barrett-Lee PJ, Berger U, et al. Growth factor expression in normal, benign, and malignant breast tissue. *Br Med J* 1988;296:1621–1624.
15. Klein G. The approaching area of the tumor suppressor genes. *Science* 1987;238:1539–1545.
16. Weinberg RA. Oncogenes, antioncogenes, and the molecular bases of multistep carcinogenesis. *Cancer Res* 1989;49:3713–3721.
17. Sager R. Tumor suppressor genes: the puzzle and the promise. *Science* 1989;246:1406–1412.
18. Sporn MB, Roberts AB. Autocrine growth factors and cancer. *Nature* 1985;313:745–747.
19. Iversen OH. Chalones. In: Baserga R, ed. *Handbook of Experimental Pharmacology*. Berlin: Springer-Verlag, 1981.
20. Massague J. The TGFβ-family of growth and differentiation factors. *Cell* 1987;49:437–438.
21. Roberts AB, Anzano MA, Lamb LC, Smith JM, Sporn MB. New class of transforming growth factors potentiated by epidermal growth factor: isolation from non-neoplastic tissue. *Proc Natl Acad Sci USA* 1981;78:5339–5343.
22. Assoian RK, Komoriya A, Meyers CA, Miller DM, Sporn MB. Transforming growth factor β in human platelets. *J Biol Chem* 1983;258:7155–7160.
23. Moses HL, Branum EL, Proper JA, Robinson RA. Transforming growth factor production by chemically transformed cells. *Cancer Res* 1981;41:2842–2848.
24. Derynck R, Jarrett JA, Chen EY, et al. Human transforming growth factor-β complementary DNA sequence and expression in normal and transformed cells. *Nature* 1985;316:701–705.
25. de Martin R, Haendler B, Hofer-Warbinek R, et al. Complementary DNA for human glioblastoma-derived T cell suppressor factor, a novel member of the transforming growth factor-β gene family. *EMBO J* 1987;6:3673–3677.
26. Madisen L, Webb NR, Rose TM, et al. Transforming growth factor-β2: cDNA cloning and sequence analysis. *DNA* 1988;7:1–8.
27. Derynck R, Lindquist PB, Lee A, et al. A new type of transforming growth factor-β, TGF-β3. *EMBO J* 1988;7:3737–3743.

28. Sporn MB, Roberts AB. Peptide growth factors are multifunctional. *Nature* 1989;332:217–219.
29. Ellingsworth LR, Nakayama D, Segarini P, Dasch J, Carillo P, Waegell W. Transforming growth factor betas are equipotent growth inhibitors of interleukin-1 induced thymocyte proliferation. *J Immunol* 1988;114:41–44.
30. Espevik T, Figari IS, Ranges GE, Palladino MA. Transforming growth factor β-1 and recombinant tumor necrosis factor reciprocally regulate the generation of lymphokine-activated killer cell activity. Comparison between natural porcine platelet-derived TGFβ-1 and TGFβ-2 and recombinant TGFβ-1. *J Immunol* 1988;140:2312–2316.
31. Ohta M, Greenberger J, Anklesaria P, Bassols A, Massague J. Two forms of transforming growth factor β distinguished by multipotential hematopoetic progenitor cells. *Nature* 1987;329:539–541.
32. Ottmann OG, Pelus LM. Differential proliferative effects of transforming growth factor β on human hematopoetic progenitor cells. *J Immunol* 1988;140:2661–2665.
33. Rosa F, Roberts AB, Danielpour D, Dart L, Sporn MB, Dawid IB. Mesoderm induction in amphibians: the role of TGF-β2-like factors. *Science* 1988;239:783–785.
34. Silberstein GB, Daniel CW. Reversible inhibition of mammary gland growth by transforming growth factor β. *Science* 1987;237:291–293.
35. Knabbe C, Lippman ME, Kasid A, et al. Evidence that transforming growth factor β is a hormonally regulated negative growth factor in human breast cancer cells. *Cell* 1987;48:417–428.
36. Zugmaier G, Ennis BE, Deschauer B, et al. Transforming growth factors type β1 and β2 are equipotent inhibitors of human breast cancer cell lines. *J Cell Physiol* 1989;141:353–361.
37. Roberts AB, Anzano MA, Wakefield LM, Roche NS, Stern DF, Sporn MB. Type β transforming growth factor: a bifunctional regulator of cellular growth. *Proc Natl Acad Sci USA* 1985;82:119–123.
38. Ranchalis JE, Gentry L, Ogawa Y, et al. Bone-derived and recombinant transforming growth factors-βs are potent inhibitors of tumor cell growth. *Biochem Biophys Res Comm* 1987;148:783–789.
39. Arrick BA, Korc M, Derynck R. Differential regulation of expression of three transforming growth factor beta species in human breast cancer cell lines by estradiol. *Cancer Res* 1990;50:299–303.
40. Arteaga CL, Tandon AK, Van Hoff DD, Osborne CK. Transforming Growth Factor β: potential autocrine growth inhibitor of estrogen receptor-negative human breast cancer cells. *Cancer Res* 1988;48:3898–3904.
41. King RJ, Wang DY, Daly RJ, Darbre PD. Approaches to studying the role of growth factors in the progression of breast tumors from the steroid sensitive to insensitive state. *J Steroid Biochem* 1989;34:133–138.
42. Shipley GD, Pittelkow MR, Wille JJ, Scott RE, Moses HL. Reversible inhibition of normal human prokeratinocyte proliferation by type β transforming growth factor-growth inhibitor in serum-free medium. *Cancer Res* 1986;46:2068–2071.
43. Kimchi A, Wang XF, Weinberg RA, Cheifetz S, Massague J. Absence of TGFβ receptors and growth inhibitory responses in retinoblastoma cells. *Science* 1988;240:196–199.
44. Stampfer MR, Bartley JC. Induction of transformation and continuous cell lines from normal human mammary epithelial cells after exposure to benzo-a-pyrene. *Proc Natl Acad Sci USA* 1985;82:2394–2398.
45. Zajchowski D, Band V, Pauzie N, Tager A, Stampfer M, Sager R. Expression of growth factors and oncogenes in normal and tumor-derived human mammary epithelial cells. *Cancer Res* 1988;48:7041–7047.
46. Valverius EM, Walker-Jones D, Bates SE, et al. Production of and responsiveness to transforming growth factor-β in normal and oncogene-transformed human mammary epithelial cells. *Cancer Res* 1989;49:6269–6274.
47. Walker-Jones D, Valverius EM, Stampfer MR, Lippman ME, Dickson RB. Stimulation of epithelial membrane antigen expression by transforming growth factor β in normal and oncogene-transformed human mammary epithelial cells. *Cancer Res* 1989;49:6407–6411.
48. Masui T, Wakefield LM, Lechner JF, LaVeck MA, Sporn MB, Harris CC. Type β transforming growth factor is the primary differentiation-inducing factor for normal human bronchial epithelial cells. *Proc Natl Acad Sci USA* 1986;83:2438–2442.
49. Cheifetz S, Weatherbee JA, Tsang LS, et al. The transforming growth factor β system, a complex pattern of cross-reactive ligands and receptors. *Cell* 1987;48:409–415.
50. Segarini PR, Rosen DM, Seyedin SM. Binding of transforming growth factor-β to cell surface proteins varies with cell type. *Mol Endocrinol* 1989;3:261–272.

51. Wakefield LM, Smith DM, Masui T, Harris CC, Sporn MB. Distribution and modulation of the cellular receptor for transforming growth factor β. *J Cell Biol* 1987;105:965–975.

52. Murthy US, Anzano MA, Stadel JM, Greig R. Coupling of TGF-β-induced mitogenesis to G-protein activation in AKR-2B cells. *Biochem Biophys Res Comm* 1988;152:1228–1235.

53. Howe PH, Bascom CC, Cunningham MR, Leof EB. Regulation of transforming growth factor β1 by multiple transducing pathways: evidence for both G protein-dependent and -independent signalling. *Cancer Res* 1989;49:6024–6031.

54. Fernandez-Pol JA, Klos DJ, Hamilton PD, Talkad VD. Modulation of epidermal growth factor expression by transforming growth factor β in a human breast carcinoma cell line. *Cancer Res* 1987;47:4260–4265.

55. Fernandez-Pol JA, Hamilton PD, Klos DJ. Transcriptional regulation of proto-oncogene expression by epidermal growth factor, transforming growth factor β1, and triiodothyronine in MDA-468 cells. *J Biol Chem* 1989;264:4151–4156.

56. Press RD, Misra A, Gillapsy G, Samols D, Goldthwait DA. Control of the expression of c-sis mRNA in human glioblastoma cells by phorbol ester and transforming growth factor β. *Cancer Res* 1989;49:2914–2920.

57. Roberts AB, Flanders KC, Kondaiah P, et al. Transforming growth factor β: Biochemistry and roles in embryogenesis, tissue repair and remodeling, and carcinogenesis. *Rec Prog Horm Res* 1988;44:157–197.

58. Chiquet-Ehrismann R, Kalla P, Pearson CA. Participation of tenascin and transforming growth factor-β in reciprocal epithelial-mesenchymal interactions of MCF-7 cells and fibroblasts. *Cancer Res* 1989;49:4322–4325.

59. Knabbe C, Zugmaier G, Dickson RB, Lippman ME. Transforming growth factor β and other growth inhibitory polypeptides in human breast cancer. *Prog Cancer Res Therapy* 1988;35:234–237.

60. Mulder KM, Ramey MK, Hoosein NM, et al. Characterization of transforming growth factor-β-resistant subclones isolated from a transforming growth factor-β-sensitive human colon carcinoma cell line. *Cancer Res* 1988;48:7120–7125.

61. Lawrence DA, Pircher R, Kryceve-Martinerie, Lullien P. Normal embryo fibroblasts release transforming growth factors in a latent form. *J Cell Physiol* 1984;121:184–188.

62. Lyons RM, Keski-Oja J, Moses HL. Proteolytic activation of latent transforming growth factor β from fibroblast-conditioned medium. *J Cell Biol* 1988;106:1659–1665.

63. Antonelli-Orlidge A, Saunders KB, Smith SR, d'Amore PA. An activated form of transforming growth factor β is produced by cocultures of endothelial cells and pericytes. *Proc Natl Acad Sci USA* 1989;86:4544–4548.

64. Sato Y, Rifkin DB. Inhibition of endothelial cell movement by pericytes and smooth muscle cells: activation of a latent transforming growth factor β-1 molecule by plasmin during coculture. *J Cell Biol* 1989;109:309–315.

65. Wakefield LM, Smith DM, Flanders KC, Sporn MB. Latent transforming growth factor β from human platelets: a high molecular weight complex containing precursor sequence. *J Biol Chem* 1988;263:7646–7654.

66. Miyazono K, Hellman U, Wernstedt C, Heldin CH. Latent high molecular weight complex of transforming growth factor β-1: purification from human platelets and structural characterization. *J Biol Chem* 1988;263:6407–6415.

67. Salomon DS, Zwiebel JA, Bano M, Losonczy I, Fehnel P, Kidwell WR. Presence of transforming growth factors in human breast cancer cells. *Cancer Res* 1984;44:4069–4077.

68. Bates SE, Dickson RB, McManaway ME, Lippman ME. Characterization of estrogen responsive transforming activity in human breast cancer cell lines. *Cancer Res* 1986;46:1707–1713.

69. Knabbe C, Hilgers W, Knust B, Danielpour D, Zugmaier G. Differential control of TGFβ-1 and TGFβ-2 in MCF-7 cells. *Proc Am Ass Can Res* 1990;31:221.

70. Danielpour D, Dart LD, Flanders KC, Roberts AB, Sporn MB. Immunodetection and quantitation of the two forms of transforming growth factor-beta (TGF-β1 and TGF-β2) secreted by cells in culture. *J Cell Physiol* 1989;138:79–86.

71. Murphy LC, Dotzlaw H. Regulation of transforming growth factor α and transforming growth factor β messenger ribonucleic acid abundance in T-47D human breast cancer cells. *Mol Endocrinol* 1989;3:611–617.

72. Knabbe C, Schmahl M, Lippman ME, Dickson RB. Induction of transforming growth factor beta by the antiestrogens droloxifene and tamoxifen in MCF-7 cells. *J Cancer Res* 1990; (Suppl 116):929.

73. Black LJ, Goode RL. Evidence for biological action of the antiestrogens LY 117018 and tamoxifen by different mechanisms. *Endocrinology* 1983;109:987–989.

74. Weatherill PJ, Wilson APM, Nicholson RI, Davies P, Wakeling AE. Interaction of the antiestrogen ICI 164,384 with the oestrogen receptor. *J Steroid Biochem* 1988;30:263–266.

75. Murphy LC, Dotzlaw H. Endogenous growth factor expression in T-47D, human breast cancer cells, associated with reduced sensitivity to antiproliferative effects of progestins and antiestrogens. *Cancer Res* 1989;49:599–604.

76. Kerr DJ, Pragnell IB, Sproul A, et al. The cytostatic effects of alpha-interferon may be mediated by transforming growth factor-beta. *J Mol Endocrinol* 1989;2:131–136.

77. Kasid A, Knabbe C, Lippman ME. Effect of v-Ha-ras oncogene transfection on estrogen-independent tumorigenicity of estrogen-dependent human breast cancer cells. *Cancer Research* 1987;47: 5733–5738.

78. Dickson RB, Kasid A, Huff K, et al. Activation of growth factor secretion in tumorigenic states of breast cancer induced by 17β-estradiol or v-Ha-ras oncogene. *Proc Natl Acad Sci USA* 1987;84:837–841.

79. Ethier SP, van de Velde RM. Secretion of a TGFβ-like growth inhibitor by normal rat mammary epithelial cells in vitro. *J Cell Physiol* 1990;142:15–20.

80. Greene GL, Sobel NB, King WJ, Jensen EV. Immunochemical studies of estrogen receptors. *J Steroid Biochem* 1984;20:51–56.

81. Derynck R, Goeddel DV, Ullrich A, et al. Synthesis of messenger RNAs for transforming growth factors α and β and the epidermal growth factor by human tumors. *Cancer Res* 1987;47:707–712.

82. Lehmann W, Graetz H, Widmayer R, Langen P. Fetal calf serum and epidermal growth factor prevent the inhibitory action of a chalone-like growth inhibitor for Ehrlich ascites mammary carcinoma cells in vitro. *Biomed Biochim Acta* 1984;43:971–974.

83. Böhmer FD, Lehmann W, Noll F, Samtleben R, Langen P, Grosse R. Specific neutralizing antiserum against a polypeptide growth inhibitor for mammary cells purified from bovine mammary gland. *Biochim Biophys Acta* 1985;846:145–154.

84. Brandt R, Pepperle M, Otto A, Kraft R, Boehmer FD, Grosse R. A 13-kilodalton protein purified from milk fat globule membranes is closely related to a mammary-derived growth inhibitor. *Biochemistry* 1988;27:1420–1425.

85. Böhmer FD, Kraft R, Otto A, et al. Identification of a polypeptide growth inhibitor from bovine mammary gland. Sequence homology to fatty acid- and retinoid-binding proteins. *J Biol Chem* 1987;262:15137–43.

86. Lehmann W, Widmaier R, Langen P. Response of different mammary epithelial cell lines to mammary derived growth inhibitor (MDGI). *Biomed Biochim Acta* 1989;48:143–151.

87. Kidwell WR, Bano M, Liu SC, Sanfilippo B, Salomon DS. Growth regulating factors from breast epithelium and milk. *Proc Am Ass Cancer Res* 1988;29:236.

88. Ervin PR Jr, Kaminski MS, Cody RL, Wicha MS. Production of mammastatin, a tissue-specific growth inhibitor, by normal human mammary cells. *Science* 1989;244:1585–1587.

89. Gaffney EV, Pigott DA, Grimaldi MA. Human serum and the growth of mammary cells. *J Natl Cancer Inst* 1979;63:913–918.

90. Dell'Aquila ML, Gaffney EV. Response of malignant mammary cell lines to a growth inhibitor partially purified from plasma-derived serum. *J Natl Cancer Inst* 1984;73:397–403.

91. Shoyab M, McDonald VL, Bradley GJ, Todaro G. Amphiregulin: a bifunctional growth-modulating glycoprotein produced by the phorbol 12-myristate 13-acetate-treated human breast adenocarcinoma cell line MCF-7. *Proc Natl Acad Sci USA* 1988;85:6528–6532.

Endocrine Dependent Tumors, edited by
Klaus-Dieter Voigt and Cornelius Knabbe.
Raven Press, Ltd., New York © 1991.

7

New Molecular Markers of Prognosis in Breast Cancer

Jeffrey A. Scott and William L. McGuire

Department of Medicine/Oncology, The University of Texas Health Science Center, San Antonio, San Antonio, Texas 78284

Breast cancer is a common disease, with more than 135,000 new cases diagnosed in the United States in 1988. Forty-two thousand women died from breast cancer in 1988 (1). Node-negative breast cancer represents about 50% of all newly diagnosed cases. Of these, only about 70% of the patients will be cured by primary therapy alone. Because of the heterogeneous population, it has become important to be able to define prognostic subgroups to select the most effective treatment and to aid in the evaluation of clinical trials.

There are several independent but interrelated factors predicting for recurrence and survival in breast cancer. These include axillary nodal status, hormonal receptors, proliferative rate, ploidy, and more recently, oncogene amplification. In this chapter, we review the newer molecular markers and compare them to more traditional prognostic factors (Table 1).

AXILLARY NODAL STATUS

For many years, it has been observed that axillary node status is the most important factor predicting recurrence and survival in breast cancer. It has been a clinical observation that most patients with negative axillary nodes were cured by the removal of the primary tumor (70% to 75%); only a minority (25% to 30%) were cured if the axillary nodes were positive.

In 1968, findings from the first clinical trial of the National Surgical Breast and Bowel Project (NSABP) showed that increasing numbers of positive axillary nodes were associated with a progressively greater incidence of treatment failures. A sharp rise occurred when four nodes or greater contained tumor. In fact, a 25% difference in 5-year survival was noted between a group of patients with one to three positive nodes and those patients with greater than or equal to four positive nodes (2). This

TABLE 1. *Prognostic factors*

Axillary node status
Hormonal receptors
Proliferative rate
Ploidy
Oncogenes

has been confirmed by several other investigators and in subsequent NSABP studies (3–5).

The San Antonio Breast Tumor Bank contains more than 5,900 cases of primary breast cancer followed up for a median of 40 months (6). Our data show a direct correlation between axillary node status and disease-free survival. The data stratify disease-free survival in patients with four or more positive lymph nodes: four to ten nodes (54%), 11–20 nodes (39%), and more than 20 nodes (27%). As in the NSABP studies there also is a direct correlation between overall survival and presence of axillary nodes (Fig. 1).

The presence and degree of involvement of tumor in axillary nodes predict recurrence and survival in primary breast cancer. Axillary nodal status remains the "gold standard" to which all other prognostic factors must be compared.

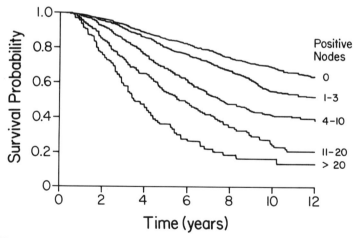

FIG. 1. Disease-free survival in more than 5,900 cases of primary breast cancer according to axillary lymph node status, median F/U of 40 months. (Adapted from Saez et al., ref. 6.)

STEROID RECEPTORS

Steroid Receptors long have been used to predict response to hormonal therapy and prognosis. Estrogen action, like most of steroid hormones, is mediated by binding to a specific nuclear protein, ER, and a subsequent interaction of this hormone-receptor complex with DNA. The use of receptor status is dependent on complex but reproducible assays of receptor content (7,8). Steroid receptors have been measured accurately by both dextran-coated charcoal or sucrose density gradient centrifugation methods (9,10).

As early as 1971, the presence of ER was used to predict response to endocrine therapy in patients with metastatic disease (11). Many investigators have noted a response to endocrine therapy in 60% of patients who exhibit the ER. This can increase to as high as 80% in those patients who are progesterone receptor-positive as well. Those patients without ER respond less than 10% to the therapy. In addition, the response to endocrine therapy in ER-positive patients is proportional to the quantitative amount of ER in the specimens.

The value of ER as a prognostic factor has been shown in studies of primary breast cancer. Knight and colleagues (12) measured ER in a series of 145 patients with operable breast cancer, and found that irrespective of age, nodal status, or size of the tumor, patients with ER-negative tumors had a higher rate of recurrence. When these data were updated (13), a higher rate of recurrence was again seen in all subsets of patients with ER-negative tumors, as well as a shorter duration of survival. Other investigators have shown that irrespective of stage, ER predicts for longer disease-free survival (DFS) and overall survival (13–16).

Because only 60% of patients with ER-positive tumors responded to endocrine therapy, an interest in progesterone receptors (PgR) arose. Progesterone receptor seemed ideal because estrogen stimulates its production in some breast cancer lines as well as in normal reproductive tissue. The distribution of PgR in a large number of breast tumor specimens can be seen in Table 2. As might be predicted, there were very few patients who were ER negative/PgR positive.

Clark and associates (10) evaluated retrospectively the relation between ER and PgR in 318 patients with Stage II breast cancer receiving adjuvant therapy. When evaluating DFS by univariate analysis, number of positive axillary nodes, size of the primary, ER and PgR correlated with time to recurrence. To evaluate the asso-

TABLE 2. *ER and PgR in 1366 human breast tumors*

Receptor Status	Premenopausal	Postmenopausal
ER+ PgR+	49%	55%
ER+ PgR−	12%	23%
ER− PgR+	9%	3%
ER− PgR−	30%	19%

Adapted from Osborne et al., ref. 13.

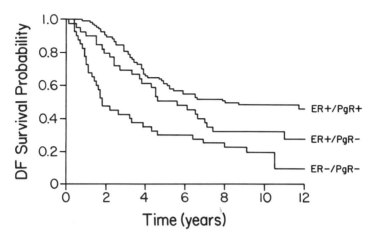

FIG. 2. Disease-free survival in 318 patients with stage II breast cancer, stratified for estrogen and progesterone receptors. (Adapted from Saez et al, ref. 6.)

ciation between the two receptors, four groups according to the ER/PgR content were chosen: ER + /PgR + , ER + /PgR − , ER − /PgR + , and ER − /PgR − . In this analysis, DFS was better for the ER + /PgR + group suggesting that PgR might be more important than the ER (Fig. 2). When DFS was analyzed by multivariate analysis, only the number of positive nodes and PgR retained significance. From hormonal receptor analysis, it can be concluded that ER and PgR predict for early recurrence and survival in Stage I and II breast cancer.

The recent cloning of a human ER complementary DNA has made possible the characterization of the ER gene on a molecular level. Hill and coworkers (17) examined in human breast cancers a single, two-allele restriction fragment length polymorphism (RFLP) using the restriction enzyme PvuII. Initial studies in human breast cancer cell lines suggested a possible association between the absence of one allele and the absence of ER expression. Subsequent analysis of allele distribution and frequency in 188 primary human breast tumor biopsies showed a significant correlation between absence of one allele and failure to express ER.

CELLULAR KINETICS

Thymide Labeling Index (TLI)

Although axillary node status is considered the single most important prognostic factor for patients with breast cancer, 30% of early breast cancer patients with histologically negative lymph nodes have recurrence of and die from their disease in 10 years (18). Although steroid receptors also are important prognostic variables, they cannot account for the varied course seen in breast cancer patients. Pathologists have known for a long time that the more mitotic figures in a tumor specimen, the more likely the tumor exhibits aggressive behavior, with subsequent shortening of the patient's survival. Because these characteristics are very difficult to quantitate, many investigators have utilized the thymidine labeling index (TLI) as a measure of proliferative rate.

The TLI is based on incubating fresh viable tumor specimens with tritiated thymidine, a precursor that incorporates specifically into DNA in cells actively synthesizing DNA. This enables the identification of S-phase cells through the use of autoradiography. The exposure time is 1 to 2 weeks, and the TLI is obtained by counting 3,000 to 10,000 cells from different specimens from the same tumor (19,20). The constraints imposed by the need of fresh tissue, by the delay in obtaining results from radiography, and by the tediousness involved in cell counting, are the main disadvantages of this procedure.

Several independent investigators have related TLI and the probability of relapse in breast cancer. Tubiani and colleagues (21) prospectively measured the TLI in 128 patients with subsequent follow-up of at least 10 years. Patients with lowest TLI had longer relapse-free and overall survival. A multivariate analysis of the prognostic factors showed that TLI was a better indicator than size of the tumor, number of involved nodes, or histologic grading. Meyer and associates (22) analyzed TLI in 227 patients with primary breast cancer. Patients with low TLI had a probability of relapse of 20% at 4 years, in contrast to 52% for patients with high TLI. There was an association between high TLI, younger age, and other poor prognostic factors. The probability of relapse was significantly related to TLI independent of axillary node status, ER content, or menopausal status. Silvestrini and coworkers (23) reviewed 127 stage I breast cancer patients. Again they found that the probability of relapse was higher in patients whose tumors had high TLI. The investigators also noted that the premenopausal group of patients had higher TLIs than the postmenopausal group, but in each group, the proliferative rate predicted for higher relapse rate.

TLI also correlates with histologic characteristics of the tumor. Meyer and associates (24) found that tumors with undifferentiated nuclei, an inflammatory response or necrosis, had a higher mean TLI. The TLI is typically increased in ER-negative tumors (25,26). An increased PgR content also has been associated with a decreased TLI.

FLOW CYTOMETRY

DNA flow cytometry (FCM) is a new approach for measuring proliferative rate by identifying S-phase cells with the use of DNA-specific fluorescent stains. Unlike TLI, which requires fresh tissue, FCM can be done on frozen pulverized tumor

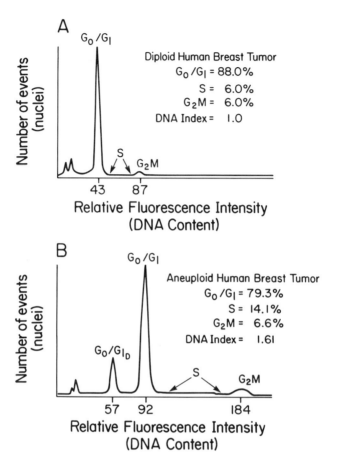

FIG. 3. DNA histograms for a diploid and aneuploid tumor specimen. The G_0/G_1 peak of the aneuploid population appears to the right of the normal diploid peak, indicating an ↑ DNA content. S-phase nuclei are located between the G_0/G_1 and G_2M peaks of the population. (Adapted from *J Natl Cancer Inst* 1985;75(3):405–410.)

specimens. After preparation of a single cell suspension from the specimen, the DNA content of 100,000 cells can be measured by FCM in a few minutes and the fraction of cells in S-phase (SPF) can be calculated (Fig. 3). An important advantage of this technique over TLI is that the analysis can be performed on frozen specimens after acetic acid fixation or on fixed paraffin-embedded blocks of tumor tissue. A good correlation between SPF by TLI and FCM has been shown (27). Poorly differentiated tumors, and ER-negative tumors tend to have higher SPF.

In a study by Moran, ER + /PgR + tumors had a mean SPF of 11% as compared to a mean of 20% in receptor negative tumors (28). The percent SPF can be a more important prognostic indicator than receptor status and cellular differentiation. The percent SPF, when low, predicted an increased time to relapse and overall survival. Multivariate analysis could not demonstrate a variable independent of the percent SPF that more significantly predicted relapse.

DNA flow cytometry also offers the advantage of determining cell populations with abnormal DNA content (aneuploid). The DNA index is a quantitative reflection of the degree of aneuploidy and can be calculated from DNA histograms. Dressler and associates (29) measured DNA content in 1184 tumors. In this series, 57% of the tumors were aneuploid. These aneuploid tumors could further be classified as simple hyperdiploid (55%), hypodiploid (3.7%), tetraploid (25%), and multiploid (8.8%). The median percent SPF for the diploid tumors was 2.6%, as opposed to 10.3% in aneuploid tumors. Receptor negative tumors were more aneuploid and had the highest median percent SPF. Other investigators also have noted that anaplastic tumors have a higher percentage of aneuploidy than well differentiated tumors (30,31).

The implication from many of the early studies is that breast cancers with a higher percent SPF and aneuploidy have a more aggressive course. Clark and coworkers (32) have investigated the impact of ploidy and percent SPF in node negative patients. Ploidy was determined in 346 specimens and patients' follow-up data were available for a median of 45 months. Patients whose tumors showed aneuploidy had a poor prognosis and could be considered at high risk for recurrence regardless of the SPF. Women with aneuploid tumors also had a shorter DFS than those with diploid tumors. Among the women with diploid tumors, a high percent SPF predicted a worse prognosis with a shorter DFS (32).

ONCOGENES

The techniques of molecular biology are shedding new insight into the subcellular pathology of malignancy. The crucial events of carcinogenesis, tumor progression, and metastatic spread are coming into focus at a molecular level. In some tumors, these advances in the laboratory are beginning to have applications at the bedside. Recently, abnormalities in the copy number and expression of several genes has been correlated with prognosis of individual patients with selected types of cancer. Molecular biology labs can provide useful predictive information and help guide therapeutic maneuvers.

Attempts to determine the prognostic significance of individual genes has focused almost entirely on abnormalities involving cellular protooncogenes. These cellular oncogenes (protooncogenes) are normal constituents of the mammalian cell, which are associated with an increased risk of malignancy when they are altered (33–35). Evidence of this association of oncogenes and the neoplastic process include sequence homology between cellular genes and genes carried by acute transforming viruses, transforming ability of these genes in transforming assays, detection of protooncogene sequences at or near the breakpoints of consistent chromosomal translocations, and amplification or overexpression of these genes in some cancers and malignant cell lines.

Amplification, mutation, deletion, and translocation all have been associated with an increased risk of malignancy. Investigators have sought prognostic correlations with many of these abnormalities. The possibility that extra gene copies or gene amplification within a tumor genome might be related to prognosis was suggested by earlier correlations between karyotypic (36) or DNA content (37–39) abnormalities and clinical outcome. The demonstration that double minute chromosomes and homogeneously staining regions are cytogenetic evidence of gene amplification gave further impetus to the search for specific genes involved in amplification (40–42). Gene amplification can be routinely demonstrated through hybridization of endonuclease-digested, size fractionated genomic DNA fragments with radiolabeled nucleotide sequences-specific probes, a technique known as Southern blotting (43).

Overexpression of cellular protooncogenes occurs in a wide variety of human malignancies (44). Overexpression can be measured by quantifying the amount of messenger RNA or amount of protein product. Messenger RNA is quantitated in a similar manner as DNA using Northern or slot blotting (45,46).

Subtle aberrations involving protooncogenes include variations in the base sequence of an allele or loss of an allele. Alleles that differ in nucleotide sequences at the cleavage site of a restriction endonuclease are detected as restriction fragment length polymorphisms (47). The loss of a single normal allele can permit expression of a recessive oncogenic allele (48). Loss of both alleles of a certain gene, or expression of an abnormal gene message, also can result in tumorigenisis, as exemplified by neuroblastoma (49).

Chromosomal rearrangements are another type of abnormality associated with oncogenes. Many hematologic malignancies are associated with characteristic chromosomal rearrangements (50). Cellular protooncogenes have been found at many of the breakpoints including the c-myc gene at the locus of the 8:14 translocation in Burkitt's lymphoma, and the c-abl gene at the point of the 9:22 translocation in chronic myelogenous leukemia (51–53).

As already reviewed, a variety of clinical and pathologic variables are known to be prognostically important in breast cancer. These include axillary lymph node status, ER and PR, cellular kinetics, and degree of aneuploidy. Other karyotypic abnormalities, including double minute chromosomes, are common in breast cancers and are correlated with a shortened survival (54,55). The presence of double-minute chromosomes suggests the importance and frequency of gene amplification. Several protooncogenes have been reported in association with breast cancer and their value in prediction of clinical behavior is just beginning to be understood. These include the HER-2/neu, c-ras, c-myc, and int-2 protooncogenes.

The HER-2/neu Oncogene

The HER-2/neu gene was isolated from three different sources using different techniques. Schechter and colleagues (56) noted the production of a protein with a relative molecular mass of 183,000 by a series of rat neuroglioblastoma cell lines induced by ethylnitrosurea. Transforming DNA isolated from these cell lines hybridized to an erb-B gene probe. The product of the erb-B gene, the epidermal growth factor receptor, was found to be antigenically related, but not identical to, the 185 kDa protein. Semba and coworkers (57) cloned two distinct genes from a human genomic library that hybridized to an erb-B probe. One was found to be the EGF receptor gene, and the other was subsequently shown to be amplified in a human salivary gland adenocarcinoma. This was the initial evidence that this gene, variously termed c-erb-2 or neu, was involved in human malignancy. An amplified gene with identical nucleotide sequence was subsequently cloned from a human breast cancer line (58). A third group, also using a viral erb-B probe isolated a cDNA coding for a 4.8kb mRNA that they named HER-2 because of its partial sequence homology with the human EGF receptor gene (59). They found that this gene was widely expressed in normal fetal and adult tissues. Subsequent studies confirmed that this new gene was distinct from the EGF receptor gene by mapping the gene to chromosome 17, unlike the EGF receptor gene that resides on chromosome 7. Subsequent studies determined that the three genes, neu, c-erb-B2, and HER-2, were identical (60,61). A fourth group using v-erb-B as a probe identified the gene in a mammary cell line, MAC 117, where it was found to be amplified five- to tenfold (58).

This gene, which we will refer to as HER-2/neu, encodes a new member of the tyrosine kinase family. Its protein product is distinct from that of EGFR gene, 185,000 daltons versus 170,000 daltons. The HER-2/neu gene generates a messenger RNA of 4.8kb compared to a mRNA of 5.8-10kb transcripts for the EGFR gene (62). The HER-2/neu protein has an extracellular domain, a transmembrane domain that includes two cysteine rich repeat clusters, and an intracellular kinase domain indicating that it is likely a cellular receptor for an as yet unidentified ligand.

Yokota and associates (63) studied 101 fresh tumors for presence of HER-2/neu amplification. They found evidence of amplification in five of 63 adenocarcinomas including two of ten breast cancers. None of the 32 other tumors, including sarcomas, squamous cell carcinoma, leukemias, and lymphomas had amplification of this gene. A second group found amplification in 16 of 95 breast cancer specimens, and that amplification was associated with overexpression of the 4.8kb mRNA (64).

Slamon and colleagues (65) undertook a large survey of clinical breast cancer specimens that were well characterized in terms of known prognostic factors. Nineteen of 103 samples showed evidence of HER-2/neu amplification, ranging from two to more than 20 copies on Southern blots. Amplification could not be correlated with hormone receptor status, size of primary tumor, or age of the patient. Gene amplification was, however, significantly more common in tumors taken from patients with more than three positive lymph nodes. This initial study indicated that it might be possible to discriminate among node-positive patients on the basis of HER-2/neu amplification. It was believed that given the correlation between number of lymph nodes positive and HER-2/neu amplification, one might predict that amplification of this gene also might have some prognostic value.

The study was extended to a second set of 86 tumors from patients with positive axillary lymph nodes and long-term clinical follow up. Amplification was found in 34/86 of these patients. A strong and highly statistically significant correlation was found between the degree of amplification and both time to disease relapse ($P = .0001$) and overall survival ($P = .0011$). Moreover, when compared in univariate analysis to other parameters, amplification of HER-2/neu was found to be superior to all other prognostic factors, with the exception of number of positive nodes (which it equaled) in predicting time to relapse and overall survival. Using multivariate analysis, amplification of the gene continued to be a strong prognostic factor, providing additional and independent predictive information on both time to relapse and overall survival in these patients, even when other prognostic factors were taken into account.

Zhou and coworkers (66) examined 98 breast cancer specimens for alterations of the HER-2/neu protooncogene. Amplification of this gene was found in 15 of 86 (17%) of primary breast cancer specimens and in three of 12 metastatic breast cancers. Amplification varied between three and 30-fold. Amplification of the gene was more common in breast cancers of stage III and IV than in stage I and II tumors ($P = .01$). Amplification of the HER-2/neu protooncogene was more common in primary tumors with metastasis to regional lymph nodes (eight of 37) than those confined to the breast (one of 21). Amplification of the HER-2/neu protooncogene was more common in primary breast cancers of stages I to III, which recurred within 3 years of mastectomy (four of 19, 32%) than in those that did not (two of 32, 6%).

Because expression of the oncogene product might be even more closely related than gene amplification to disease progression, Tandon and associates (67) have examined expression of the HER-2/neu oncogene protein for its prognostic potential in both node-positive and node-negative patients. Using Western blot analysis, expression of the HER-2/neu oncogene was determined in 728 primary human breast cancer specimens. In 378 node-negative patients, HER-2/neu expression failed to predict disease outcome. However, in 350 node-positive patients, those with higher expression of the HER-2/neu oncogene had statistically shorter disease-free survival ($P = .0014$) and overall survival ($P < .0001$) than patients with lower expression of the gene. Higher expression of the HER-2/neu oncogene was found in patients without estrogen and progesterone receptors and in those patients with greater than three positive lymph nodes. Higher expression of HER-2 oncogene protein was associated with a lower 5-year DFS and overall survival when patients were strati-

TABLE 3. *HER-2 expression in axillary node-positive breast cancer*

Positive nodes	Her-2 expression	N	5-yr DFS	5-yr OS
1–3	Low	136	60 ± 5	81 ± 4
	High	91	35 ± 13	42 ± 13
4–10	Low	67	48 ± 6	67 ± 6
	High	21	34 ± 10	39 ± 12
>10	Low	23	19 ± 5	45 ± 7
	High	17	24 ± 12	36 ± 13

fied for number of positive lymph nodes. The differences in survival diminished in patients with $>10+$ lymph nodes (Table 3). A significant correlation was seen between amplification of the HER-2/neu oncogene and protein expression. Multivariate analysis in these patients showed that expression of the HER-2/neu oncogene is a significant independent predictor of both DFS and overall survival in node positive breast cancer patients.

The c-myc Protooncogene

The c-myc protooncogene has been one of the most closely studied of all of the known protooncogenes (68,69). It was initially detected through hybridization with the analogous transforming gene carried by the avian myeloblastosis virus. Its importance in human malignancy was first suspected because of its involvement in the translocations characteristic of Burkitt's Lymphoma (33,68). The c-myc gene does not demonstrate transforming ability *in vitro* and point mutations are detected rarely.

The c-myc protein products are localized to the nucleus, where they participate in the progression of cells from G_0 to G_1 phase in response to certain mitogens (69). In some transformed cells, c-myc is expressed continuously. Transgenic mice carrying a deregulated myc gene develop breast cancer during pregnancy. High levels of myc mRNA were detected in both the cancers and a variety of apparently normal tissue in these mice (70).

Although there are data suggesting that the c-myc oncogene might be functionally important in some breast cancers, the relationship between c-myc and prognosis is not known. In 1984, Kozbor and associates (71) reported finding amplification of c-myc on one of five human breast cancer cell lines. Approximately eight- to 16-fold amplification was associated with overexpression of c-myc mRNA. A second breast cancer cell line was later shown to have amplification, which contained copies of the c-myc gene. After serial culture, the extra c-myc genes were found to have integrated into chromosomes (72).

Escot and colleagues (73) surveyed 121 primary human breast cancer specimens for evidence of c-myc amplification. In 25, there was a two- to five-fold amplification and in 13 patients there was a five- to 16-fold amplification. Overexpression of c-myc mRNA was found in patients with and without amplification. Amplification or rearrangement of the c-myc gene was not correlated with known prognostic variables, such as tumor grade, receptor status, or axillary lymph node involvement. The relationship between this gene and prognosis is not known.

The H-ras Protooncogene

The most frequently detected transformation-inducing genes in human solid tumors are members of the ras family of cellular oncogenes (74). Mutations in the ras gene have been found in approximately 15% of tumors, yielding a gene product (p21) with increased transforming ability (75,76). Transfected DNA from about 15% of human cancers has the ability to transform cultured NIH 3T3 cells (77). In fact, it is now known that about 90% of all human genes identified in this transforming assay are members of the ras family. These genes (H-ras, K-ras, and N-ras) have similar nucleotide sequences and code for proteins with a molecular weight of 21 kDa. Normal cellular ras genes do not appear to have transforming ability when transfected; all transforming ras genes have point mutations, which usually involve codon 12 or 61 (78,79).

Normal ras genes have been shown to transform the 3T3 cell line when they were overexpressed or amplified. Overexpression has been achieved by linking the ras gene to retroviral clements (80). It is not known whether H-ras amplification plays a role in spontaneous cancers, but overexpression of ras p21 protein has been reported (81–85).

Kasid and coworkers (86), transfected the v-ras oncogene into MCF-7 breast cancer cells. In contrast to the parental cell line, MCF-7$_{ras}$ cells no longer responded to exogenous estrogen in culture and their growth was minimally inhibited by exogenous antiestrogens. When tested in the nude mouse, the MCF-7$_{ras}$ cells were fully tumorigenic in the absence of estrogen supplementation. This showed that cells acquiring an activated oncogene were able to bypass the hormonal regulatory signals that trigger the neoplastic growth of a human breast cancer cell line. Oncogene activation might be one method that human breast cancer cells might alter their hormone-dependent phenotype.

Several investigators have noted the frequent overexpression of H-ras mRNA or p21 protein in breast cancers (44,87,88). Methods for determination included detection of increased amounts of H-ras mRNA or increased amounts of p21. Ohuchi and coworkers (89, 90), attempted to define the role of H-ras 21 in the development of breast cancers. On average, 18% of hyperplastic lesions reacted with an anti-p21 monoclonal antibody. This rose sequentially to 33% in hyperplasia with atypia, 52% in carcinoma *in situ*, and 60% in invasive carcinoma. Fifteen-year follow-up studies revealed a generally higher level of ras p21 in hyperplasia from patients who subsequently developed carcinoma, as compared to those from patients without carcinoma development. Carcinomas from postmenopausal patients generally demonstrated higher levels of ras p21 than those from premenopausal patients, but no significant difference in ras p21 expression in carcinomas between estrogen-receptor rich and estrogen-receptor poor patients was found.

Lundy and associates (91) reported on 41 breast cancers that were studied for H-ras expression. The primary tumors from ten of 21 patients with negative axillary lymph nodes stained positive of p21 antigen. In contrast, 19 of 20 primary tumors from women with axillary node metastasis were positive for p21 antigen. No correlation was found between estrogen receptor status and p21 antigen ($P = .03$).

Clair and colleagues (92) reviewed the association of H-ras p-21 oncogene with the progression and prognosis of breast cancer. The investigators found that 37 of 54 (69%) human breast cancer specimens contained p21 levels two- to tenfold greater than control breast tissue. Greater than fivefold increases over control occurred more frequently in patients with T_3 and T_4 (60%) disease compared to those with T_1 or T_2 (21%) primary tumors ($P<.05$). As with previous studies, p21 levels were positively correlated with involvement of axillary lymph nodes at time of primary therapy. These investigators were able to show a relation with tumor recurrence and p21 antigen. Eight of nine patients (89%) with tumors expressing low p21 antigen levels were disease free for more than 4 years after primary treatment, whereas only 5 of 9 patients (56%) with high p21 tumors remained disease free ($P<.05$). These results suggest that a quantitative enhancement of p21 oncogene is associated with both the progression and prognosis of breast cancer. These findings, however, are based on a small number of patients with various types of therapy and further study in larger groups is warranted.

Lidereau and coworkers (93) have noted at least 20 DNA restriction fragment length polymorphisms at the H-ras locus in human breast cancers. Peripheral leukocytes from these breast cancer patients contain the same H-ras alleles as the corresponding tumor specimens, implying that these are inherited polymorphisms rather than somatic mutations. Four common alleles accounted for 91% of all H-ras RFLPs in a normal population. The most frequent of these four alleles was significantly less common in breast cancer patients ($P<.001$). In contrast, 16 rare alleles were seen significantly more common in breast cancer patients ($P<.001$). Not all breast cancer patients had rare H-ras alleles, however, and their presence could not be associated with any clinical or pathologic characteristics of the patients or their tumors.

Theillet and coworkers (88), showed that deletion of an allele at the H-ras locus had important clinico-pathologic correlations. They noted increased expression of H-ras in 16 of 22 invasive ductal carcinomas of the breast. There was no increase in the expression of the K-ras or N-ras protooocogene. No amplification or rearrangement of the ras oncogene was noted. In tumor DNAs from 14 of 51 patients, heterozygous for the H-ras-1 related BamHI restriction fragments, one allele was lost. Correlation with clinicopathological data showed, however, that loss of one H-ras-1 allele in breast carcinoma DNAs is significantly linked to histologically Grade III tumors, the lack of estrogen and progesterone receptors, and the subsequent occurrence of distant metastasis. These results indicated that loss of one H-ras-1 allele correlated with more aggressive primary carcinomas of the breast. Further study is needed to determine whether the evaluation of H-ras structure can provide independent prognostic information in breast cancer.

The int-2 Protooncogene

The development of transforming virus-induced cancers in mice has been linked to expression of a gene related to the human int-2 gene. In the mouse, int-2 is induced by MMTV. The virus integrates into cellular DNA and activates previous silent genomic areas. Expression of the int-2 protooncogene encodes for a 27,000 dalton molecule, which is related to a fibroblast growth factor. The int-2 gene is apparently expressed during embryonic development but not in adult tissues.

In a series of 104 human primary breast cancer specimens, 16% had amplification of int-2. Int-2 amplification was significantly more common in patients who had known metastatic disease (94). Int-2 also has been found to be amplified in primary lung and colon tumors as well as in a variety of metastatic tumor.

CONCLUSION

Breast cancer presents a challenge to the oncologist. It is a major health problem worldwide. One of the biggest contributions to its care has been an increased public awareness leading to earlier diagnosis. However, as we near the end of the twentieth century, we still do not have a cure for metastatic or recurrent disease. Although adjuvant therapy is accepted as standard care in primary breast cancer, neither the particular therapeutic modalities involved nor the specific subset to which it should be directed are well defined. The major role of prognostic factors are to define those breast cancer patients at higher risk of recurrence who could benefit from additional therapy, and also to provide stratification factors to evaluate such therapy in clinical trials.

There are several independent but interrelated factors that predict for relapse and survival in breast cancer. Axillary node status remains the major prognostic factor for long-term survival. Estrogen and progesterone receptors predict for responsiveness to hormonal therapy and correlates with longer survival and disease-free interval in stage I and II breast cancer.

Several newer molecular markers that increase our predictive abilities are available. Studies have shown a correlation between a high TLI (or high S-phase fraction by flow cytometry) and a higher relapse rate in premenopausal and postmenopausal women with breast cancer. Aneuploidy also has been associated with a poorer prognosis. These prognostic factors are interrelated as ER-negative and PgR-negative tumors commonly are aneuploid with high SPF.

The role of oncogenes in the pathogenesis of breast cancer is just beginning to be elucidated. The fact that alterations in oncogenes can be related to prognosis in breast cancer provides an important link between the molecular level and the clinical behavior of the tumor.

Future trials will need to stratify on the basis of newer prognostic factors. Other than oncongenes, these factors can be obtained readily at the time the tumor is resected and the axillary nodes dissected.

Acknowledgment

This work was supported by NIH Grant CA30195

REFERENCES

1. CA-A Journal for Clinicians. In: Holleb IA, ed. *Cancer Statistics 1988*, 38(1).
2. Fischer B, Ravdin RG, Ausman RK, Slack NH, Moore GE. Survival adjuvant therapy in cancer of the breast. *Ann Surg* 1968;168:337-356.

3. Fisher B, Bauer M, Wickerham L. Relation of number of positive axillary nodes to the prognosis of patients with primary breast cancer. *Cancer* 1983;52:1551-1557.
4. Fisher B, Carbone P, Economou SG. L-phenylalanine mustard in the management of primary breast cancer: a report of early finding. *N Engl J Med* 1975;292:117-122.
5. Fisher B, Montague E, Redmond C. Comparison of radical mastectomy with alternative treatments for primary breast cancer: a first report of results from a prospective randomized clinical trial. *Cancer* 1977;39:2827-2829.
6. Saez RA, Clark GM, McGuire WL. Prognostic factors in cancer of the breast. In: Veronesi U, ed. *Bailliere's Clinical Oncology Volume 2 — Breast Cancer*. London: Bailliere Tindall, 1988;103-115.
7. King RJ. Quality control of estradiol receptor analysis: The United Kingdom experience. *Cancer* 1980;46:2822-2824.
8. Oxley DK. Hormone receptors in breast cancer: analytical accuracy of contemporary assays. *Arch Pathol Lab Med* 1987;108:20-23.
9. McGuire WL, De La Garza M, Chamness GC. Evaluation of estrogen receptor assays in human breast cancer tissue. *Cancer Res* 1977;37:637-639.
10. Clark GM, McGuire WL, Hubay CA, Pearson OH, Marshall JS. Progesterone receptors as prognostic factors in stage II breast cancer. *N Engl J Med* 1983;309:1343-1347.
11. Jensen EV, Block GE, Smith S, Kyser K, DeSombre E. Estrogen receptors and breast cancer response to adrenalectomy. *NCI Monogr* 1971;34:55-70.
12. Knight WA III, Livingston RB, Gregory EJ, McGuire WL. Estrogen receptor as an independent prognostic factor for early recurrence in breast cancer. *Cancer Res* 1977;37:4669-4671.
13. Osborne CK, Yochmowitz MG, Knight WA III, McGuire WL. The value of estrogen and progesterone receptors in the treatment of breast cancer. *Cancer* 1980;46:2884-2888.
14. Hahnel R, Woodings T, Vivian AB. Prognostic value of estrogen receptors in primary breast cancer. *Cancer* 1979;44:671-675.
15. Crowe JP, Hubay CA, Pearson OH, Marshall JS. Estrogen receptor status as a prognostic indicator for stage I breast cancer patients. *Breast Cancer Res Treat* 1982;2:171-176.
16. Valagussa P, Bignami P, Buzzoni R, Rilke F. Are estrogen receptors (ER) alone a reliable prognostic factor in node negative breast cancer. *Proc Am Soc Clin Oncol* 1984;C-511:130.
17. Hill SM, Fuqua SAW, Chamness GC, Greene GL, McGuire WL. Estrogen receptor expression in human breast cancer associated with an estrogen receptor gene restriction fragment length polymorphism. *Cancer Res* 1989;49:145-148.
18. Harris JR, Hellman S, Canellos GP, Fischer B. Cancer of the breast. In: DeVita VT, Rosenberg SA, eds. *Cancer Principles and Practice of Oncology*. Philadelphia: Lippincott, 1985;1119-1177.
19. Tannock I. Cell kinetics and chemotherapy. A critical review. *Cancer Treat Rep* 1978;62:1117-1133.
20. Meyer JS, Province M. Proliferative index of breast carcinoma by thymidine labeling: prognostic power independent of stage, estrogen and progesterone receptors. *Breast Cancer Res Treat* 1988;12:191-204.
21. Tubiani M, Pejovich MH, Chavaudra N, Contesso G, Malaise EP. The long term prognostic significance of thymidine labelling index in breast cancer. *Int J Cancer* 1984;33:441-445.
22. Meyer JS, Friedman E, McCrate MM, Bauer WC. Prediction of early course of breast carcinoma by thymidine labeling. *Cancer* 1983;51:1879-1886.
23. Silvestrini R, Daidone MG, Di Fronzo G, Morabito A, Valagussa P, Bonadonna G. Prognostic implication of labeling index versus estrogen receptors and tumor size in node-negative breast cancer. *Breast Cancer Res Treat* 1986;7:161-169.
24. Meyer RW, Pregy MU, Babcock DS, McDivitt RW. Breast carcinoma cell kinetics, morphology, stage and host characteristics: a thymidine labeling study. *Lab Invest* 1986;54:41-51.
25. Coulson PB, Thornthwaite JT, Woolley EV, Sugarbaker EV, Seckinger D. Prognostic indicators including DNA histogram type, receptor content, and staging related to human breast cancer patient survival. *Cancer Res* 1984;44:4187-4196.
26. Hedley DW, Rugg CA, Ng ABP, Taylor IW. Influence of cellular DNA content on disease-free survival of stage II breast cancer patients. *Cancer Res* 1984;44:5395-5398.
27. McDivitt RW, Stone KR, Craig RB, Meyer JS. A comparison of human breast cancer cell kinetics measured by flow cytometry and thymidine labeling. *Lab Invest* 1985;52:287.
28. Moran RE, Black MM, Alpert L, Straus MJ. Correlation of cell cycle kinetics, hormone receptors, histopathology, and nodel status in human breast cancer. *Cancer* 1984;54:1586-1590.
29. Dressler LG, Seamer LC, Owens MA, Clark GM, McGuire WL. DNA flow cytometry and prognostic factors in 1331 frozen breast cancer specimens. *Cancer* 1988;61:420-427.

30. Olszewski W, Darzynkiewicz Z, Rosen PP, Schwartz MK, Melamed MR. Flow cytometry of breast carcinoma: I. relation of DNA ploidy level to histology and estrogen receptor. *Cancer* 1981;48:980–984.
31. Olszewski W, Darzynkiewicz Z, Rosen PP, Schwartz MK, Melamed MR. Flow cytometry of breast cancer: II. Relation of tumor cell cycle distribution to histology and estrogen receptor. *Cancer* 1981;48:985–988.
32. Clark GM, Dressler LG, Owens MA, Pounds G, Oldaker T, McGuire WL. Prediction of relapse or survival in patients with node-negative breast cancer by DNA flow cytometry. *N Engl J Med* 1989; 320:627–633.
33. Barbacid M. Human oncogenes. In: De Vita Jr VT, Hellman S, Rosenberg SA, eds. *Advances in Oncology*. Philadelphia: Lippincott, 1986;322.
34. Bishop JM. Cellular oncogenes and retroviruses. *Ann Rev Biochem* 1983;52:301–354.
35. Bishop JM. The molecular genetics of cancer. *Science* 1987;235:305–311.
36. Sandberg AA. The Chromosome in Human Cancer and Leukemia. New York: Elsevier-Holland, 1980.
37. Barlogie B, Johnston DA, Smallwood L, Raber MN, et al. Prognostic implications of ploidy and proliferative activity in human solid tumors. *Cancer Genet Cytogenet* 1982;6:17–28.
38. Friedlander ML, Hedley DW, Taylor IW. Clinical and biological significance of aneuploidy in human tumors. *J Clin Pathol* 1984;37:961–974.
39. Merkel DE, Dressler LG, McGuire WL. Flow cytometry, cellular DNA content, and prognosis in human malignancy. *J Clin Oncol* 1987;5:1690–1703.
40. Gebhart E, Bruderlein S, Augustus M, Sieberg E, Feldner J, Schmidt W. Cytogenetic studies on human breast carcinomas. *Breast Cancer Res Treat* 1986;8:125–138.
41. Barker PE. Double minutes in human tumor cells. *Cancer Genet Cytogenet* 1982;5:81–94.
42. Cowell JK. Double minutes and homogenously staining regions: gene amplification in mammalian cells. *Ann Rev Genet* 1982;16:21–59.
43. Southern EM. Detection of specific sequences among DNA fragments separated by gel electrophoresis. *J Mol Biol* 1975;98:503–517.
44. Slamon DJ, deKernion JB, Verma IM, Cline MJ. Expression of cellular oncogenes in human malignancies. *Science* 1984;224:256–262.
45. Alwine JC, Kemp DJ, Start GR. Method for detection of specific RNAs in agarose gels by transfer to diazo-benzyloxy methyl paper and hybridization with DNA probes. *Proc Natl Acad Sci USA* 1977;74:5350–5359.
46. Thomas PS. Hybridization of denatured RNA transferred or dotted to nitrocellulose paper. Recombinant DNA C. In: Wu R, Grossman L, Moldave K, eds. *Methods in enzymology*. New York: Academic Press, 1983;255–265.
47. White R. DNA polymorphisms: new approaches to the genetics of cancer. *Cancer Surv* 1982; 1:175–186.
48. Sager R. Genetic suppression of tumor formation: a new frontier in cancer research. *Cancer Res* 1986;46:1573–1580.
49. Lee WH, Bookstein R, Hong F, Young LJ, Shew JY, Lee EH. Human retinoblastoma susceptibility gene: cloning identification, and sequence. *Science* 1987;235:1394–1399.
50. Rowley JD. Biochemical implications of consistent chromosome rearrangements in leukemia and lymphoma. *Cancer Res* 1984;44:3159–3168.
51. Favera R, Bregni M, Erikson J, Paterson D, Gallo RC, Croce CM. Human c-myc oncogene is located on the region of chromosome 8 that is translocated in Burkitt's lymphoma cells. *Proc Natl Acad Sci USA* 1982;79:7824–7827.
52. Taub R, Kirsch I, Morton C, et al. Translocation of the c-myc gene into the immunoglobulin heavy chain locus in human Burkitt's lymphoma and murine plasmacytoma cells. *Proc Natl Acad Sci USA* 1982;79:7837–7841.
53. Keisterkamp N, Stephenson JR, Groffen J, et al. Localization of the c-abl oncogene adjacent to a translocation breakpoint in chronic myelogenous leukemia. *Nature* 1983;306:239–242.
54. Trent JM. Cytogenetic and molecular biologic alterations in human breast cancer: a review. *Breast Cancer Res Treat* 1985;5:221–229.
55. Gebhart E, Bruderlein S, Tulusan AM, von Maillot K, Birkmann J. Incidence of double minutes, cytogenetic equivalents of gene amplification, in human carcinoma cells. *Int J Cancer* 1984;34:369–373.

56. Schechter AL, Stern DR, Vaidyanathan L, et al. The neu oncogene: an erb-B-related gene encoding a 185,000-M tumor antigen. *Nature* 1984;312:513–516.
57. Semba K, Kamata N, Toyoshima K, Yamamoto T. A v-erb related protooncogene, c-erb-2, is distinct for the c-erb-1/epidermal growth factor-receptor gene and is amplified in human salivary gland adenocarcinoma. *Proc Natl Acad Sci USA* 1985;82:6497–6501.
58. King CR, Kraus MH, Aaronson SA. Amplification of a novel v-erbB related gene in human mammary carcinoma. *Science* 1985;229:974–976.
59. Coussens L, Yang-Feng TL, Liao YC, et al. Tyrosine kinase receptor with extensive homology to EGF receptor shares chromosome locations with neu oncogene. *Science* 1985;230:1132–1139.
60. Schechter AL, Humg MC, Vaidyanathan L, et al. The neu gene: an erbB-homologous gene distinct from and unlinked to the gene encoding the EGF receptor. *Science* 1985;229:976–978.
61. Fukashige S, Matsusara K, Yoshida M, et al. Localization or a novel v-erb-related gene, c-erb-B2, on human chromosome 17 and its amplification in a gastric cancer cell line. *Mol Cell Biol* 1986; 6(3):955–958.
62. Ullrich A, Coussens L, Hayflick JS, et al. Human epidermal growth factor receptor cDNA sequence and aberrant expression of the amplified gene in 431 epidermoid carcinoma cells. *Nature* 1984;309: 418–421.
63. Yokota J, Yamamoto T, Toyoshima K, et al. Amplification of c-erbB-2 oncogene in human adenocarcinomas in vivo. *Lancet* 1986;1:765–766.
64. Van De Vijver M, Van De Bersselaar R, Devilee P, Cornelisse C, Peterse J, Nusse R. Amplification of the new (c-erbB-2) oncogene in human mammary tumors is relatively frequent and is often accompanied by amplification of the linked c-erbA oncogene. *Mol Cell Biol* 1987;7:2019–2023.
65. Slamon DJ, Clark GM, Wong SW, Levin WJ, Ullrich A, McGuire WL. Human breast cancer: correlation of relapse and survival with amplification of the HER-2/neu oncogene. *Science* 1987; 235:177–182.
66. Zhou D, Battifora H, Yokota J, Yamamoto T, Cline MJ. Association of multiple copies of the c-erbB-2 oncogene with spread of breast cancer. *Cancer Res* 1987;47:6123–6125.
67. Tandon AK, Clark GM, Chamness GC, Ullrich A, McGuire WL. HER-2/neu oncogene protein and prognosis in breast cancer. *J Clin Oncol* 1989;7:1120–1128.
68. Robertson M. Message of myc in context. *Nature* 1984;309:585–587.
69. Campisi J, Grey HE, Pardee AB, Dean M, Soneshein GE. Cell cycle control of c-myc but not c-ras expression is lost following chemical transformation. *Cell* 1984;36:241–247.
70. Stewart TA, Pattengale PK, Leder P. Spontaneous mammary adenocarcinomas in transgenic mice that carry and express MTV-myc fusion genes. *Cell* 1984;38:627–637.
71. Kozbor D, Croce CM. Amplification of the c-myc oncogene in one of the five human breast cancer cell lines. *Cancer Res* 1984;44:438–441.
72. Modjtahedi N, Lavialle C, Poupon MF, et al. Increased level of amplification of the c-myc oncogene in tumors induced in nude mice by a human breast adenocarcinoma cell line. *Cancer Res* 1985;45:4372–4379.
73. Escot C, Theillet C, Lidereau R, et al. Genetic alteration of the c-myc protooncogene in human primary breast carcinomas, *Proc Natl Acad Sci USA* 1986;83:4834–4838.
74. Land HG, Parada G, Weinburg R. Cellular oncogenes and multistep carcinogenesis. *Science* 1984; 222:771–778.
75. Pulciani S, Santos E, Lauver A. Oncogenes in solid human tumors. *Nature* 1982;300:539–542.
76. Fujita J, Srivastava S, Kraus M. Frequency of molecular alterations affecting ras proto-oncogenes in human urinary tract tumors. *Proc Natl Acad Sci USA* 1985;82:3849–3855.
77. Der C, Krontiris T, Cooper G. Transforming genes of human bladder and lung carcinoma cell lines are homologous to the ras genes of Harvey and Kirsten sarcoma viruses. *Proc Natl Acad Sci USA* 1982;79:3637–3649.
78. Tabin CJ, Bradley SM, Bargmann CI, Weinberg RA, Papageorge AG. Mechanisms of activation of a human oncogene. *Nature* 1982;300:143–149.
79. Reddy EP, Reynolds RK, Santos E, Baracid M. A point mutation is responsible for the acquisition of transforming properties of the T24 human bladder carcinoma oncogene. *Nature* 1982;300:149–152.
80. Chang EH, Furth ME, Scolnick EM, Lowy DR. Tumorigenic transformation of mammalian cells induced by a normal human gene homologous to the oncogene of Harvey murine sarcoma virus. *Nature* 1982;297:479–483.

81. Hand PH, Thor A, Wunderlich D, Muraro R, Caruso A, Schlom J. Monoclonal antibodies of predefined specificity detect activated ras gene expression in human mammary and colon carcinomas. *Proc Natl Acad Sci USA* 1984;81:5227–5231.

82. Spandidos DA, Kerr IB. Elevated expression of the human ras oncogene family in premalignant and malignant tumours of the colon. *Br J Cancer* 1984;49:681–688.

83. Thor A, Hand PH, Wunderlich D, Caruso A, Muraro R, Schlom J. Monoclonal antibodies define differential ras gene expression in malignant and benign colonic diseases (letter). *Nature* 1984;311: 562–565.

84. Debortoli ME, Abou-Tssa H, Haley BE, Cho-Chung YS. Amplified expression of p21 ras protein in hormone dependent rodents. *Biochem Biophys Res Commun* 1985;127:699–706.

85. Viola MV, Fromowitz F, Oravez S, Deb S, Schlom J. Ras oncogene p21 is increased in premalignant lesions and high grade bladder carcinoma. *J Exp Med* 1985;161:1213–1218.

86. Kasid A, Lippman ME, Papageorge AG, Lowry DR, Gellmann EP. Transfection of v-ras-H DNA into MCF-7 human breast cancer cells bypasses dependence on estrogen for tumorigenicity. *Science* 1985;228:725–728.

87. Spandidos DA, Agnantis NJ. Human malignant tumours of the breast, as compared to their respective normal tissue, have elevated expression of Harvey ras oncogene. *Anticancer Res* 1984;4:269–272.

88. Theillet C, Lidereau R, Escot C, et al. Loss of a c-H-ras-1 allele and aggressive human primary breast carcinomas. *Cancer Res* 1986;46:4776–4781.

89. Thor A, Ohuchi N, Hand PH, et al. Ras gene alterations and enhanced levels of ras p21 expression in a spectrum of benign and malignant human mammary tissues. *Lab Invest* 1986;55:603–615.

90. Ohuchi N, Thor A, Page DL, Hand HP, Halter SA, Schlom J. Expression of the 21,000 molecular weight ras protein in a spectrum of benign and malignant human mammary tumors. *Cancer Res* 1986;46:2511–2519.

91. Lundy J, Grimson R, Mishriki Y, et al. Elevated ras oncogene expression correlates with lymph node metastasis in breast cancer patients. *J Clin Oncol* 1986;4:1321–1325.

92. Clair T, Miller WR, Cho-Chung YS. Prognostic significance of the expression of a ras protein with molecular weight of 21,000 by human breast cancer. *Cancer Res* 1987;47:5290–5293.

93. Lidereau R, Escot C, Theillet C, et al. High frequency of rare alleles of the human c-H-ras-1 protooncogene in breast cancer patients. *J Natl Cancer Inst* 1986;77:697–701.

94. Lidereau R, Callahan R, Dickson C, Peters G, Escot C, Ali IU. Amplification of the int-2 gene in primary human breast tumors. *Oncogene Res* 1988;2(3):285–291.

Endocrine Dependent Tumors, edited by
Klaus-Dieter Voigt and Cornelius Knabbe.
Raven Press, Ltd., New York © 1991.

8

Endocrine Aspects of Endometrial Cancer

R. Vihko and V. Isomaa

*Biocenter and Department of Clinical Chemistry, University of Oulu,
SF-90220 Oulu, Finland*

The functions of the human endometrium are strictly hormone-regulated during the reproductive years. The central issue is an interplay between estradiol and progesterone, the former steroid stimulating proliferation of the endometrial epithelium, the latter being essential for the differentiation of, and secretion by the estradiol-stimulated tissue. Evidence has been accumulating showing that excessive estradiol stimulation, frequently associated with a lack of cyclic progesterone secretion, characterizes the categories of women at increased risk for endometrial cancer (1,2). This phenomenon frequently can be observed in women not exposed to exogenous estrogens,and also in women who have been subjected to such treatment modalities (3). The protective effect toward endometrial cancer of contraceptive preparations of the estrogen-progestin combination type (4) is completely in line with the thesis of the estrogen-progestin interplay being protective toward endometrial cancer.

This chapter deals mainly with the effects of steroid hormones and their antagonists on endometrial tissue, whether normal, hyperplastic, or malignant, as reflected by the concentrations of the receptors for these classes of steroids. In addition, data will be presented concerning endometrial 17β-hydroxysteroid dehydrogenase (17-HSD), a progestin-induced protein present in the endometrial epithelial cells. Clinical aspects of female sex steroid receptors (SRs) and 17-HSD assays also will be discussed.

ENDOCRINE REGULATION OF ENDOMETRIAL FUNCTION

Steroid Receptors

In early studies, synthesis of tritiated steroids having sufficiently high specific activity allowed to study their distribution in steroid target tissues of laboratory animals at physiological hormone concentrations. This approach led to the discovery of estrogen receptors (ERs) (5) and, shortly after, some physicochemical characteristics of the rat cytosol ER were determined, using ligand-binding assays and sucrose gradient ultracentrifugation of fractionated uterine tissue (6,7). When the methods were applied to human endometrium, high concentrations of ERs were observed in tissue samples taken during the proliferative phase of the menstrual cycle (8,9).

Characterization of progestin receptors (PRs) from mammalian sources proved to be more difficult than that of ERs. The major reasons for the difficulties were the rapid dissociation of the receptor-progesterone complex, the lability of the receptor protein, and the presence of corticosteroid binding globulin-like proteins in uteri of several mammalian species (10). The development of several synthetic progestins with high affinity for progestin receptors greatly facilitated the study of the latter in the human uterus (11,12). After being identified in normal human tissues, ERs and PRs also were detected in several neoplastic tissues, and receptor determinations have been used in numerous studies to predict the therapeutic response to a variety of treatments in patients suffering from breast, or gynecological cancers (more details later in this chapter).

Over the last few years, a considerable amount of data has been accumulating concerning the structure, the intracellular localization, and the function of steroid receptors in both normal and pathological uterine tissues. Estrogen and progestin receptors also have been purified and characterized from human sources and highly specific monoclonal antibodies against them have been developed (13–16). These antibodies have allowed the development of immunohistochemical methods for ER and PR assays (17–19). These novel techniques have the benefit of being able to show the heterogeneity of tissues with respect to the presence and concentrations of the receptors. The availability of immunocytochemical techniques also has shown that estrogen and progestin receptors reside in the target cell nuclei (15,17,20). During homogenization of the tissues, part of the receptors are recovered in the cytosol fraction. Receptors in this "loosely bound" fraction are referred to as cytosol receptors in this chapter, whereas the more "tightly bound" receptors, residing in the nuclear fraction following tissue homogenization, are referred to as nuclear receptors.

Recently, cDNAs encoding human ERs (21,22) and PRs (23) have been cloned and sequenced, and the primary structure of the receptor proteins determined.

Steroid Receptors During Normal Menstrual Cycle

The concentrations of ERs and PRs in the human endometrium undergo characteristic variations throughout the menstrual cycle in response to changes in the circulating steroid hormone concentrations. These changes have been characterized by ligand-binding studies of the cytosol and nuclear fractions of uterine homogenates from premenopausal women. As shown in Fig. 1, in normally cycling women, cytosol endometrial ER concentrations are highest during the early proliferative phase, and lowest near the end of the menstrual cycle (8,9,24–26). The maximal nuclear ER concentrations are seen later during the proliferative phase and persist until the early luteal phase (8,25). The highest concentrations of the cytosol PRs are

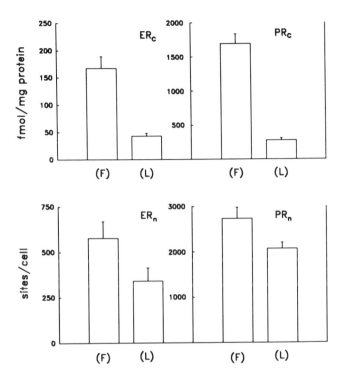

FIG. 1. Cytosol estrogen (ERc) and progestin (PRc) receptor concentrations, and nuclear estrogen (ERn) and progestin (PRn) receptor concentrations during the normal menstrual cycle. The measurements were carried out using ligand-binding assays. F = follicular phase, L = luteal phase. (Data from refs. 26, 28)

present during the preovulatory period of the cycle and they are rapidly decreased subsequent to ovulation. The nuclear progestin receptor concentration peaks immediately after ovulation (8,9,25). These data, together with other observations concerning the interrelationships between estrogen and progestin and sex steroid receptor levels in various animal models, led to the suggestion that estradiol stimulates the synthesis of ERs and PRs in the human endometrium, whereas progesterone leads to their depletion (10,27).

The last few years have seen the appearance of monoclonal antibodies directed against ERs and PRs. Using immunohistochemical techniques, these antibodies have allowed to directly visualize the localization of receptors within individual cells. These studies have confirmed that the concentrations of SRs are markedly changed during the normal menstrual cycle and they have considerably extended our knowledge of receptor distribution in different cell types. In all these studies, both ERs and PRs have been found to be localized within the nuclei of cells. In the case of ERs, an increase in the number of positively stained cells is observed during the follicular phase. The maximal ER staining in nuclei of endometrial cells is present during the late follicular phase and, during that time, staining is seen in the

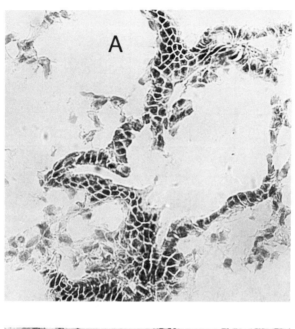

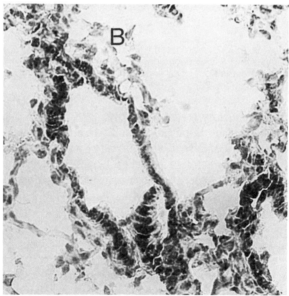

FIG. 2. Immunocytochemical assays of estrogen **(A)** and progestin **(B)** receptors in the human endometrium. (From Mäentausta et al., in preparation.)

majority of the glandular epithelial cells (Fig. 2). Specific staining also is detected in about half of the endometrial stromal cells and the intensity of this staining approximates that of the glandular epithelium (18,20,29). The vascular spaces lined by endothelial cells remain unstained (29). In the midluteal phase, a dramatic reduction in the number and staining intensity of positively stained cells is observed. The decrease of staining intensity seems to be more pronounced in the glandular epithelium than in the stromal cells (18,20,29). In the myometrium, the staining of ERs seems to follow a pattern similar to that observed in the endometrium (20). In the postmenopausal endometrium, staining of ERs is relatively strong in most epithelial cell nuclei, and strong staining also is seen in stromal cell nuclei, but fewer stromal cells are stained (29).

The changes in endometrial PRs detected by immunohistochemical analysis during the menstrual cycle show parallelism with those seen for ERs. However, the changes in progesterone receptors are more complex. The variation of PRs is most marked in the epithelium, where very strong PR immunostaining is demonstrated in the late proliferative phase and after ovulation days 1 to 3 of the early secretory phase (15,17,20). After that, PR immunoreactivity decreases very rapidly in the epithelial cell nuclei, and remains weak, or absent, during the mid- and late-secretory phase. In contrast, stromal cell nuclei remain quite strongly immunostained throughout the secretory phase (15,17,20). Myometrial smooth muscle cell nuclei also are strongly stained during the late follicular phase and staining decreases during the luteal phase (17,20). Overall, the changes in epithelial PR concentrations correlate with changes in endogenous estrogen and progesterone levels, reflecting sex steroid sensitivity, whereas stromal and myometrial PRs might be, at least in part, constitutively synthesized (17).

Effects of Estrogens, Antiestrogens, Progestins and Antiprogestins on Endometrial Steroid Receptors

The effects of exogenous steroids on the endometrial sex SR concentrations frequently can be deduced from the receptor changes just described in relation to the menstrual cycle. Estrogen administration leads to increases in ER and PR concentrations in the endometrium (9,30), whereas, as shown in Fig. 3, the administration of progesterone, or synthetic progestins, leads to an opposite effect (31,32). Effects of tamoxifen administration on human endometrium have been reported to mimic those of estrogen (33). Fig. 3 shows that tamoxifen has no effect on the medroxyprogesterone acetate-induced decreases in total cellular estrogen and progestin receptor concentrations during short-term experiments. The same is true during long-term experiments (34).

Recently, steroids with an antiprogestin effect have been synthesized (35). These compounds, such as RU 486 (mifepristone), are characterized by high affinity-binding to progesterone receptors, which are then unable to interact with the target cell genome to produce a progesterone-like effect (36). In contrast, shedding of the non-pregnant endometrium takes place rapidly after RU 486 administration (37),

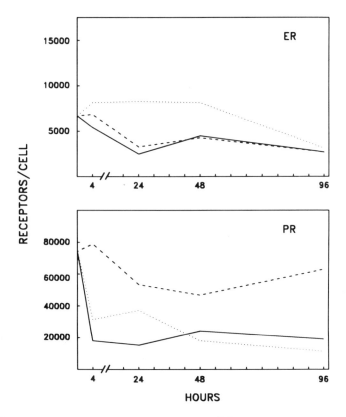

FIG. 3. Total cellular estrogen (ER) and progestin (PR) receptor concentrations during medroxyprogesterone acetate (dotted line), tamoxifen (dashed line) and their simultaneous (solid line) administration. (From Neumannová et al., ref. 31.)

and clinical studies during early pregnancy have demonstrated that appropriate doses of RU 486 lead to pregnancy interruption (35). Studies on rhesus monkey decidua have demonstrated an increase in the estrogen receptor concentration following RU 486 administration. This was interpreted to indicate the opposition of estrogen receptor depletion associated with high circulating concentrations of progesterone (38).

17β-Hydroxysteroid Dehydrogenase

17β-Hydroxysteroid dehydrogenase (17-HSD) catalyzes the reversible interconversion of neutral and phenolic 17-hydroxy- and 17-ketosteroids. In addition to steroidogenic tissues, this enzyme activity is present in several target tissues of steroid hormone action. In the human endometrium, the principal activity of 17-HSD is to catalyze the conversion of estradiol to a less active estrogen, estrone (39). This activity is regulated by progestins and, therefore, progesterone and synthetic progestins can affect intracellular estrogen concentrations. Because progestins increase the activity of 17-HSD, thereby leading to increased estrone concentrations at the expense of the more active estradiol, this enzyme might have a key role in the regulation of the exposure of the endometrial cells to estrogens (39).

In one series of studies, we investigated the effects of synthetic steroids on endometrial 17-HSD activity in normal and pathological endometrium. Medroxyprogesterone acetate administration to normally cycling women during the follicular phase resulted in a rapid increase in the activity of endometrial 17-HSD. By 96 hours of treatment, the increase in 17-HSD activity was 10 to 15 fold (31). The induction was, however, relatively short lived (about 7 to 10 days) and, despite continued progestin administration, was followed by a decrease in enzyme activity. A period of 2 to 3 weeks of continuous progestin administration was sufficient to completely terminate the acute progestin effect reflected by the high 17-HSD activity in the endometrium (32,34). These data, along with the endometrial histology, seem to imply that progestin action comprises two phases: an acute stimulation of endometrial activity, followed by the depression of endometrial metabolism, ultimately leading to the atrophy of this tissue.

Studies on the regulation of 17-HSD activities in the human endometrium have made it possible to better understand the mechanisms of action of certain synthetic steroids used clinically for the treatment of certain gynecological disorders. Danazol, a derivative of ethinyl testosterone, has several different endocrine effects and it interacts with a number of SRs, including human PRs (28). When danazol was given to normally cycling women, its effects on the activities of 17-HSD were similar to those seen with progestin administration (32). In addition, we studied the effects of gestrinone, a synthetic trienic 19-norsteroid, on endometrial 17-HSD and a typical progestin effect, the induction of 17-HSD, was observed (40). In all these studies, the induction of 17-HSD activity was associated with changes in the endometrial ER and PR concentrations and the changes were typical of progesterone action.

To get more detailed information on the regulation and biological properties of 17-HSD, we recently purified the enzyme from human placental tissue and raised polyclonal antibodies against it (41). The antibodies detected an immunologically similar antigen in the human endometrium. To localize 17-HSD in human tissue, we developed immunohistochemical techniques and, to immunologically quantitate the enzyme protein, we established a radioimmunoassay using the polyclonal antibodies. Immunostaining of 17-HSD was low, or absent, in the endometrial specimens taken during the follicular phase. In the midluteal phase, a strong staining was detected in the glandular epithelium that gradually disappeared during the late luteal phase. When the enzyme protein concentration was quantified using the established radioimmunoassay, a several-fold increase in 17-HSD concentration was observed during the luteal phase as compared to that observed during the follicular phase. These data are in line with, and confirm, the data obtained previously with measurements of the catalytic activity of the enzyme. Recently, the cDNA of the placental enzyme was cloned and sequenced in our laboratory (42), and the data were later confirmed in another laboratory (43). The human gene for 17-HSD was found to reside on chromosome 17, at the level of bands Q12-Q21 (44). These molecular biological approaches can be expected to shed more light on the endocrine regulation of 17-HSD.

STEROID RECEPTORS AND 17-HSD IN ABNORMAL HUMAN ENDOMETRIUM

Endometriosis Tissue

Histopathologically, endometriosis lesions resemble normal endometrium. Furthermore, the disease displays a cyclicity of symptoms in relation to the menstrual cycle, and different modalities of endocrine treatment have been used with success, at least in some patients. In particular, progestins (45), danazol and gestrinone, the two latter having progestin-like effects (28,40) have been used and, recently, gonadotropin-releasing hormone analogs have proved successful (46). It is interesting to observe that there are certain similarities and dissimilarities when variables related to female sex steroid action are compared in endometrial tissue and endometriosis lesions. Although ERs and PRs have been present in most of the endometriosis lesions studied (32,47–49), their concentrations have been very much lower than in endometrial specimens from the same subjects. A remarkable difference is in the response to progestin action. During normal cycles, there is no increase of 17-HSD activity in the endometriosis lesions during the luteal phase (50), and neither medroxyprogesterone acetate, nor danazol, nor gestrinone administration lead to increases in the activity of this enzyme (40,50). This is in sharp contrast to what takes place in the endometrial tissue. Furthermore, no depletion of cytosol ERs and PRs was observed during these treatments, which again is in contrast to what takes place in normal endometrium. Presently, the mechanisms behind this apparent progestin-refractory state of endometriosis lesions are enigmatic.

Endometrial Hyperplasia

The development of endometrial hyperplasia is characterized by an unopposed estrogen action and the tissue should, therefore, contain elevated, or at least not decreased, concentrations of sex steroid receptors compared to the normal endometrium. The data available for ERs partially support this assumption. Gurpide and Tseng (51) found the cytosol ER concentrations in endometrial hyperplasia to be similar to those of proliferative endometrium. Data from this laboratory also show that cytosol ER levels tend to be high in hyperplastic endometrium, although not significantly higher than in the normal endometrial tissue (38). In some studies, however, it has been reported that the cytosol ER concentration of hyperplastic endometrium is lower than in normal tissue (24), but these findings have not been confirmed. More recently, immunohistochemical analyses of estrogen receptors in hyperplastic endometrium have shown that hyperplastic endometrium without cytological atypia contains high ER contents in both the epithelial and stromal components, (52) similar to those found in proliferative endometrium. In contrast to this, ER levels in the epithelium of endometrial intraepithelial neoplasia (hyperplasia with cytological atypia) are low and resemble the situation seen in endometrial adenocarcinoma specimens (52).

The finding showing that stromal cells also contain ERs supports the hypothesis that epithelial-stromal interactions might play a role in the induction and growth of epithelial tumors (53).

The concentrations of cytosol PRs in hyperplastic endometrium measured by biochemical assays have been reported not to differ significantly from those in normal tissue (9,54). Although the mean PR concentrations are not statistically different, most endometrial hyperplasia specimens have high PR levels. Immunohistochemical studies of PRs show a similar PR distribution pattern to that of ERs in endometrial hyperplasia. The PR content is high in the epithelium of hyperplastic tissue without cytological atypia, and low in the epithelium of endometrial intraepithelial neoplasia. The stromal cell nuclei also are positively stained for PRs, but the overall staining intensity is lower than in the epithelial cell component (55). The combined analysis of ERs and PRs in the epithelium of hyperplasia suggests that the ERs are functional in this tissue and that it is sensitive to estradiol. Presently, it seems that progestin induction of 17-HSD has not been assayed in hyperplastic endometrial tissue, but the responsiveness of endometrial hyperplasia to progestin treatment suggests that progestin action is undisturbed in this tissue.

Endometrial Carcinoma

It has been amply demonstrated that the concentrations of ERs and PRs in endometrial carcinoma are generally lower than those in the proliferative normal endometrium (9,26,56), and there is a strong correlation between cytosol ER and PR concentrations in the malignant tissue (26). A fraction of the malignant endometrial specimens have been classified as receptor-negative. In different studies, different decision limits have been used as to whether a specimen has been classified as cytosol estrogen, or progestin receptor-positive, or negative. Because different techniques have been used in receptor assays, and that sound reference methods are not available, there are relatively large variations in the data concerning the presence and concentrations of female sex SRs in malignant tissues. Using biochemical techniques for receptor measurements, cytosol ERs and PRs in endometrial adenocarcinoma have been found to be simultaneously present in 41% to 80% of the samples, estrogen receptors alone in 5% to 32%, progestin receptor alone in 2.5% to 18%, and both receptors simultaneously absent in 11% to 36% of the specimens (9,57–60). Occasionally, even higher frequencies for the presence of cytosol ERs and PRs have been given (61). Especially when correlating endometrial cancer female sex steroid receptor concentrations with other prognostic indicators, it has been found useful to classify the specimens into categories comprising either receptor-rich, or receptor-poor tumors (60,62–64). Obviously for methodological reasons, the decision limits of the receptor concentrations can vary in different studies.

In contrast to the situation concerning cytosol receptors, the concentrations of nuclear female sex SRs tend to be higher in malignant tissue than in normal tissue (26). As a result of this, the ratios of cytosol to nuclear ERs and PRs are significantly higher in normal proliferative endometrium than in endometrial adenocarcinoma (26).

Biochemical assays from cytosol and nuclear fractions of whole tissue homogenates do not determine receptor localization among different tissue components. Therefore, the immunohistochemical analysis of ERs and PRs provides an attractive approach to study hormone dependency in carcinoma specimens. These techniques have demonstrated a marked tumor cell and tissue heterogeneity in the staining patterns of receptors within carcinoma specimens. However, there seems to be a relatively good correlation between biochemical and immunohistochemical measurements of female sex SRs, both in the case of ERs (65,66), and in that of PRs (67). In about 20% of the samples, biochemical and immunohistochemical techniques give different results. The most likely explanation for these discrepancies is the contamination of tumors by adjacent benign endometrial glands, stroma, or myometrium that might occur in the biochemical assays. This is supported by findings showing that there is no statistically significant relationship between ER and PR levels in the malignant epithelium and in adjacent benign tissue (68).

The induction of endometrial 17-HSD activity has been observed in endometrial adenocarcinoma tissues. After a one-week medroxyprogesterone acetate, or danazol treatment, a significant increase in the activity of 17-HSD was observed in carcinoma specimens (69), and the posttherapy 17-HSD activities significantly correlated with the pretreatment cytosol PR concentrations in both treatment groups. Both treatments also decreased the proliferative activity and increased the secretory activity of the malignant epithelial endometrial cells. These data on female sex SRs and 17-HSD indicate that, at least in the majority of endometrial adenocarcinomas, essential features of female sex steroid action have been retained.

Clinical Correlations of Steroid Receptor Measurements

During the last few years, a number of reports have appeared relating ER and PR concentrations to a number of clinical and histopathological variables. Subsequently, these receptor assays have been in use in a number of centers for more than ten years, and data also are accumulating on their importance in the prediction of the clinical outcome of patients with endometrial cancer. Altogether, the aim in these studies has been to evaluate whether SR assays could be used in the process of planning treatment strategies for individual patients.

Essential features of hormone dependency have been retained in the majority of endometrial adenocarcinomas. In this connection, it is pertinent to point out that the endocrine milieu of a patient seems to have an influence on the endocrine-related characteristics of her adenocarcinoma and, consequently, also on her clinical outcome. We found that patients younger than 50 years old, and having a tumor of clinical stage I or II, had a higher 17-HSD activity in their tumor tissue than did corresponding patients of 50 years, or older (70). In a comparable patient group, Ehrlich and associates (71) found that patients of less than 50 years old had tumors that were predominantly progesterone receptor-positive, whereas the contrary was true for older patients. These findings might be explained by the production of ovarian hormones in the patients of less than 50 years of age. We also found that obesity has an influence on the endocrine-related variables of endometrial adenocarcinoma tissue (70). In clinical stages I and II, tumors in the patients weighing more than 198 lbs had significantly higher concentrations of estrogen and PRs than those in other women. This finding possibly relates to the ability of fat tissue to convert adrenal androgens into estrogens (72,73). Taken together, the endocrine characteristics of endometrial carcinoma tissue in young and obese patients might explain the fact that these patients have a better clinical outcome than other patients (59, 63).

Steroid Receptors and Clinical Advancement

Most of the available data shows that the early clinical stages of endometrial cancer are more frequently female sex steroid receptor-positive than are the more advanced stages (59,70,71,74). Furthermore, the receptor concentrations in stage I and II tumors have been reported to be higher than in advanced, or recurrent diseases. Compared to clinical stage I, nuclear ER and PR concentrations are lower in stages III and IV of the disease (70). It seems that the degree of myometrial invasion is not related to endocrine variables of the tumor (58,70).

Steroid Receptors and Histopathological Grade

There are extensively overlapping receptor concentrations in each histopathological grade category of endometrial cancer, indicating different characteristics for these two types of risk indicators. However, it has been repeatedly shown that the cytosol female sex SR concentrations decrease in relation to the loss of differentiation (58, 64,70,75–77). A limited amount of recent data from immunohistochemical studies are in line with these observations (55,65–68). Evidence also has been presented indicating that the activity of 17-HSD is lower in anaplastic endometrial cancer specimens than in more differentiated ones (70,78). In addition, well-differentiated tumors have responded to progestin therapy with increased 17-HSD activity, whereas more poorly differentiated tumors have not (79). Together, these findings support the view of a decreased sensitivity of anaplastic endometrial malignancies to hormonal therapy.

Steroid Receptors and Response to Treatment

In unselected endometrial cancer patients with advanced, or recurrent disease, approximately one-third show an objective response to progestin treatment (80–83). Recently, Ehrlich and associates (71) have summarized published data on the response rate of endometrial cancer to progestins. Seventy-two percent (41 of 57) of the patients who had PR-positive tumors responded, whereas only 12% (11 of 95) presenting PR-negative tumors responded. Measurements of ERs have not been quite so accurate in predicting responses (80). The limited amount of data available on the application of female sex SR assays to predicting responses to cytotoxic chemotherapy suggest that ER and PR-poor tumors have a significantly greater response rate than receptor-rich tumors (84).

Steroid Receptors and Disease-Free Interval

Only limited data are available on this topic, but they all basically convey the same message as shown in Fig. 4. The disease-free interval is significantly longer in the patient group having one, or both of the receptors present in relatively high concentrations (58,64,70). In the studies of Kauppila and coworkers (71) and Creasman and colleagues (58), adjuvant progestin treatment was used, but not in the study of

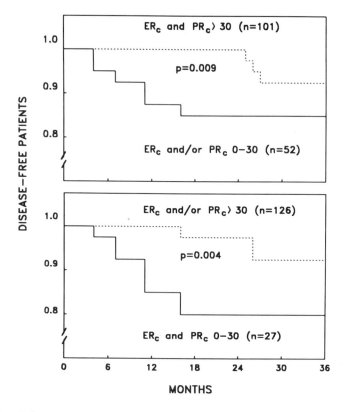

FIG. 4. Cumulative proportions of disease-free patients with clinical stage I endometrial cancer. After primary treatment, all patients received p.o. medroxyprogesterone acetate, at a dose of 100 mg a day for 2 years. The patients were grouped on the basis of cytosol estrogen (ERc) and progestin receptor concentrations (PRc), as indicated. (Data from Kauppila et al., ref. 70.)

Utaaker and associates (64). The upper panel of Fig. 4 shows that there was no case of recurrent disease during the two years of medroxyprogesterone acetate adjuvant treatment in the category of patients with ER- and PR-rich tumors, all the recurrences detected in this group appearing soon after the termination of the treatment. It is tempting to suggest that this phenomenon was because of some kind of arresting effect of progestin on tumor growth. Another possibility is that this phenomenon is simply because of the slow progression of tumors rich in receptors. In contrast to patients with receptor-rich tumors, all recurrences in patients with receptor-poor tumors appeared during medroxyprogesterone acetate administration. Taken together, these findings suggest that adjuvant medroxyprogesterone acetate should be given to patients with receptor-rich tumors, in the form of a long-term treatment.

Steroid Receptors and Survival

A number of studies show that low concentrations, or an absence of cytosol female sex steroid receptors are indicators of an increased risk of a fatal outcome to the

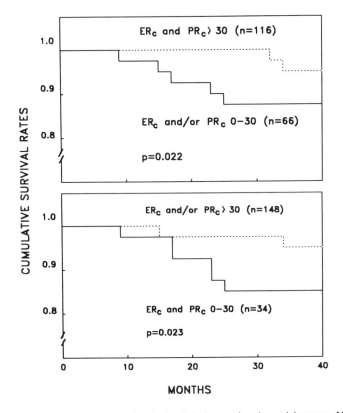

FIG. 5. Cumulative survival rates in patients with clinical stage I endometrial cancer. After primary treatment, all patients received p.o. medroxyprogesterone acetate, at a dose of 100 mg a day for 2 years. The patients were grouped on the basis of cytosol estrogen (ERc) and progestin receptor (PRc) concentrations, as indicated. (Data from Kauppila et al., ref. 70.)

disease (58,60,62,70,74,85). Our studies (60,70), and those of Palmer and colleagues (63) and Chambers and associates (62), show that the maximum prognostic information from receptor measurements is obtained using decision limits for concentrations that are relatively high.

Figure 5 shows survival data in clinical stage I endometrial cancer patients from our study (70). A relatively low death rate characterizes the categories of receptor-rich tumors, and death from endometrial malignancy took place relatively late in these cases, always several months after the termination of adjuvant medroxyprogesterone acetate treatment. This is in contrast to what is seen in the receptor-poor categories (Fig. 5). These findings are in line with our results on the disease-free interval already described, and they further emphasize the importance of extended adjuvant medroxyprogesterone acetate administration in patients with receptor-rich malignancies.

At this point, it should be emphasized that the real benefit of an indiscriminate use of adjuvant progestin treatment in endometrial carcinoma has been unproven. Recently, Vergote and coworkers (86) carried out a randomized, controlled clinical study on whether adjuvant progestin treatment improved the chances of survival in patients with stage I or II endometrial cancers, and they concluded that there is little to gain from adjuvant progestin therapy in this low-risk category of endometrial cancer. However, the authors point out that the number of patients included in their study might not have been sufficiently high to show a significant improvement of survival in this patient group. Interestingly, they found that, in grade 2 tumors, the relapse rate tended to be lower in the progestin treatment group than in the controls. This was not the case for patients with grade 3 tumors. This might be related to the possibility of higher PR levels in grade 2 tumors than in grade 3 tumors, but receptor measurements were not reported in the study of Vergote and associates (86).

Conclusions

Used together with clinical and histopathological indicators of prognosis, endocrine indicators such as female sex SRs give some promise of being useful for categorizing patients with endometrial carcinoma, at least as far as prognosis and treatment modalities are concerned. In clinical stage I patients, poor prognosis can be predicted by an anaplastic structure of the malignancy, and low tissue concentrations of ER, PR, or of both simultaneously. Progestin treatment is effective in about one-third of the patients with advanced, or recurrent endometrial carcinoma, whereas adjuvant progestin treatment has not been shown to be beneficial in unselected groups of patients. It is possible that adjuvant progestin treatment should be restricted to patients with receptor-rich, early stage tumors, and should take the form of a long-term (several years) treatment.

Acknowledgments

The studies on endometrial cancer in this laboratory were supported by grants from the Research Council for Medicine of the Academy of Finland and the Finnish

Cancer Foundation. The Department of Clinical Chemistry is a WHO Collaborating Centre supported by the Ministries of Education, Health and Social Affairs, and of Foreign Affairs, Finland.

REFERENCES

1. Gambrell RD. Role of hormones in the etiology and prevention of endometrial and breast cancer. *Acta Obstet Gynecol Scand Suppl* 1982;106:37–46.
2. Nisker JA, Ramzy I, Collings JA. Adenocarcinoma of the endometrium and abnormal ovarian function in young women. *Am J Obstet Gynecol* 1978;130:546–550.
3. Smith DC, Prentice R, Thompson DJ, Herrman WL. Association of exogenous estrogen and endometrial carcinoma. *N Engl J Med* 1975;293:1164–1167.
4. Centers for Disease Control Cancer and Steroid Hormone Study. Oral contraceptive use and the risk of endometrial cancer. *J Am Med Ass* 1983;249:1600–1604.
5. Jensen EV, Jacobsen HI. Basic guides to the mechanism of estrogen action. *Rec Progr Horm Res* 1962;18:387–414.
6. Jensen EV, Suzuki T, Kawashima T, Stumpf WE, Jungblut PW, DeSombre ER. A two-step mechanism for the interaction of estradiol with rat uterus. *Proc Natl Acad Sci USA* 1968;59:632–638.
7. Toft D, Gorski I. A receptor molecule for estrogen: isolation from the rat uterus and preliminary characterization. *Proc Natl Acad Sci USA* 1966;55:1574–1581.
8. Bayard F, Damilano S, Robel P, Baulieu EE. Cytoplasmic and nuclear estradiol and progesterone receptors in human endometrium. *J Clin Endocrinol Metab* 1978;46:635–648.
9. Jänne O, Kauppila A, Kontula K, Syrjälä P, Vihko R. Female sex steroid receptors in normal, hyperplastic and carcinomatous endometrium. The relationship to serum steroid hormones and gonadotropins and changes during medroxy-progesterone acetate administration. *Int J Cancer* 1979; 24:545–554.
10. Jänne O, Kontula K, Vihko R, Feil PD, Bardin CW. Progesterone receptor and regulation of progestin action in mammalian tissues. *Med Biol* 1978;56:225–248.
11. Jänne O, Kontula K, Vihko R. Progestin receptors in human tissues: concentrations and binding kinetics. *J Steroid Biochem* 1976;7:1061–1068.
12. Philibert D, Raynaud JP. Binding of progesterone and R 5020, a highly potent progestin, to human endometrium and myometrium. *Contraception* 1974;10:457–466.
13. Clarke CL, Zaino RJ, Feil PD, et al. Monoclonal antibodies to human progesterone receptor: characterization by biochemical and immunochemical techniques. *Endocrinology* 1987;121:1123–1132.
14. Greene GL, Fitch FW, Jensen EV. Monoclonal antibodies to estrophilin: probes for the study of estrogen receptors. *Proc Natl Acad Sci USA* 1980;77:157–161.
15. Press MF, Udove JA, Greene GL. Progesterone receptor distribution in the human endometrium. Analysis using monoclonal antibodies to the human progesterone receptor. *Am J Pathol* 1988;131: 112–124.
16. Vu Hai MT, Jolivet A, Ravet V, et al. Novel monoclonal antibodies against human uterine progesterone receptor. Mapping of receptor immunogenic domains. *Biochem J* 1989;260:371–376.
17. Bergeron C, Ferenczy A, Toft DO, Schneider W, Shyamala G. Immunocytochemical study of progesterone receptors in the human endometrium during the menstrual cycle. *Lab Invest* 1988;59: 862–869.
18. Garcia E, Bouchard P, DeBrux J, et al. Use of immunocytochemistry of progesterone and estrogen receptors for endometrial dating. *J Clin Endocrinol Metab* 1988;67:80–87.
19. Press MF, Greene GL. An immunocytochemical method for demonstrating estrogen receptor in human uterus using monoclonal antibodies to human estrophilin. *Lab Invest* 1984;50:480–486.
20. Lessey BA, Killam AP, Metzger A, Haney AF, Greene GL, McCarty KS. Immunohistochemical analysis of human uterine estrogen and progesterone receptors throughout the menstrual cycle. *J Clin Endocrinol Metab* 1988;67:334–340.
21. Green S, Walter P, Kumar V, et al. Human oestrogen receptor cDNA: sequence, expression and homology to v-erb A. *Nature* 1986;320:134–139.
22. Walter P, Green S, Greene G, et al. Cloning of the human estrogen receptor cDNA. *Proc Natl Acad Sci USA* 1985;82:7889–7893.
23. Misrahi M, Atger M, d'Auriol L, et al. Complete amino acid sequence of the human progesterone receptor deduced from cloned DNA. *Biochem Biophys Res Commun* 1987;143:740–748.

24. Evans LH, Martin JD, Hähnel R. Estrogen receptor concentration in normal and pathological human uterine tissues. *J Clin Endocrinol Metab* 1974;38:23–32.
25. Levy C, Robel P, Gautray JP, Debrux J, Baulieu EE, Euchenne B. Estradiol and progesterone receptors in human endometrium: normal and abnormal menstrual cycles and early pregnancy. *Am J Obstet Gynecol* 1980;136:646–651.
26. Neumannova M, Kauppila A, Vihko R. Cytosol and nuclear estrogen and progestin receptors and 17betahydroxysteroid dehydrogenase activity in normal and carcinomatous endometrium. *Obstet Gynecol* 1983;61:181–188.
27. Baulieu EE, Atger M, Best-Belpomme M, et al. Steroid hormone receptors. *Vitam Hormon* 1975; 33:639–736.
28. Kokko E, Jänne O, Kauppila A, Rönnberg L, Vihko, R. Danazol has progestin-like actions on the human endometrium. *Acta Endocrinol* 1982;99:588–593.
29. Press MF, Nousek-Goebl N, King WJ, Herbst AL, Greene GL. Immunohistochemical assessment of estrogen receptor distribution in the human endometrium throughout the menstrual cycle. *Lab Invest* 1984;51:495–503.
30. Kreitmann B, Bugat R, Bayard F. Estrogen and progestin regulation of the progesterone receptor concentration in human endometrium. *J Clin Endocrinol Metab* 1979;49:926–929.
31. Neumannova M, Kauppila A, Kivinen S, Vihko R. Short-term effects of tamoxifen, medroxy-progesterone acetate, and their combination on receptor kinetics and 17β-hydroxysteroid dehydrogenase in human endometrium. *Obstet Gynecol* 1985;66:695–700.
32. Vihko R, Isotalo H, Kauppila A, Rönnberg L, Vierikko P. Hormonal regulation of endometrium and endometriosis tissue. In: Raynaud JP, Ojasoo T, Martini L, eds. *Medical Management of Endometriosis*, New York: Raven Press, 1984;79–89.
33. Mortel R, Levy C, Wolff JP, Nicolas JC, Robel P, Baulieu EE. Female sex steroid receptors in post-menopausal endometrial carcinoma and biochemical response to an antiestrogen. *Cancer Res* 1981; 41:1140–1147.
34. Kokko E, Jänne O, Kauppila A, Vihko R. Effects of tamoxifen, medroxyprogesterone acetate, and their combination on human endometrial estrogen and progestin receptor concentrations, 17β-hydroxysteroid dehydrogenase activity, and serum hormone concentrations. *Am J Obstet Gynecol* 1982;143:382–388.
35. Baulieu EE, Segal SJ, eds. *The antiprogestin steroid RU486 and human fertility control.* New York: Plenum Press, 1985.
36. Baulieu EE. Contragestion and other clinical applications of RU486, an antiprogesterone at the receptor. *Science* 1989;245:1351–1357.
37. Garzo VG, Liu J, Ulmann A, Baulieu EE, Yen SSC. Effects of an antiprogesterone (RU486) on the hypothalamic-hypophyseal-ovarian-endometrial axis during the luteal phase of the menstrual cycle. *J Endocrinol Metab* 1988;66:508–517.
38. Haluska GJ, West NB, Novy MJ, Brenner RM. Uterine estrogen receptors are increased by RU486 in late pregnant Rhesus Macaques but not after spontaneous labor. *J Clin Endocrinol Metab* 1990; 70:181–186.
39. Tseng L. Hormonal regulation of steroid metabolic enzymes in human endometrium. In: Thomas JA, Singhal RL, eds. *Advances in Sex Hormone Research*. Baltimore: Urban & Schwarzenberg, 1980;329–361.
40. Kauppila A, Isomaa V, Rönnberg L, Vierikko P, Vihko R. Effect of gestrinone in endometriosis tissue and endometrium. *Fertil Steril* 1985;44:466–470.
41. Mäentausta O, Peltoketo H, Isomaa V, Jouppila P, Vihko R. Immunological measurement of human 17β-hydroxysteroid dehydrogenase. *J Steroid Biochem* 1990; (in press).
42. Peltoketo H, Isomaa V, Mäentausta O, Vihko R. Complete amino acid sequence of human placental 17β-hydroxysteroid dehydrogenase deduced from cDNA. *FEBS Lett* 1988;239:73–77.
43. Luu, The V, Labrie C, et al. Characterization of cDNA for human estradiol 17β-dehydrogenase and assignment of the gene to chromosome 17: evidence of two mRNA species with distinct 5'-termini in human placenta. *Mol Endocrinol* 1989;3:1301–1309.
44. Winqvist R, Peltoketo H, Isomaa V, Grzeschick KH, Mannermaa A, Vihko R. The gene for 17betahydroxysteroid dehydrogenase maps to human chromosome 17, bands q12-21, and shows an RFLP with SCAI. *Hum Genet*, (in press).
45. Roland M, Leisten D, Kane R. Endometriosis therapy with medroxyprogesterone acetate. *J Reprod Med* 1976;17:249–252.
46. Lemay A, Maheux R, Huot C, Blancet J, Faure N. Efficacy of intranasal or subcutaneous luteneiz-

ing hormone-releasing hormone agonist inhibition of ovarian function in the treatment of endometriosis. *Am J Obstet Gynecol* 1988;158:233–236.

47. Bergqvist A, Rannevik G, Thorell J. Estrogen and progesterone cytosol receptor concentration in endometriotic tissue and intrauterine endometrium. *Acta Obstet Gynecol Scand, Suppl* 1981;101: 53–58.

48. Jänne O, Kauppila A, Kokko E, Lantto T, Rönnberg L, Vihko R. Estrogen and progestin receptors in endometriosis lesions: comparison with endometrial tissue. *Am J Obstet Gynecol* 1981; 141:562–566.

49. Tamaya T, Motoyama T, Ohone Y, Ide N, Tsurusaki T, Okada J. Steroid receptor levels and histology of endometriosis and adenomyosis. *Fertil Steril* 1979;31:396–400.

50. Vierikko P, Kauppila A, Rönnberg L, Vihko R. Steroidal regulation of endometriosis tissue: lack of induction of 17β-hydroxysteroid dehydrogenase activity by progesterone, medroxyprogesterone acetate, or danazol. *Fertil Steril* 1985;43:218–224.

51. Gurpide E, Tseng L. Potentially useful tests for responsiveness of endometrial cancer to progestagen therapy. In: Brush MG, King RJB, Taylor RW, eds. *Endometrial Cancer*. London: Bailliere Tindall, 1978:252–257.

52. Bergeron C, Ferenczy A, Shyamala G. Distribution of estrogen receptors in various cell types of normal, hyperplastic, and neoplastic human endometrial tissues. *Lab Invest* 1988;58:338–345.

53. Cunha GR, Chung LWK, Shannon JM, Taguchi O, Fujii H. Hormone-induced morphogenesis and growth: role of mesenchymal-epithelial interactions. *Rec Progr Horm Res* 1983;39:559–598.

54. Rodrigues J, Sen KK, Seski SC, Menon M, Johnson TR, Menon KMJ. Progesterone binding by human endometrial tissue during the proliferative and secretory phases of the menstrual cycle and by hyperplastic and carcinomatous endometrium. *Am J Obstet Gynecol* 1979;133:660–665.

55. Bergeron C, Ferenczy A, Toft DO, Shyamala G. Immunocytochemical study of progesterone receptors in hyperplastic and neoplastic endometrial tissues. *Cancer Res* 1988;48:6132–6136.

56. Young PC, Ehrlich CE, Cleary RE. Progesterone binding in human endometrial carcinomas. *Am J Obstet Gynecol* 1976;125:353–358.

57. Creasman WT, McCarty KS Sr, Barton TK, McCarty KS Jr. Clinical correlates of estrogen- and progesterone-binding proteins in human endometrial adenocarcinoma. *Obstet Gynecol* 1980;55: 363–370.

58. Creasman WT, Soper JT, McCarty KS Jr, McCarty KS Sr, Hinshaw W, Clarke-Pearson L. Influence of cytoplasmic steroid receptor content on prognosis of early stage endometrial carcinoma. *Am J Obstet Gynecol* 1985;151:922–932.

59. Kauppila A, Kujansuu E, Vihko R. Cytosol estrogen and progestin receptors in endometrial carcinoma of patients treated with surgery, radio-therapy and progestin. Clinical correlates. *Cancer* 1982;50:2157–2162.

60. Vihko R, Alanko A, Isomaa V, Kauppila A. The predictive value of steroid hormone receptor analysis in breast, endometrial and ovarian cancer. *Med Oncol Tumor Pharmacothr* 1986;3:197–210.

61. Lindahl B, Alm P, Fernö M, Norgren A, Tropé A. Plasma steroid hormones, cytosol receptors, and thymidine incorporation rate in endometrial carcinoma. *Am J Obstet Gynecol* 1984;149:607–612.

62. Chambers JT, MacLusky N, Eisenfield A, Kohorn EI, Lawrence R, Schwartz PE. Estrogen and progestin receptor levels as prognosticators for survival in endometrial cancer. *Gynecol Oncol* 1988;31:65–77.

63. Palmer DC, Muir IM, Alexander AI, Cauchi M, Bennett RC, Quinn MA. The prognostic importance of steroid receptors in endometrial carcinoma. *Gynecol Oncol* 1988;72:388–393.

64. Utaaker E, Iversen OE, Skaarland E. The distribution and prognostic implications of steroid receptors in endometrial carcinomas. *Gynecol Oncol* 1987;28:89–100.

65. Budwit-Novotny DA, McCarty KS, Cox EB, et al. Immunohistochemical analyses of estrogen receptor in endometrial adenocarcinoma using monoclonal antibody. *Cancer Res* 1986;46:5419–5425.

66. Pertschuk LP, Beddoe AM, Gorelic LS, Shain SA. Immunocytochemical assay of estrogen receptors in endometrial carcinoma with monoclonal antibodies. Comparison with biochemical assay. *Cancer* 1986;57:1000–1004.

67. Zaino RJ, Clarke CL, Mortel R, Satyaswaroop PG. Heterogeneity of progesterone receptor distribution in human endometrial adenocarcinoma. *Cancer Res* 1988;48:1889–1895.

68. Segreti EM, Novotny DB, Soper JT, Mutch DG, Creasman WT, McCarty KS. Endometrial cancer:

histologic correlates of immunohistochemical localization of progesterone receptor and estrogen receptor. *Obstet Gynecol* 1989;73:780–785.

69. Kauppila A, Isotalo H, Kivinen S, Stenbäck F, Vihko R. Short-term effects of danazol and medroxyprogesterone acetate on cytosol and nuclear estrogen and progestin receptors, 17β-hydroxysteroid dehydrogenase activity, histopathology, and ultrastructure of human endometrial adenocarcinoma. *Int J Cancer* 1985;35:157–163.

70. Kauppila A, Isotalo HE, Kivinen ST, Vihko R. Prediction of clinical outcome with estrogen and progestin receptor concentrations and their relationships to clinical and histopathological variables in endometrial cancer. *Cancer Res* 1986;46:5380–5384.

71. Ehrlich CE, Young PCM, Stehman FB, Sutton GP, Alford WM. Steroid receptors and clinical outcome in patients with adenocarcinoma of the endometrium. *Am J Obstet Gynecol* 1988;158:796–807.

72. Longcope C. Steroid production in pre- and postmenopausal women. In: Greenblatt RB, Mahesh VB, McDonough PG, eds. *The Menopausal Syndrome*, 1974;615–629.

73. Siiteri PK, MacDonald PC. Role of extraglandular estrogen in human endocrinology. In: Greep RP, Astwood ED, eds. *Handbook of Physiology*. Baltimore: American Physiology Society, 1973;615–629.

74. Liao BS, Twiggs LB, Leung BS, Yu WCY, Potish RA, Prem KA. Cytoplasmic estrogen and progesterone receptors as prognostic parameters in primary endometrial carcinomas. *Obstet Gynecol* 1986;67:463–467.

75. Martin PM, Rolland PH, Gammere M, Serment H, Toga M. Estradiol and progesterone receptors in normal and neoplastic endometrium: correlations between receptors, histopathological examinations and clinical responses under progestin therapy. *Int J Cancer* 1979;23:321–329.

76. McCarty KS Jr, Barton TK, Fetter BF, Creasman WT, McCarty KS Sr. Correlation of estrogen and progesterone receptors with histologic differentiation in endometrial adenocarcinoma. *Am J Pathol* 1979;96:171–184.

77. Quinn MA, Cauchi M, Fortune D. Endometrial carcinoma: steroid receptors and response to medroxyprogesterone acetate. *Gynecol Oncol* 1985;21:314–319.

78. Pollow K, Mainz B, Grill HJ. Estrogen and progesterone receptors in endometrial cancer. In: Jasonni VM, Nenci I, Flamigni C, eds. *Progress in Cancer Research and Therapy: Steroids and Endometrial Cancer*. New York: Raven Press, 1983;37–60.

79. Pollow K, Schmidt-Gollwitzer M, Pollow B. Progesterone- and estradiol-binding proteins from normal human endometrium and endometrial carcinoma: a comparative study. In: Wittliff JL, Dapunt O, eds. *Steroid Receptors and Hormone-Dependent Neoplasia*. New York: Masson Publishing USA, 1980;69–94.

80. Kauppila A. Progestin therapy of endometrial, breast and ovarian carcinoma. A review of clinical observations. *Acta Obstet Gynecol Scand* 1984;63:441–450.

81. Kohorn EJ. Gestagens and endometrial cancer. *Gynecol Oncol* 1976;4:398–411.

82. Piver MS, Barlow JJ, Lurain JR, Blumenson LE. Medroxyprogesterone acetate (Depo-Provera) vs hydroxyprogesterone caproate (Delalutin) in women with metastatic endometrial adenocarcinoma. *Cancer* 1980;45:268–272.

83. Reifenstein EC. Hydroxyprogestagen caproate therapy in advanced endometrial cancer. *Cancer* 1971;27:485–502.

84. Kauppila A, Jänne O, Kujansuu E, Vihko R. Treatment of advanced endometrial adenocarcinoma with a combined cytotoxic therapy. Predictive value of cytosol estrogen and progestin receptor levels. *Cancer* 1980;46:2162–2167.

85. Martin JD, Hähnel R, McCartney AJ, Woodings TL. The effect of estrogen receptor status on survival in patients with endometrial carcinoma. *Am J Obstet Gynecol* 1983;147:322–324.

86. Vergote I, Kjorstad K, Abeler V, Kolstad P. A randomized trial of adjuvant progestagen in early endometrial cancer. *Cancer* 1989;64:1011–1016.

Endocrine Dependent Tumors, edited by
Klaus-Dieter Voigt and Cornelius Knabbe.
Raven Press, Ltd., New York © 1991.

9

Current Trends in Diagnosis and Treatment of Renal, Upper Urinary Tract, and Bladder Carcinomas

Arnulf Stenzl and Jean B. deKernion

*Division of Urology, UCLA School of Medicine,
Los Angeles, California 90024*

RENAL CELL CARCINOMA

Epidemiology

Renal cell carcinoma (RCC) is a relatively rare tumor, accounting for approximately 3% of all adult cancers. The tumor is more common among urban dwellers and males. The male-to-female ratio is approximately 2:1, and the tumor occurs primarily in the fifth to seventh decades of life. Careful postmortem studies on hospital inpatients have shown that a significant number of cases are not diagnosed during life. A series of 16,294 autopsies performed in Malmo, Sweden, revealed 350 cases of RCC, 235 of which were unrecognized during life (1). These occult tumors are being detected with increasing frequency, because of increased use of a variety of investigative procedures, including ultrasound, computerized tomography and magnetic resonance imaging (MRI). Frohmüller and associates (2) also noted a shift to a smaller tumor size when comparing 225 patients treated between 1982 and 1985 to 415 patients treated from 1966 to 1980. Increased diagnosis of subclinical disease with improved patient selection must be considered when an increasing incidence of RCC is reported and when survival data are compared with historical controls.

No definitive relationship between occupational and industrial carcinogens and renal carcinoma has been documented. Male cigarette smokers exposed to industrial contaminants of cadmium have been reported to have a slightly increased risk of developing the tumor (3). Subjecting RCC to cytogenetic analysis, trisomy or tetrasomy of chromosome 7 was found to be the most frequent abnormality, the rest were chromosome 3 abnormalities (4). Chromosome 3 abnormalities also have been reported for Von Hippel-Lindau disease (5), an autosomal dominant disorder with inherited susceptibility to various forms of cancer, particularly RCC. Renal cancer occurs frequently bilaterally in this disease, and identical chromosomal abnormalities in the tumors in both kidneys have been observed.

Oncogenes, altered versions of a group of normal genes that are present in all cells, also might play an important role in the carcinogenesis of renal cancer. The mechanisms that create aberrant protooncogenes are varied and include point mutations, DNA-amplification, deletion, translocation, and altered gene expression. The loss of genes on chromosome 11 as well as changes in regions of chromosome 3 appear to be specifically related to RCC (6,7).

Electron microscopic studies have identified the proximal tubular cell as the origin of renal cell carcinoma. The electron microscopic features characteristic of renal adenocarcinoma, which are shared with cells of the proximal convoluted tubules, include a brush border of tightly packed microvilli, membrane-associated vesicles involved in pinocytosis, membrane coatings of extracellular material, infoldings of the plasma membranes, and an abundance of tortuous and elongated mitochondria. Although the mitochondria might be normal, many are atypical with bizarre arrangements and elongation, branching, and vacuolation of cristae (8). Brush border antigens on renal tumors, characteristic of proximal tubular cells, and the absence of the distal tubular Tamm-Horsfall antigen have been demonstrated and are an additional evidence of the proximal tubular cell as the origin of renal cell carcinoma (9).

Evaluation

Clinical Symptoms

The clinical presentation of RCC is diverse and has given the disease its reputation as one of the great mimics of medicine. Pain and hematuria, either macroscopic or microscopic, are the most common presenting symptoms. The classic triad of hematuria, pain, and a palpable mass is not common, constituting only 5% of one large series reported by Riches and colleagues (11). Weight loss, fever, night sweats and the sudden development of a varicocele in the male resulting from obstruction of the gonadal vein also are common findings. Hypertension is known to occur and heart failure can result from arteriovenous fistulae within the tumor bed, or from the presence of tumor reaching the atrium via the vena cava. Symptoms because of metastatic disease occur frequently; 23% of patients have metastases at presentation. Approximately 30% of patients present with a paraneoplastic syndrome consisting of a variety of perplexing, seemingly unrelated symptoms that can occur early in the natural history of the disease, which can make diagnosis difficult. The occurrence of these symptoms is not necessarily indicative of the presence of metastases (11–13).

Hematogenous spread of RCC is the most important and most frequent route. Invasion can occur at the level of intrarenal or hilar vessels, with venous invasion and growth along the renal vein and eventually into the vena cava, a particular feature of this tumor. Imaging of the extent of venous involvement is an important aspect of surgical management because inadvertent ligation of a vein containing tumor can result in pulmonary tumor embolism (14). The correlation between venous extension, presence of metastases and prognosis will be discussed later. The reported incidence of metastases to lymph nodes varies from 6% to 32% (15); the highest incidence of 32% represented a study with probably the most careful pathologic investigation of all lymph node tissue (16). The regional lymphatic drainage of the right kidney is basically circumvena-caval. Lymphatic vessels also can cross the vena cava and end in the interaortocaval nodes. The left renal lymphatics drain into a periaortic group of nodes, but there is no significant drainage to the interaortocaval area. Once the disease has spread to the regional lymph nodes the lymphatic drainage becomes diffuse, and retroperitoneal, abdominal, and mediastinal lymph nodes can be involved (15).

In a review of the literature, Ritchie and associates (12) found that the incidence of metastases in 3,159 patients with RCC at the time of presentation was 23.0%. Tumor stage, size, architectural pattern, cell type and nuclear grade seem to be significantly correlated to the incidence of metastases. The most common site is lung and mediastinum, followed by bone, skin, liver, and brain (17). The many unusual sites of metastases seen with renal adenocarcinoma can be explained by a high frequency of hematogenous metastases, a particular feature of this tumor (18). Some of the unusual sites of metastases reported include the iris, epididymis, gallbladder, urinary bladder, subungual skin, and corpus cavernosum (12).

At UCLA, survival figures for 181 patients with metastatic disease were 73% at six months, 48% at one year, and 9% at five years (19). Patients in this series were treated with a variety of regimens including various interferons. The natural course of patients with untreated, advanced disease was demonstrated in a series of 443 patients reported by Riches (20). The approximate survival rates were 4.4% at three years and 2.7% at five years.

A characteristic of patients with longer survival is a diploid or near-diploid DNA content of the tumor cells. A statistically significant difference in survival has been noted after 14 months of a follow-up study in patients with metastases and diploid or near-diploid tumors when compared with aneuploid tumors (21).

Analysis of the cause of death in patients with renal cell carcinoma reveals that the tumor itself is not always responsible. Hadju and associates reported that the tumor was a major cause of death in approximately 50% of patients (22). Hellsten and colleagues found that metastatic renal cell carcinoma was the cause of death in only 21% of their postmortem series, whereas cardiovascular disease was responsible for 44% of the deaths (1).

Paraneoplastic Syndromes

Renal cell carcinoma is associated with diverse paraneoplastic syndromes. In about 30% of patients, specific genitourinary symptoms are absent, and systemic effects—paraneoplastic syndromes and ectopic hormone production—often are the initial presenting symptoms. The kidney is normally involved in the production of renin, erythropoietin, prostaglandins, and 1,25-dihydroxy-cholacalciferol. The production of at least the first three has been described in association with renal adenocarcinoma (23). In addition, and possibly of greater significance, renal carcinomas are capable of elaborating ectopic factors including parathormone, insulin, glucagon, enteroglucagon, chorionic gonadotropin, and ferritin (24,25).

Hypernephroma can produce hypertension through a variety of mechanisms including hyperreninemia, renal arteriovenous fistulae, polycythemia, hypercalcemia, ureteral obstruction, and elevated intracranial pressure secondary to cerebral metastases. The secretion of renin by renal carcinoma has been reported in both clear and granular cell tumors and usually in lesions of low histologic grade. In these cases, a decline of elevated blood pressure and plasma renin levels was noted to occur following nephrectomy. Tumor-tissue renin determinations further confirmed renin production by the tumors (25–27).

Nonmetastatic hepatic dysfunction in patients with renal carcinoma is referred to as "Stauffer syndrome." It is characterized by focal hepatic necrosis, altered liver function tests, fever and weight loss, but no hepatic metastases (28). When the syndrome is the presenting sign of renal carcinoma, the diagnosis might be delayed because of the nonlocalizing, nonurologic nature of the symptoms. The effect of nephrectomy on the abnormal liver function tests might be of prognostic value. In patients whose liver function studies returned to normal following nephrectomy, 88% were alive and well after one year. Humoral mediators were found to play an important role in the pathogenesis of the Stauffer's syndrome (29).

The incidence of fever in association with hypernephroma is about 20%, and temperature levels in 90% of patients are generally below 39 C. Ectopic adrenocorticotrophic hormone production and Cushing's syndrome and the extopic production of prolactin with nonpuerperal galactorrhea have occurred only rarely in patients with RCC.

Hypercalcemia, perhaps the most common systemic metabolic aberration associated with cancers in general, has been reported in 3% to 13% of patients with renal carcinoma. The etiology of the hypercalcemia of cancer, however, is varied, and mutiple factors including osteoclast activating factor, 1,25-dihydroxyvitamin D, prostaglandins, direct erosion of bone by tumor cells, parathyroid hormone, and colony-stimulating factors have all been implicated (34). The structure of a tumor-secreted peptide corresponding to the amino-terminal region of the parathyroid hormone-related protein was analyzed and found to be a potent human hypercalcemic factor, acting on bone and kidney, and stimulating 1,25 dihydroxy vitamin D3 (31).

Pseudohyperparathyroidism, the syndrome of hypercalcemia with normal parathyroid glands in the presence of cancer without osseous metastases, has been noted in patients with renal carcinoma. Pseudohyperparathyroidism is often found in association with hypernephroma. Documentation that parathormone or a parathormone-like peptide is responsible for the hypercalcemia has been provided by immunoassay of tumor extracts.

Erythropoietin (EP), a glycoprotein produced by the renal cortex in response to hypoxia, is the principal factor regulating erythropoiesis and is believed to act by inducing erythrocyte differentiation. The mechanisms that have been proposed to account for the increased EP levels, which have been reported in more than 40% of patients with renal adenocarcinoma, include synthesis of EP by the neoplastic cells themselves or enhanced EP production by the nonmalignant portion of the kidney in response to tumor-induced hypoxia (32).

Ectopic chorionic gondotropin, insulin, glucagon, enteroglucagon production, as well as disorders of iron metabolism and iron transport, have all been noted in patients with renal carcinoma.

Imaging of Renal Tumors

Exact delineation of the extent of local spread and regional metastases, especially to the lymph nodes, still eludes the clinician and evaluation for the presence of distant metastases is important in view of the fact that cure is an unrealistic goal in these patients. The recommended staging modality for renal cancer and currently the standard modality in most institutions is computed tomography (CT). It is useful in demonstrating local invasion of the primary lesion, detecting regional and distant enlarged lymph nodes, pulmonary and hepatic metastases. Lesions as small as 5–10 mm are accurately displayed and with state-of-the-art equipment clear differentiation between cystic and solid lesions is obtained in more than 93% of cases (33,34). Unfortunately CT cannot always show the real tumor extent, and a number of false-positive scans can be expected when CT suggests direct extension into muscle or liver. Metastases in normal-sized lymph nodes usually are not detected either, because nodal architecture is not visualized. Lymph node metastases therefore are not accurately diagnosed unless the nodes are large and the tumor is far advanced (2). Further improvement in assessment of local extension with CT can be achieved with contrast-controlled ultrafast scans (20 scans/second) (35).

Magnetic resonance imaging (MRI) appears to produce imaging equivalent to that of CT without the requirement of contrast injection. The imaging of regional lymph nodes might be more accurate because of the clear visualization of the major vessels and the indentations produced by adenopathy. Furthermore, extension into the renal vein or vena cava appears to be more accurately determined by MRI (33,36,37).

Angiography and lymphography, once widely used for staging, have been replaced in most cases by CT and MRI. Arteriography is indicated when a partial nephrectomy is planned to map the arterial supply or as part of a tumor embolization. Radionuclide bone scans generally will not visualize skeletal metastases in a patient who does not have skeletal system symptoms and has a normal alkaline phosphatase (38,39).

Tumor-thrombus extension into the vena cava must be determined preoperatively to plan the surgical approach and to avoid entering the tumor when dividing the renal vein (40). The vena cavogram is perhaps the most accurate method of assessment, although false positives can occur because of external compression of the cava. Ultrasound and MRI are helpful adjuncts to the detection of thrombus within the lumen of the vena cava and might replace the vena cavogram as the screening test of choice in most patients (2,37).

Computed tomography has been compared with other diagnostic studies. It has been suggested that its reliability in the detection of local spread, although imperfect, makes it currently the single most important staging modality, representing the most effective diagnostic and staging modality for renal cell carcinoma (2,40,41). Furthermore, the detection of small tumors is perhaps more accurate with the CT scan, as reported by several authors, (33,34,41). Besides CT, a cost-effective evaluation in a patient with distant metastases should further include only physical examination, routine chest radiography, liver function tests, and determination of serum calcium (39).

Staging

The most common staging system in the United States until recently had been instituted by Flocks and Kadesky and modified by Robson and associates (42). The limitation of the system becomes evident when it is noted that important physical findings with very different prognoses are placed in the same stage. For example,

TABLE 1A. *TNM clinical staging system*

T	Primary Tumor
TX	Primary tumor cannot be assessed
T0	No evidence of primary tumor
T1	Tumor 2.5 cm or less in greatest dimension, limited to the kidney
T2	Tumor more than 2.5 cm in greatest dimension, limited to the kidneys
T3	Tumor extends into major veins or invades adrenal gland or perinephric tissues but not beyond Gerota's fascia
T3a	Tumor invades adrenal gland or perinephric tissues but not beyond Gerota's fascia
T3b	Tumor grossly extends into renal vein(s) or vena cava
T4	Tumor invades beyond Gerota's fascia
N	Regional lymph nodes
N_O	No identifiable nodes in a specified clinical assessment
N1	Metastasis in a single lymph node, 2 cm or less in greatest dimension
N2	Metastasis in a single node, 2 cm but not more than 5 cm, or in multiple lymph nodes none more than 5 cm in greatest dimension
N3	Metastasis in a lymph node more than 5 cm in greatest dimension
M	Distant metastasis
M_O	Tumors without distant metastasis
M1	Tumors with distant metastasis
G —	Histopathologic grading
G1	Well-differentiated
G2	Moderately differentiated
G3–G4	Undifferentiated, anaplastic

(The regional lymph nodes are the hilar, abdominal paraaortic, and paracaval nodes. Laterality does not affect the N categories.)

TABLE 1B. *Comparison of Robson's staging with TNM staging system*

Stage I	T1	N_O	M_O
Stage II	T2	N_O	M_O
Stage III	T1	N1	M_O
	T2	N1	M_O
	T3a	N_O, N1	M_O
	T3b	N_O, N1	M_O
Stage IV	T4	Any N	M_O
	Any T	N2, N3	M_O
	Any T	Any N	M1

patients with all levels of renal vein, vena caval, and lymph node involvement are placed in stage III, suggesting that there is equal survival for all patients with stage III tumors. The tumor-nodes-metastasis (TNM) system proposed and lately revised by the American Joint Commitee for Cancer Staging and End Results Reporting separates venous involvement from lymph node invasion, and quantitates each of them (Table lA) (43). Primary tumors limited to the kidney and less than 2.5 cm in diameter are termed T_1, more than 2.5 cm but still limited to the kidney are classified as T_2. Tumors extending into the capsule are grouped with those extending into the renal vein in the T_3 category but are separated by subclasses (T_{3a}, T_{3b}). T_4 are those tumors extending beyond Gerota's fascia. The quantitation of the extent of lymph node involvement is another important refinement of the TNM system: N_0—no identifiable nodes in a specified clinical assessment, N_1—metastasis in a single lymph node 2 cm or less in greatest dimension, N_2—metastasis in a single lymph node more than 2 cm but not more than 5 cm, or multiple lymph nodes, none more than 5 cm in greatest dimension, N_3—metastasis in a lymph node more than 5 cm in greatest dimension. M_0 describes tumors without distant metastasis, M_1 those with distant metastasis. Histopathological grading ranges from G_1 (well differentiated) to G_4 (undifferentiated).

The new TNM system, however, is complicated, and the optimal way to combine groups is controversial. Table lB compares the categories of the two systems.

Treatment

Management of Localized Renal Carcinoma

Surgery remains the only method of cure for resectable renal cancer and should be done whenever the tumor appears to be confined to the kidney. The long-term results of surgery, even for tumors confined within the renal parenchyma, are disappointing and lead to clinical experimentation with preoperative and postoperative adjuvant treatment modalities. Angioinfarction of the renal artery either as definitive treatment or as a preoperative adjunct has been advocated in patients with a poor surgical risk or with large vascular tumors (44). Improved survival with angioinfarction has not been demonstrated and most surgical procedures can be performed safely without it. The postinfarction syndrome (severe abdominal pain, ileus, sepsis, and dislocation of the infarcting material) is disabling and can be life threatening.

Radical nephrectomy is the gold standard of treatment for renal malignancies. The term radical nephrectomy is applied for en-bloc removal of the whole kidney with its intact tumor, the adrenal, the perirenal fat and the surrounding Gerota's fascia. The renal vein is ligated early during the surgery to prevent tumor emboli. A concomitant regional lymph node dissection is done in most institutions.

Partial nephrectomy is indicated in patients with renal carcinoma in a solitary kidney, or with bilateral renal tumors, to avoid chronic hemodialysis. Some authors have shown that the long-term results of patients following partial nephrectomy for renal carcinoma under certain circumstances was equivalent to the traditional approach of radical nephrectomy (45,46).

Vena cava tumor extension is now recognized as a surgically treatable manifestation of renal carcinoma. Direct caval wall invasion rarely occurs, but can be treated by partial excision of the vena cava with the tumor thrombus. If the defect cannot be covered with a patch graft, the vena cava is ligated (40).

Management of Metastatic Renal Cancer

Approximately 25% of new patients with RCC will have radiographic evidence of metastases at the time of presentation (47). In carefully selected patients with a solitary metastasis a radical nephrectomy with surgical removal of the solitary metastasis is justified. A palliative nephrectomy might become necessary in patients with multiple metastases and disabling or life-threatening symptoms from their primary tumor such as blood loss secondary to trauma or gross hematuria, heart failure because of hypertension or arterio-venous shunting, uncontrollable pain, or significant compression of adjacent organs by the local tumor mass (48).

Interestingly, there are rare reports about remissions after angioinfarction of primary renal tumors. Complete or partial response of metastatic disease in 12 of 49 patients (24%) after angioinfarction has been reported by Wallace and associates (49). The authors speculated that the necrosis of the primary tumor released tumor-associated antigens, precipitating an ensuing immune response that was responsible for the effect on the distant metastases.

Immunotherapy

The unusual natural history of renal carcinoma, including spontaneous regression of the primary tumor, regression of metastases after removal of the primary tumor, delayed growth of metastatic lesions, and varying tumor-doubling times, suggests that host-immune factors might be important in the immune surveillance of this tumor. Although many studies of immune function have been conducted in patients with renal cancer, no firm evidence has been found to implicate host immunity as the regulating factor in tumor growth.

A fundamental principle in tumor immunology is the concept that tumors are antigenic in the host. There is ample evidence now that tumor associated antigens exist in renal cancer. With monoclonal antibodies produced in a mouse against human renal carcinoma cell lines several cell-surface antigenic systems were detected. By selecting and expanding a particular B-cell clone production of vast amounts of pure antibody to a single antigen was made possible.

Interferon and Interleukin-2 are cytokines with reported antitumor effects in RCC. Interferons are potent cell-growth inhibitors and immunostimulants. Various forms have shown some effectiveness in the treatment of RCC, especially pure recombinant alpha-Interferon 2_a and 2_b (50). The response rate of patients with metastases of the lung and mediastinum can be as high as 40%. Quesada noted in his studies that most of the responding patients were men with a good performance status whose primary tumor had been resected, whose metastases were confined to the chest, and whose overall tumor load was small. No remission was observed in 60 patients with unresected primary tumors or recurrent local masses (51). Interleukin-2 (IL-2), a lymphokine produced by interleukin-1, a macrophage product, has been shown to induce lysis of natural killer cell resistant RCC-cell lines and fresh RCC specimens. In a more recent study, recombinant IL-2 was used to stimulate and multiply lymphokine activated killer (LAK) cells. The susceptibility of human fresh renal tumor cell suspensions, as well as short-term renal tumor cultures, to lysis by LAK cells could be demonstrated (52). Rosenberg and colleagues expanded and activated lymphocytes of tumor patients with IL-2 and reinfused these to the patients with an additional IL-2 therapy. In 36 patients he reports a complete or partial response of 33% (53).

The role of tumor necrosis factor in the immune response of renal cancer is not clear: it is a protein secreted by macrophages with a biologic activity against tumor cells in culture in the presence of other agents like dactinomycin. It seems to mediate the killing of tumor targets themselves (54).

Hormonal Therapy

Progestational drugs have been approved in the United States for the management of metastatic renal cell carcinoma. Treatment in the form of megestrol acetate (Megace, 40 mg three times a day) or medroxyprogesterone acetate (Provera) is well tolerated and often produces at least some subjective symptomatic relief. The antitumor effect of these substances has not been substantiated in randomized trials, but response rates (minimal or partial) in up to 30% of the patients have been observed (48). Currently little evidence has been published in support of the true efficacy of hormone therapy in renal carcinoma.

Prognosis

Accumulated data indicate that the prognosis of renal adenocarcinoma is a function of the anatomic distribution of disease in the host at risk. Thus, with the surgical removal of the tumor, the most important risk factor is gone. However, once the disease becomes disseminated, survival is related to the biology of the disease and there appears to be a direct correlation between histologic factors and biologic aggressiveness of the tumor. The presence or absence of metastatic disease at the time of nephrectomy is seen as the single most important factor in determining survival: 10% of patients with metastatic disease at the time of nephrectomy will survive more than 3 years, and the average survival is only 6 to 9 months (55). Secondary metastases appearing after removal of the primary neoplasm have a better prognosis than metastases present at the time of diagnosis. In a review of the literature regarding prognosis of patients with lymph node metastases Marshall (5) noted an incidence of 17.4% in 2,000 cases. The overall 5-year survival rate, including patients with different tumor stages, and with or without regional lymphadenectomy, was 16% (15 of 95 patients).

Because there is considerable evidence that this tumor grows slowly, the unfavorable outcome is not attributable solely to aggressiveness, but in part to silent growth until the tumor reaches a relatively large size, with metastases frequently being responsible for the presenting symptoms. The patient's delay in seeking medical care until after symptoms occur also contributes to the generally poor outcome. Perinephric invasion was shown to have an adverse effect on the patient's chances for survival as well as on regional lymph node metastases. This has been demonstrated by significantly longer periods of survival and more survivors at 5 and 10 years for those patients without invasion (55).

The biologic behavior of renal cell cancer often is unpredictable. It is, for example, the second most likely tumor (following melanoma) to undergo spontaneous regression. Spontaneous regression of the primary RCC, however, is a very rare phenomenon. In a review from the literature of 1,139 cases of RCC, Bloom estimated the frequency of spontaneous regression to be 0.3% (56).

Involvement of the renal vein; extension through Gerota's facia; extension to renal lymph nodes; involvement of contiguous organs; multiple distant metastases; and certain histologic features such as high grade, aneuploidy, and cell type have all been associated with a poor prognosis (48)

Approximately 5% of the patients undergoing radical nephrectomy for RCC have extension of tumor thrombus into the inferior vena cava. Radical nephrectomy and removal of intracaval tumor thrombus in those patients (N = 32) without evidence of lymph node involvement and distant metastases led to 5- and 10-year survival rates of 68.8 and 60.2%, respectively (40). Venous tumor thrombosis in conjunction with metastasis, on the other hand, had a poor prognosis: no survival extended beyond 4.8 years. Extension of the tumor to the main vein was associated with a significant increase in postsurgical local recurrence and metastases, whereas involvement of smaller veins was of no prognostic significance (57).

The size of tumor seems to be related indirectly to survival, and tumors 3 to 4 cm in size have been known to become widely metastatic. Extension through Gerota's fascia and into the perinephric fat was a greater concern prior to the widespread adoption of the current radical nephrectomy. Even with the standard radical nephrectomy, however, extension beyond Gerota's fascia decreases the five-year survival rate to approximately 45%. Tumor involvement of contiguous organs is seldom associated with five-year survival rates, even after radical excision. Patients with persistent or recurrent local tumor (with or without metastases) have a much poorer prognosis compared with those with distant metastases without local tumor recurrence (58,59).

Several correlations between morphologic parameters and survival have been found. Medeiros and associates detected a decrease in disease free survival (DFS) with an increasing nuclear grade (60). Several authors demonstrated the adverse effects of higher tumor stages on DFS (10,58–60). Within a given stage of RCC, a higher microscopic grade shows a less favorable prognosis, although this is not as pronounced as in other tumors. No significant difference in survival has been found in patients with tumors containing clear cells and those with tumors containing granular cells. However, tumors composed mainly of spindle cells seem to have a worse prognosis (58,60).

UROTHELIAL CANCER OF THE UPPER URINARY TRACT

Epidemiology

Carcinoma of the renal pelvis and ureter are relatively rare, accounting for less than 1% of all genitourinary tumors. They are more frequent in men than in women with a male to female ratio of 2:1. The peak incidence is in the sixth and seventh decade, occurrances in younger people or children is rare. Histologically, approximately 90% of urothelial tumors of the upper urinary tract are transitional cell carcinomas (TCC), around 10% are squamous cell carcinomas, and less than 1% adenocarcinomas (61). TCC tends to be part of a general dysplasia affecting the entire urothelium and causing multiple tumors. In 50% of patients with TCC, another urothelial tumor is diagnosed either before, at the same time, or after detection of the primary tumor in the upper urinary tract. These tumors occur mostly in the bladder or in the ipsilateral ureter (20% to 30%) in conservatively treated patients with preservation of the ureter, 1% to 2% of the patients with TCC develop a tumor in the contralateral ureter or renal pelvis.

Cigarette smoking seems to be an important etiologic factor of urothelial tumors of the upper urinary tract and the bladder. Long-term abuse of analgesics containing phenacetin or acetaminophen is connected with an increased incidence of TCC in the renal pelvis. Leukoplakia and chronic irritation of the urothelium by urolithiasis or chronic urinary tract infection has been associated with squamous cell carcinoma and adenocarcinoma. Squamous cell carcinoma also can be caused by schistosomiasis in parts of the world where Schistosoma is endemic. In certain parts of Eastern Europe with a high incidence of the so-called Balkan nephropathy (Danubian endemic familial nephropathy) (62), TCC accounts for half of all renal tumors. This suggests a strong association between this nephropathy of unknown origin and TCC.

Evaluation

Clinical Symptoms

Gross hematuria is the initial symptom in the majority of the patients with urothelial tumors of the upper urinary tract. The second most common presenting symptom is flank pain. Occasionally a pelvic or abdominal mass can be palpated. Upper urinary tract tumors might be an incidental finding of a urologic evaluation for another not directly related reason.

Imaging

Radiographic Studies

Excretory urography is the most important study for the diagnosis of papillary tumors of the upper urinary tract, which comprise around 85% of all tumors. These tumors usually are visualized as negative filling defects in the pelvocaliceal system or ureter. Unfortunately urinary calculi, blood clots, ectopic or sloughed renal papillae, extrinsic vascular compression, lymphatic cysts, cystic pyelo-ureteritis, and various forms of strictures cause filling defects as well, which can be undistinguishable from urothelial tumors.

Retrograde ureteropyelography is used for patients who are either allergic to intravenous contrast material, or in whom further delineation of the upper urinary tract after excretory urography is necessary. A crescent-shaped rim of contrast material around the lower half of a filling defect, together with a dilatation of the ureter just distal to the filling defect constitute the so-called "goblet sign," pathognomonic of a ureteral tumor (63).

CT, MRI, Ultrasonography

Computer tomography can be helpful in the evaluation of bulky tumors, lymph node involvement, or distant metastases. Magnetic resonance imaging is helpful in patients allergic to contrast material. However, no larger study has yet shown its advantage over CT for staging of upper urinary tract tumors. Ultrasonography might be helpful in outlining a papillary tumor in a dilated urinary tract.

Cytology

Cytology is useful for the diagnosis and follow-up of urothelial tumors of the upper and lower urinary tract. For evaluation of the upper urinary tract, urine specimens must be obtained by ureteral catheterization. This usually is done in conjunction with retrograde pyelography before injection of the contrast material. The overall accuracy for urinary cytology in this area is 80% for the detection of carcinoma in situ, and 50% for papillary tumors (63).

Brush biopsy using a wire brush through a 6Fr ureteral catheter with or without ureteroscopic guidance reveals more useful material for histocytological examination. It is, however, a much more invasive procedure and should only be done in case of inconclusive noninvasive procedures (64).

Endoscopy

With the development of actively flexible ureterorenoscopes and new percutaneous nephrostomy techniques, ureterorenoscopy is increasingly used for diagnosis and occasionally for treatment of upper tract urothelial tumors. With a diameter in the range of 8.5 to 12 Fr, a total usable length of up to 65 cm, a working channel and an active deflection mechanism of 180 degrees. Ureterorenoscopes have become more and more useful in the management of upper tract urothelial cancer (65). With some experience retrograde instrumentation of the upper urinary tract also is possible in patients with a urinary diversion (66).

Staging

Urothelial tumors of the upper urinary tract commonly are staged according to the Jewett-Strong staging system for the bladder (Table 2). Recently the TNM clinical staging system (43) has been introduced for ureter and pelvis classifying separately tumor (T), lymph nodes (N), metastases (M), and grade (G) (Table 3). Both the traditional four-grade system (1 = well, 2 = moderately, 3 = poorly differentiated, 4 = undifferentiated) and the WHO three-grade system (1 = well, 2 = moderately, 3 = poorly differentiated and undifferentiated) have been used for histological grading in the last decade.

TABLE 2. *Marshall modification of Jewett-Strong classification for bladder cancer*

0	Includes: no tumor, or no definitive tumor specimen
	carcinoma *in situ*
	papillary tumors without invasion
A	Invasion of lamina propria
B1	Superficial muscle invasion
B2	Deep muscle invasion
C	Invasion of perivascular fat
D1	Invasion of prostate, vagina, or uterus; fixed to pelvic or abdominal wall pelvic nodes
D2	Distant metastases
	Nodes above aortic bifurcation

Treatment

Nephroureterectomy and excision of a bladder cuff is the treatment of choice for higher grade or multiple urothelial tumors in the upper urinary tract. In patients with grade 4 (or grade 3 in the 3-grade system) tumors of the renal pelvis. Nephrectomy alone might be considered because of the short life expectancy that makes a recurrance in the ureteral stump unlikely. In certain selected cases of grade 1 tumors a more conservative approach can be considered, consisting of partial nephrectomy for caliceal tumors, or wide excision of the tumor bearing ureter with ureteroureterostomy, ureteral reimplantation into the bladder, or replacement of the ureter by an ileal segment.

In recent years attempts were made to treat small, low-stage, and low-grade tumors endoscopically with fulguration or resection using either electrocautery or laser (65,68). The number of patients who can be treated endoscopically is small, and further clinical experience and longer follow-up is necessary.

Chemotherapy can be used as an adjuvant to surgery in high grade tumors or with concomitant nodal disease (69). It might be attempted in metastatic disease, but the results are poor. Currently the most promising regimen consists of Methotrexate, vinblastine, adriamycin (doxorubicin) and cisplatin (M-VAC). Instillation therapy via a ureteral catheter has been applied with limited success for treatment of carcinoma in situ, but created a higher complication rate than in the bladder (67).

Prognosis

Survival rate for patients with urothelial tract tumors of the upper urinary tract is correlated with both tumor grade and stage. Five-year survival rates for patients with noninvasive paillary tumors lie between 88% and 100% whereas those with deeply invasive tumors have 5-year survival rates ranging from 0% to 34%. All patients with metastatic disease at the time of initial presentation succumb to their disease within 3 years (70).

BLADDER CANCER

Epidemiology

Cancer of the bladder is the fifth leading cancer in men and the tenth leading cancer in women (71). In the United States there are approximately 45,000 new cases of bladder cancer every year. It is about three times as common in males as in females.

Overall, bladder cancer is more common in whites than in nonwhites, but the rate for nonwhite women is higher than for white women. The probability for male newborn of eventually developing bladder cancer has been estimated as 3%, for female newborn about 1% (71). Distribution of tumors by age shows the greatest incidence in male patients 65 to 79 years, and female patients 70 to 79 years old.

Between 90% and 95% of the tumors are TCCs, and the rest are squamous cell carcinomas and at rare occasions adenocarcinomas.

According to some studies, more than 50% of bladder cancers in males, and more than 35% in females in the United States are the result of either cigarette smoking or industrial exposure to carcinogens (72). Several case-control studies reported a two-fold relative risk for cigarette smokers compared with nonsmokers, with dose dependent steadily higher risks (73).

Arylamines compose the class of chemical carcinogens most strongly related to bladder cancer. In 1895 Rehn reported on cases of bladder cancer in workers exposed to anilin in a German chemical dye factory. Since then several arylamines, including beta-Naphtylamine and benzidine, have been shown in clinical and experimental studies to be human bladder carcinogens. Patients at risk are workers in the textile dye and rubber industries, hair dressers and painters (73).

Evaluation

Clinical Symptoms

The presenting symptoms in the majority of patients is hematuria. At least 75% of patients with bladder cancer have either gross or microscopic hematuria, which can be persistent, intermittent, or even a one time event. Frequently hematuria is accompanied by vesical irritability symptoms in the form of frequency, urgency, and dysuria.

Urinary Cytology

One of the characteristics of urothelial malignancies is a lack of intercellular cohesiveness. Malignant cells shed into the bladder lumen can be detected in the sediment of centrifuged or Millipore-filtered urine samples. The diagnostic accuracy is improved either by obtaining multiple specimen, or by vigorous lavage of the bladder with normal saline through a catheter or a cystoscope (74). Only a small percentage of patients have false positive results, but approximately 20% of grade 3, 50% of grade 2, and more than 70% of grade 1 tumors have false negative results. Lower-grade tumors are least likey to shed cells, and their cells, if present, also are the least atypical cells. These tumors, therefore account for almost all false negative results.

Flow Cytometry

The DNA content of cells obtained from voided urines, bladder lavage, or single-cell preparations of tumor biopsy specimens can be determined by using this technique. Patients with tumor cells that contain aneuploid quantities of DNA are more likely to have invasive tumors, and they have a high recurrence rate when no adjuvant therapy is applied (75). Flow cytometry also is significantly more sensitive than repeated urine cytologic examinations (76).

Radiographic Studies

The cystogram phase of an intravenous urography (IVU) might reveal a radiolucent filling defect, which might represent a neoplasm or a filling defect. It also might show an unanticipated abnormality in the upper urinary tract, which then can be further investigated by retrograde pyelography, barbotage for cytology, brush biopsy and ureteropyeloscopy at the time of cystoscopy. An IVU therefore should always be done before cystoscopy. Concomitant upper tract tumors have been reported in 2% to 5% of patients with bladder cancer.

CT gives additional information in staging of patients with invasive bladder tumors. Tumors larger than 1 cm are visualized, whereas smaller tumors are not imaged because they have a similar density to that of urine. CT is valuable for the detection of metastatic adenopathy where a sensitivity of over 80% is reported (77). Small nodes, however, are not detectable by CT.

Ultrasonography and MRI

These two fairly new imaging modalities differ from conventional radiographic studies by producing a picture of the tissue composition rather than its contrast outline. Transabdominal ultrasound can show large bladder tumors and their extension, but fails to detect a fair amount of early tumors, especially those of nonpapillary origin. In an older study, 100% of intravesical tumors larger than 5mm were imaged successfully, whereas only 60% of papillary tumors between 2 and 5 mm were detected (78). The recent development of a high frequency (10 mHz) transurethral ultrasonography probe adapted to a standard cystoscope offers additional staging information. It fails, however, to accurately differentiate bladder wall layers. Ta/Tl tumors tend to be overstaged, and the amount of perivesical extent can sometimes not be assessed (79).

MRI, a rather new imaging technique, can have some benefit in the future for staging of invasive tumors. With the currently available equipment and software, MRI cannot adequately diagnose and stage microscopic, in situ, or superficially invading bladder tumors. These can be picked up better with conventional clinical methods such as cystoscopy, bladder biopsy, and urinary cytology (80). The accuracy of MRI for the staging of deeply invasive tumors is reported between 50% and 90% and seems highly dependent on the type of machine, the software, and imaging technique used (81).

Cystoscopy

Cystoscopy is the most important diagnostic study for bladder cancer. With few exceptions, for example, a trauma, a single episode of urinary tract infection, or documented interstitial cystitis in women, all patients with hematuria should undergo a cystoscopic examination. Most of the time, especially when using flexible cystoscopes, this can be done as an outpatient procedure without anesthesia. In patients with evident bladder tumors this must be done with some type of regional or general anesthesia to biopsy the tumor and perform an adequate bimanual examination. A palpable tumor on bimanual examination generally indicates that at least the muscular wall of the bladder has been penetrated. Even with tumor biopsies and bimanual examination inaccuracies in staging of 50% can be expected (75).

Tumor Markers

Three major categories of tumor markers exist for bladder cancer: blood group antigens, immunohistochemical markers, and cell surface markers.

The deletion of antigens for blood groups ABO on transitional cell carcinoma cells serves as a useful marker for predicting the invasive and metastatic potential. Whereas these antigens are often present with low-grade tumors, they are absent in 99% of high grade invasive tumors. Superficial tumors that lack the ABH antigen (H antigen is present on the cell surface of patients with blood type 0) have a much higher rate of later invasion than tumors where the antigen is present. The T antigen is another blood-group antigen that is present on normal urothelial cells. It is masked by other molecules and becomes evident with a loss of differentiation of tumors. Several monoclonal antibodies against tumor associated antigens have been developed. Several authors developed monoclonal antibodies to distinct antigens in superficial as well as high stage bladder cancers (82). Chopin and associates developed a monoclonal antibody (E7) to a cell surface glycoprotein on TCC cells that has been used to detect bladder associated antigens in the urine of patients with TCC. Most higher grade tumors can be detected, but less than a third of grade 1 tumors can be picked up (83,84).

Carcinoembryonic antigens in urine and serum are useful markers for the detection of adenocarcinomas of the bladder. Nearly 90% of these patients have elevated CEA values (85). Elevated urinary levels of CEA also have been found in 60% to 100% of patients with urinary tract infections. A variety of other tumor markers have been described or used in clinical trials, but so far no cost effective and clinically reliable marker has evolved.

Staging

Currently two staging systems are mainly used for bladder cancer. Marshall's modification (86) of the Jewett-Strong classification (see Table 2) is based on a large

TABLE 3. *TNM clinical staging system for ureteropelvic tumors*

TX	Primary tumor cannot be assessed
T0	No evidence of primary tumor
Tis	Carcinoma *in situ*
Ta	Papillary noninvasive carcinoma
T1	Tumor invades subepithelial connective tissue
T2	Tumor invades muscularis
T3	Tumor invades beyond muscularis into periureteric or peripelvic fat or renal parenchyma
T4	Tumor invades adjacent organs or through the kidney into the perinephric fat

From Hermanek and Sobin, ref. 43.
N, M, and G classification as in Table 1A.

TABLE 4. *TNM clinical staging system for bladder carcinoma*

TX	Primary tumor cannot be assessed
T0	No evidence of primary tumor
Tis	Carcinoma *in situ*: "flat tumor"
Ta	Noninvasive papillary carcinoma
T1	Tumor invades subepithelial connective tissue
T2	Tumor invades superficial muscle (inner half)
T3	Tumor invades deep muscle or perivesical fat
T3a	Tumor invades deep muscle (outer half)
T3b	Tumor invades perivesical fat
T4	Tumor invades any of the following: prostate, uterus, vagina, pelvic wall, abdominal wall

N, M, and G classification as in Table 1A.

series of autopsy studies of Jewett and Strong 40 years ago. More recently the Union Internationale contre le Cancer (UICC) introduced the TNM clinical staging system (43), which has been revised several times (Table 4).

The TNM system allows a classification of tumors based on the assessment of the extent of the primary tumor (T), the involvement of lymph nodes (N), and the existence of metastases (M). Some authors, however, prefer a simpler form of classification (87).

With both staging systems a considerable staging error between clinical and pathological staging is encountered. Patients with muscle invasive disease (T2/T3a or B) were understaged in 31% to 46% of the cases whereas overstaging varied between 20% and 50%.

Treatment

Management of Superficial Bladder Cancer

Superficial bladder cancer is defined as transitional cell cancer limited to mucosa and submucosa of the bladder (clinical stages Ta, Tis, Tl or O, A). It accounts for approximately 75% to 80% of all newly diagnosed bladder cancers.

The initial step in the treatment of superficial bladder cancer is almost always transurethral resection. In larger tumors the superficial portion of the tumor should be resected first and sent as a separate specimen, followed by a resection of the deep portion of the tumor including underlying bladder wall musculature. Routine cold cup biopsies from normal appearing bladder mucosa adjacent to the tumor and from distant selected sites are performed to rule out concomitant carcinoma in situ. In men these biopsies should include the prostatic urethra. Some authors have expressed concern that random biopsies are inefficient and might even cause tumor cell implantation, and therefore, in lieu, recommended vital staining with hematoporphyrine derivatives, methylene blue, or acridine orange (88).

Laser Therapy

Lately, several studies reported better results in the removal of superficial bladder carcinomas with Laser (68,89). The most useful laser for this purpose seems to be the neodymium yttrium-aluminium-garnet (Nd:YAG) laser. It enables a noncontact thermal destruction of tumors with virtually no acute or delayed bleeding. Patients are able to perceive the laser energy when it is applied to the bladder through a rigid or flexible cystoscope, but there is much less discomfort than with electrocautery and treatment can be performed on an outpatient ambulatory basis. The greatest potential complication with the Nd:YAG laser is forward scattering of the energy that can result in damage of adjacent small bowel, even though the bladder itself may remain structurally intact.

Intravesical Therapy

Intravesical therapy can be used to prevent tumor recurrence after complete endoscopic removal of TCC, to eradicate residual TCC after incomplete resection, and in the treatment of carcinoma in situ. Drugs instilled into the bladder ensure that the antineoplastic agent is in contact with the jeopardized or tumor containing urothelium, while systemic side effects are minimized. Most of the treatment courses consist of six to eight weekly instillations, sometimes followed by a maintenance therapy with monthly instillations. The most commonly used drugs include thiotepa, epodyl, mitomycin C, doxorubicin (Adriamycin), and BCG (Bacille Calmette-Guerin) (90).

Thiotepa is one of the oldest chemotherapeutic agents used for instillation therapy. The usual weekly dose for this alkylating agent is 30 to 60 mg diluted in a concentration of 1 mg/ml. Thiotepa has the lowest molecular weight and therefore the greatest absorption and systemic toxicity of the commonly used intravesical chemotherapeutic agents. The main toxicity is myelosuppression, and a complete blood count must be obtained at regular intervals during thiotepa treatment. The complete response rate for thiotepa is 35% to 45%.

Epodyl also is an alkylating agent, but it has a higher molecular weight than thiotepa and therefore causes less myelosuppression. It has a greater incidence, however, for chemical cystitis. It is instilled in a 1% solution weekly for 12 weeks, and thereafter can be applied monthly, if indicated. Its response rate is similar to thiotepa.

Mitomycin C is an antitumor antibiotic with a high molecular weight. The absorption through the bladder mucosa is extremely low and myelosuppression is uncommon, so that there is no need to monitor the patient's blood count. The most likely side effect is chemical cystitis and genital or palmar rash. The usual dose is 20 to 40 mg weekly for 8 weeks. A complete tumor response is reported in approximately 40%, and a partial response in up to another 40% of patients. Mitomycin seems to be more effective with high-grade tumors than other agents (91).

Doxorubicin (Adriamycin) is an antineoplastic anthracycline antibiotic with a high molecular weight. Dose schedules vary, most studies use a dose of 30 to 50 mg at either weekly, biweekly, or monthly intervals. The overall complete response rate is about 40%, and the partial response rate approximately 35%. Chemical cystitis occurs in at least 25% of patients after doxorubicin therapy, and 5% to 10% experience a decrease in bladder capacity (90).

Intravesical BCG has shown to be effective in recent years in regression of residual papillary tumors as well as prophylaxis against tumor recurrence. Various different BCG strains including Tice, Pasteur, Connaught, Tokyo, Moreau, and Glaxo strains have been used. The viability and density of bacilli per milligram of vaccine can vary considerably among the different strains as well as within the same strain, and can have an impact on response to treatment. The Glaxo strain seems to be ineffective according to some reports (92). A complete response is achieved in 56% of patients with existing superficial tumors. In a UCLA series, 67% of patients with previously rapidly recurrent tumors had no recurrence during a follow-up of 10–26 months (93). BCG is also cost effective. The price for the drug is comparable to thiotepa, which is by far the cheapest among the chemotherapeutic agents. BCG, however, has more frequent side effects than other intravesical agents. In the UCLA series using the Tice strain, 85% of the patients had irritative bladder symptoms, 20% had severe cystitis requiring discontinuance of treatment in some, and 20% had low-grade fever following treatment. Occasionally polyarthritis, flu-like symptoms, and ureteral stricture or fibrosis in the presence of vesico-ureteral reflux was seen. Recently granulomatous prostatitis, tuberculous granulomas in other organs, and systemic infection secondary to BCG (so-called "BCGiosis") have been reported, especially in immuno-compromised patients (94).

Carcinoma in Situ

Carcinoma in situ (CIS) can be defined by the presence of malignant cells confined to the flat, nonpapillary bladder urothelium. These lesions are sometimes called severe atypia or grade III dysplasia. These anaplastic cells are weakly cohesive and freely shed into the urine, thus accounting for the high detection rate with urinary cytology. Coincident involvement of the prostatic urethra and the ureters is common. CIS is a frequent finding in mucosal biopsies adjacent to and/or distant from obvious papillary tumors. As an entity itself it is rather rare, accounting for approximately 2% to 3% of all bladder cancers. The mucosal area(s) might or might not be visible endoscopically, and symptoms like dysuria, frequency, and suprapubic pain might be the only clinical signs. The risk of developing invasive bladder cancer has been estimated to be from 12% to 80%, depending on the degree of bladder involvement, presence and duration of symptoms, and the presence of previous or coexisting papillary tumors.

Unless urethral or ureteral involvement is present, visible areas of CIS should be treated endoscopically with fulguration or resection followed by intravesical instillation therapy. The selection of the appropriate intravesical agent for CIS is somewhat arbitrary. The most effective agents seem to be BCG and mitomycin C, whereas doxorubicin and thiotepa are less efficient, both in terms of treatment and prevention of tumor recurrence (90).

In case of treatment failure twice using at least two intravesical agents, or CIS in the ureters or in the urethra, cystectomy is recommended.

Partial and Radical Cystectomy

Any form of cystectomy is fortunately seldomly required for patients with superficial bladder tumors. It might become necessary in patients with widespread (papillary) tumors that are not resectable, and that have not responded to at least two intravesical agents. Partial cystectomy is reserved for patients with primary, solitary tumors, which can be resected with a 2 cm tumor-free margin, and without concomitant CIS (95). In the vast majority these criteria cannot be fulfilled and a radical cystectomy with creation of an ileal conduit, a continent urinary diversion, or a ureterosigmoidostomy is indicated.

Management of Muscle-Invasive Bladder Cancer

Treatment of low-grade TCC solely invading into bladder-wall musculature (T2,T3a or B1,B2) might be attempted with vigorous transurethral resection. The failure rate, however, is high, and the possibility of a staging error lies around 40%. External or interstitial radiation, and preoperative or intraoperative radiotherapy have not been of any value and currently have no proven role in either downstaging or definitive treatment of the primary tumor or its distant metastases.

Adjuvant cisplatin-based combination chemotherapy given either preoperatively ("neo-adjuvant") or postoperatively seems to be promising in patients with localized, deeply invasive tumors (96–98). The preferred regimens consist of cisplatin combined either with methotrexate, vinblastine, and adriamycin (M-VAC) or with adriamycin and cyclophosphamide (CISCA).

Cystectomy

A bilateral pelvic lymph node dissection and radical cystectomy is the treatment of choice for all high-grade muscle-infiltrating and all bladder wall penetrating tumors. The reported 5-year survival rate for stage T2 (= B1) tumors after cystectomy ranges from 31% to 50%, for T3a (= B2) from 31% to 40%, and for T3b (= C) from 13% to 21% (99).

Several ways to create an intestinal urinary reservoir have been described using either ileum or colon or both. The selection and length of bowel used for the creation of an intestinal reservoir has a major impact on life quality and morbidity. Exclusion of larger bowel segments, as exercised in some methods (100,101) might lead to a short bowel syndrome with nutritional disorders and metabolic disturbances.

Ureterosigmoidostomy was the standard method of ureteral disposal until 1950, when Bricker (102) reported his experiences with the uretero-ileo-cutaneous diversion and at the same time Gilchrist and associates reported about the use of an ileocecal segment as bladder substitute (103). Kock's description of a continent ileostomy in the late sixties eventually led to the development of an ileal pouch used as a continent urinary reservoir (104). The early and late complication rate is relatively high (up to 30%) requiring one or several reoperations (105). On the other hand, these continent urinary diversions improve patients' quality of life because of a better body image and more independence in their physical activity. At UCLA a continent right colonic pouch was developed and is currently used with excellent results (106).

Chemotherapy

Five percent of all patients with bladder cancer present with metastatic lesions at the time of diagnosis. In addition, about 50% of patients with initially localized muscle-infiltrating tumors (T2-4, M0, N0 or stage B, C) will develop extravesical spread even if the primary tumor is controlled by treatment.

Definitive systemic chemotherapy is reserved for patients with metastatic disease (N + , M + or stage D). Based on studies with single agent chemotherapy (none of them reaching a combined partial and complete remission rate of more than 30%) several combination regimens have been developed. M-VAC (methotrexate, vinblastine, adriamycin, cisplatin), CMV (cisplatin, methotrexate, vinblastin), and CISCA (cisplatin, cyclophosphamide, adriamycin) administered either intravenously or intraarterially have shown activity against metastatic bladder cancer, and disappearance of metastatic disease of three years or more have been demonstrated (107).

REFERENCES

Renal Cell Carcinoma

1. Hellsten S, Berge T, Wehlin L. Unrecognized renal cell carcinoma: pathological and diagnostic aspects. *Scand J Urol Nephrol* 1981;8:269–272.
2. Frohmueller HGW, Grups JW, Heller V. Comparative Value of Ultrasonography, Computerized Tomography, Angiography and Excretory Urography in the Staging of Renal Cell Carcinoma. *J Urol* 1987;138:482–484.

3. Kolonel LN. Association of cadmium with renal cancer. *Cancer* 1976;37:1782–1787.

4. Weaver DJ, Michalski K, Miles J. Cytogenetic analysis in renal cell carcinoma: correlation with tumor aggressiveness. *Cancer Res* 1988;48:2887–2889.

5. Seizinger BR, Rouleau GA, Ozelius LJ, et al. Von Hippel-Lindau disease maps to the region of chromosome 3 associated with renal cell carcinoma. *Nature* 1988;332:268–269.

6. Pathak S, Strong LC, Ferrell RE, Trinidade A. A familial renal cell carcinoma with a 3;11 chromosome translocation limited to tumor cells. *Science* 1982;217:939–941.

7. Kovacs G, Szucs S, De Riese W, Baumgartel H. Specific chromosome aberration in human renal cell carcinoma. *Int J Cancer* 1987;40:171–178.

8. Tannenbaum M. Ultrastructural pathology of human renal cell tumors. *Pathol Annual* 1971;6:249–277.

9. Wright G Jr, Schellhammer PF, Faulconer RI. Isolation of a soluable tumor-associated antigen from human renal cell carcinoma by gradient acrylamide gel electrophoresis. *Cancer Res* 1977; 37:4228–4232.

10. Stenzl A, deKernion JB. Pathology, biology, and clinical staging of renal cell carcinoma. *Sem Oncol* 1989;16:1 (Suppl 1) 3–11.

11. Riches EN, Griffiths IH, Thackray AC. New growth of kidney and ureter. *Br J Urol* 1951;23:297–356.

12. Ritchie AWS, deKernion JB. The natural history and clinical features of renal carcinoma. *Sem Nephrol* 1987;7:131–139.

13. deKernion JB. Renal tumors. In: Walsh PC, ed. *Campbell's Urology, 5th ed., vol 2.* Philadelphia: Saunders, 1986;1294–1342.

14. Friedland GW. Staging of genitourinary cancer: the role of diagnostic imaging. *Cancer* 1987;60:450–458.

15. Marshall FF. Lymphadenectomy for Renal Cell Carcinoma. In: deKernion JB, Pavone-Macaluso M, eds. *Tumors of the Kidney.* Baltimore: Williams & Wilkins, 1986;87–97.

16. Hulten L, Rosencrantz M, Seeman T, Wahlquist L, Ahren C. Occurrence and localization of lymph node metastases in renal carcinoma. A lymphographic and histopathological investigation in connection with nephrectomy. *Scand J Urol Nephrol* 1969;3:129–134.

17. Khoury S, Saul A: Metastatic renal adenocarcinoma. In: deKernion JB, Pavone-Macaluso, eds. *Tumours of the kidney.* Baltimore: Williams & Wilkins, 1986;194–204.

18. Bennington JL. Histopathology of renal adenocarcinoma. In: Sufrin G, Beckley SA, eds. UICC Technical Report Series, No. 10. *Renal Adenocarcinoma* 1980;49:61–77.

19. Maldazys JD, deKernion JB. Prognostic factors in metastatic renal carcinoma. *J Urol* 1986; 136:376–379.

20. Riches E. The natural history of renal tumors. *Tumors of the Kidney and Ureter.* Edinburgh: Livingstone, 1964;124–134

21. Ljunberg B, Sternline R, Roos G. Prognostic value of deoxyribonucleic acid content in metastatic renal cell carcinoma. *J Urol* 1986;136:801–804.

22. Hajdu SI, Thomas AC. Renal cell carcinoma at autopsy. *J Urol* 1967;97:978–982.

23. Chrisholm GD. Nephrogenic ridge tumors and their syndromes. *Ann NY Acad Sci* 1974;240:403.

24. Pavelic K, Popovic M. Insulin and glucagon secretion by renal adenocarcinoma. *Cancer* 1981;48:98–100.

25. Mufti GH, Hamblin TJ, Stevens J. Basic isoferritin and hypercalcemia in renal cell carcinoma. *J Clin Pathol* 1982;35:1008–1010.

26. Dahl T, Eide I, Fryjordet A. Hypernephroma and hypertension. *Acta Med Scand* 1981;209:121–124.

27. Hollifield JS, Page DL, Smith C, et al. Renin-secreting clear cell carcinoma of the kidney. *Arch Intern Med* 1975;135:859–864.

28. Boxer RJ, Waisman J, Lieber MM, et al. Nonmetastatic hepatic dysfunction associated with renal cell carcinoma. *J Urol* 1978;119:468–471.

29. Sherwood ER, Keer HN, Fike W, Smith D, et al. The role of colony stimulating factor(s) in the pathogenesis of nephrogenic hepatic dysfunction (Stauffer's) syndrome. Read at the AUA annual meeting in Boston, June 3–7, 1988.

30. Mundy JR, Ibbotson KF, D'Souza SM, et al. The hypercalcemia of cancer. *N Engl J Med* 1984; 310:1718–1727.

31. Kemp BE, Moseley JM, Rodda CP, et al. Parathyroid hormone-related protein of malignancy: active synthetic fragments. *Science* 1987;238:1568–1570.

32. Erslev AJ, Caro J. Physiologic and molecular biology of erythropoietin. *Med Oncol Tumor Pharmacother* 1986;3:159–164.

33. Fein AB, Lee JKT, Balfe DM, et al. Diagnosis and staging of renal cell carcinoma: a comparison of MR imaging and CT. *AJR* 1987;148:749–753.

34. Amendola MA, Bree RL, Pollack HM, et al. Small renal carcinomas: resolving a diagnostic dilemma. *Radiology* 1988;166:637–641.

35. Lang EK. Comparison of dynamic and conventional computed tomography and ultrasonography in the staging of renal cell carcinoma. *Cancer* 1984;54:2205–2214.

36. Patel SK, Stack CM, Turner DA. MRI in staging of renal cell carcinoma. *Radiographics* 1987;7:703–728.

37. Hricak H, Theoni RF, Carroll PR, et al. Detection and staging of renal neoplasms: a reassessment of MR Imaging. *Radiology* 1988;166:643–649.

38. Zabbo A, Novick AC, Risius B, Montie JE. Digital subtraction angiography for evaluating patients with renal cell carcinoma. *J Urol* 1985;134:252–259.

39. Lindner A, Goldman DG, deKernion JB. Cost effective analysis of prenephrectomy radioisotope scans in renal cell carcinoma. *Urology* 1983;22:127–129.

40. Libertino JA, Zinman L, Watkins E. Long-term results of resection of renal cell carcinoma with extention into inferior cava. *J Urol* 1987;137:21–24.

41. Raval B, Lamki N. Computed tomography in detection of occult hypernephroma. *CT* 1983;7:199–207.

42. Robson CJ, Churchhill BM, Anderson W. The results of radical nephrectomy for renal cell carcinoma. *Trans Am Assoc Genitourin Surg* 1968;60:122.

43. International union against cancer. In: Hermanek P, Sobin LH, eds. *TNM Classification of Malignant Tumors, ed 4*. New York: Springer-Verlag, 1987.

44. Swanson D, et al. Angioinfarction plus nephrectomy for metastatic renal cell carcinoma-an update. *J Urol* 1983;130:449.

45. Smith RB, deKernion RB, Ehrlich RM, Skinner DG, Kaufmann JJ. Bilateral renal cell carcinoma and renal cell carcinoma in the solitary kidney. *J Urol* 1984;132:450.

46. Zincke H, Engen DE, Henning KM. Treatment of renal cell carcinoma by in situ partial nephrectomy and extracorporeal operation with autotransplantation. *Mayo Clin Proc* 1985;60:651–662.

47. Skinner DG, Colvin RB, Vermillon CD, et al. Diagnosis and management of renal cell carcinoma: a clinical and pathologic study of 309 cases. *Cancer* 1971;28:1165–1177.

48. deKernion JB: Management of renal adenocarcinoma. In: deKernion JB, Paulson DF, eds. *Genitourinary Cancer Management*. Philadelphia: Lea & Febiger, 1987.

49. Wallace S, Chuang VP, Swanson D, et al. Embolization of renal carcinoma: experience with 100 patients. *Radiology* 1981;138:563–570.

50. Sarna G, Riglin R, deKernion JB. Interferon in renal cell carcinoma: The UCLA experience. *Cancer* 1987;59:610–612.

51. Quesada JR. Biologic Response Modifiers in the therapy of metastatic renal cell carcinoma. *Sem Oncol* 1988;18(4):396–407.

52. Belldegrun A, Muul LM, Rosenberg SA. Interleukin 2 expanded tumor-infiltrating lymphocytes in human renal cell cancer: isolation, characterization, and antitumor activity. *Cancer Res* 1988; 48:206–214.

53. Rosenberg SA, Lotze MT, Muul LM, et al. A progress report on the treatment of 157 patients with advanced cancer using lymphokine activated killer cells and interleukin-2 or high dose interleukin-2 alone. *N Engl J Med* 1987;316:889–897.

54. Reinman R, Henriksen-DeStefano D, Tsujimoto M, et al. Tumor necrosis facto is an important mediator of tumor cell killing by human monocytes. *J Immunol* 1987;138:635–640.

55. Paulson DF. Prognostic factors in renal adenocarcinoma. EORTC Genitourinary Group Monograph 5: Progress and controversies in Oncological Urology II. New York: Liss, 1988;359–378.

56. Bloom HG. Hormone-induced and spontaneous regression of metastatic renal cancer. *Cancer* 1973;32:1066–1071.

57. Hoehn W, Hermanek P. Invasion of veins in renal cell carcinoma: frequency, correlation, and prognosis. *Eur Urol* 1983;9:276–280.

58. O'Dea MJ, Zincke H, Utz DC, Bernatz PE. The treatment of renal cell carcinoma with solitary mestastases. *J Urol* 1978;120:148.

59. deKernion JB, Ramming KD, Smith RB. The natural history of metastatic renal cell carcinoma: a computer analysis. *J Urol* 1978;120:148–152.

60. Medeiros LJ, Gelb AB, Weiss LM. Renal cell carcinoma: prognostic significance of morphologic parameters in 121 cases. *Cancer* 1988;61:1639–1651.

Upper Urinary Tract Carcinoma

61. Richie JP. Carcinoma of the renal pelvis and ureter. In: Skinner DG, Lieskovsky G, eds. *Diagnosis and Management of Genitourinary Cancer*. Philadelphia: Saunders, 1988; 323–336.
62. Markovic B. Endemic nephritis and urinary tract cancer in Yugoslavia, Bulgaria and Romania. *J Urol* 1972;107:212–219.
63. McDonald MW, Zincke H. Urothelial tumors of the upper urinary tract. In: deKernion JB, Paulson DF, eds. *Genitourinary Cancer Management*. Philadelphia: Lea & Febiger, 1987;1–32.
64. Gill WB, Lu CT, Thomsen S. Retrograde brushing: a new technique for obtaining histologic and cytologic material from ureteral, renal pelvic and renal caliceal lesions. *J Urol* 1973;109:573.
65. Huffmann JL, Morse MJ, Herr HW. Ureteropyeloscopy: the diagnostic and therapeutic approach to the upper tract urothelial tumors. *World J Urol* 1985;3:58–63.
66. Fuchs AM, Stenzl A, Fuchs GJ. Instrumentation of the upper urinary tract after supravesical urinary diversion. *J Urol* 1989;141:235A.
67. Studer UE, Casanova G, Kraft R, Zingg EJ. Percutaneous Bacillus Calmette Guerin perfusion of the upper urinary tract for carcinoma in situ. *J Urol* 1989;142:975–977.
68. Smith JA. Lasers In Urologic Surgery. In: Stamey TA, ed. *Monographs in Urology*, 1989;10:37–47.
69. Scher HI, Yagoda HW, Herr HW, et al. Neoadjuvant M-VAC (Methotrexate, Vinblastine, Doxorubicin and Cisplatin) for extravesical urinary tract tumors. *J Urol* 1988;139:475–476.
70. Petersen RO. *Urologic Pathology*. Philadelphia: Lippincott, 1986;205.

Bladder Carcinoma

71. Silverberg E. Statistical and epidemiologic data on urologic cancer. *Cancer* 60(suppl): 1987;692–717.
72. Doll R, Peto R. The causes of cancer: quantitative estimates of avoidable risks of cancer in the United States today. *JNCI* 1981;66:1191–1308.
73. Ross RK, Paganini-Hill A, Henderson BE. Epidemiology of bladder cancer. In: Skinner DG, Lieskovsky G, eds. *Diagnosis and Management of Genitourinary Cancer*. Philadelphia: Saunders, 1988;23–31.
74. Koss LG, Dietch D, Ramanathan R, Sherman AB. Diagnostic value of cytology of voided urine. *Acta Cytol* 1985;29:810–806.
75. Olsson CA. Management of invasive carcinoma of the bladder. In: deKernion JB, Paulson DF, eds. *Genitourinary Cancer Management*. Philadelphia: Lea & Febiger, 1987;1–32.
76. Badalament RA, Kimmel M, Gay H, et al. The sensitivity of flow cytometry compared with conventional cytology in the detection of superficial bladder carcinoma. *Cancer* 59:1987;2078–2085.
77. Boswell WD. Diagnostic imaging in genitourinary cancer. In: Skinner DG, Lieskovsky G, eds. *Diagnosis and Management of Genitourinary Cancer*. Philadelphia: Saunders, 1988;237–263.
78. Brun B, Gammelgard J, Christoffersen J. Transabdominal dynamic ultrasonography in detection of bladder tumors. *J Urol* 1984;132:19.
79. Resnick MI, Kursh ED. Transurethral ultrasonography of the urinary bladder. *World J Urol* 1988;6:22–26.
80. Wood DP, Lorig R, Pontes JE, Montie JE. The role of magnetic resonance imaging in the staging of bladder carcinoma. *J Urol* 1988;140:741–744.
81. Hricak H. Editorial comment. *J Urol* 1988;140:744.
82. Brosman SA. Tumor markers in transitional cell carcinoma. In: Paulson DF, ed. *Problems in Urology, Vol 2*. 1988; (3), 283–296.
83. Chopin DK, deKernion JB, Rosenthal DL, et al. Monoclonal antibodies against transitional cell carcinoma for detection of malignant urothelial cells in bladder washing. *J Urol* 1985;134:260.

84. Liu BCS, Neuwirth H, Zhu LW, et al. Detection of onco-fetal bladder antigen in urine of patients with transitional cell carcinoma. *J Urol* 1987;136:1258.
85. Wahren B, Nilsson BO, Zimmerman R. Urinary CEA for prediction of survival time and recurrance in bladder cancer. *Cancer* 1982;50:139.
86. Marshall VF. Relation of preoperative estimate to pathologic demonstration of extent of vesical neoplasms. *J Urol* 1952;68:714–723.
87. Lieskovsky G, Ahlering T, Skinner DG. Diagnosis and staging of bladder cancer. In: Skinner DG, Lieskovsky G, eds. *Diagnosis and Management of Genitourinary Cancer*. Philadelphia: Saunders, 1988;264–280.
88. Smith JA, Middleton RG. Bladder cancer. In: Smith JA, ed. *Lasers in urologic surgery*. Chicago: Year Book Medical Publishers, 1985;52–62.
89. Breisland HO, Seland P. A prospective randomized study on neodymium:YAG laser irradiation versus TUR in the treatment of urinary bladder cancer. *Scand J Urol Nephrol* 1986;20:209.
90. Maldazys JD, deKernion JB. Management of superficial bladder tumors and carcinoma in situ. In: deKernion JB, Paulson DF, eds. *Genitourinary Cancer Management*. Philadelphia: Lea & Febiger, 1987;33–58.
91. Soloway MS. Intravesical therapy for bladder cancer. *Urol Clin N Am* 1988;15:661–669.
92. Morales A. Long term results and complications of intracavitary bacillus Calmette-Guerin therapy for bladder cancer. *J Urol* 1984;132:457–459.
93. deKernion JB, Huang M, Lindner A, et al. The management of superficial bladder tumors and carcinoma in situ with intravesical bacillus Calmette-Guerin. *J Urol* 1985;133:598.
94. Lamm DL, Stogdill VD, Stogdill BJ, Cirspen RG. Complications of Bacillus Calmette-Guerin immunotherapy in 1278 patients with bladder cancer. *J Urol* 1986;135:272.
95. Stenzl A, deKernion JB. Overview: partial cystectomy. In: Whitehead ED, ed. *Current operative urology*. Philadelphia: Lippincott, 1990 (in press).
96. Scher HI, Yagoda A, Herr HW, et al Neoadjuvant M-VAC (methotrexate, vinblastine, doxorubicin and cisplatin) effect on the primary bladder lesion. *J Urol* 1988;139:470–474.
97. Logothetis CJ, Johnson DE, Chong C, et al. Adjuvant cyclophosphamide, doxorubicin, and cisplatin chemotherapy for bladder cancer: an update. *J Clin Oncol* 1988;6:1590–1596.
98. Stenzl A, deKernion JB, Blyth B. Management of non-resectable transitional cell carcinoma by combined preoperative chemotherapy and cystectomy. Read at the 65th Annual Meeting of the Western Section of the American Urological Association, Scottsdale, Arizona 1989.
99. Skinner DG, Lieskovsky G. Management of invasive and high grade bladder cancer. In: *Diagnosis and Management of Genitourinary Cancer*. Philadelphia: Saunders, 1988;297.
100. Boyd SD. Quality of life survey of urinary diversion patients: comparison of ileal conduits versus continent Kock ileal reservoirs. *J Urol* 1987;138:1386–1389.
101. Thuroff JW, Alken P, Riedmiller H, Engelmann U, Jacobi GH, Hohenfellner R. The Mainz Pouch (mixed augmentation ileum and cecum) for bladder augmentation and continent diversion. *J Urol* 1986;136:17–26.
102. Bricker EM. Bladder substitution after pelvic evisceration. *Surg Clin N Amer* 1950;30:1511–1521.
103. Gilchrist RK, Merricks JW, Hamlin MH, Rieger IT. Construction of a substitute bladder and urethra. *Surg Gynec Obst* 1950;90:752–760.
104. Kock NG. The development of the continent ileal reservoir (Kock pouch) and application in patients requiring urinary diversion. In: King LR, Stone AR, Webster GD, eds. *Bladder reconstruction and continent urinary diversion*. Chicago: Year Book Medical Publishers, 1986;269–289.
105. Skinner DG, Lieskovsky G, Boyd SD. Continent urinary diversion: a 5 1/2 year experience. *Ann Surg* 1988;208:337–344.
106. Stenzl A, deKernion JB. Overview: Radical Cystectomy. In: Whitehead ED, ed. *Current operative urology*. Philadelphia: Lippincott, 1990 (in press).
107. Whitmore WF: Toward the rational management of bladder cancer: an overview. *Urology* 1988;31 (2,Suppl.):5–8.

Subject Index

Subject Index